Medical Informatics

Medical Informatics

Edited by Cole Webb

hayle medical
New York

Hayle Medical,
750 Third Avenue, 9th Floor,
New York, NY 10017, USA

Visit us on the World Wide Web at:
www.haylemedical.com

ISBN: 978-1-63241-836-4

Cataloging-in-Publication Data

Medical informatics / edited by Cole Webb.
p. cm.
Includes bibliographical references and index.
ISBN 978-1-63241-836-4
1. Medical informatics. 2. Bioinformatics. 3. Medicine--Data processing.
4. Information storage and retrieval systems--Medicine. I. Webb, Cole.
R858 .M43 2020
610.28--dc23

Table of Contents

Preface

This book has been an outcome of determined endeavour from a group of educationists in the field. The primary objective was to involve a broad spectrum of professionals from diverse cultural background involved in the field for developing new researches. The book not only targets students but also scholars pursuing higher research for further enhancement of the theoretical and practical applications of the subject.

Medical informatics is the information engineering that deals with the use and management of healthcare information. It ensures the optimization of the acquisition, retrieval, storage and use of such information, in order to foster greater cooperation and collaboration among the different healthcare providers of a patient. It serves a critical role in healthcare reform. It is applied to the fields of dentistry, nursing, pharmacy, occupational therapy, clinical medicine, etc. An important application of this is the concept of integrated data repository, which incorporates different sources of clinical data to render support for solving problems of identity management, comparability of data, protection of confidentiality, etc. This book elucidates new techniques and applications of medical informatics in a multidisciplinary manner. It explores all the important aspects of this discipline in the present day scenario. It will prove to be immensely beneficial to students and researchers in this field.

It was an honour to edit such a profound book and also a challenging task to compile and examine all the relevant data for accuracy and originality. I wish to acknowledge the efforts of the contributors for submitting such brilliant and diverse chapters in the field and for endlessly working for the completion of the book. Last, but not the least; I thank my family for being a constant source of support in all my research endeavours.

Editor

Combining information from a clinical data warehouse and a pharmaceutical database to generate a framework to detect comorbidities in electronic health records

Emmanuelle Sylvestre[1,2,3,4*], Guillaume Bouzillé[1,2,3,4], Emmanuel Chazard[5], Cécil His-Mahier[1,2,3,4], Christine Riou[1,2,3,4] and Marc Cuggia[1,2,3,4]

Abstract

Background: Medical coding is used for a variety of activities, from observational studies to hospital billing. However, comorbidities tend to be under-reported by medical coders. The aim of this study was to develop an algorithm to detect comorbidities in electronic health records (EHR) by using a clinical data warehouse (CDW) and a knowledge database.

Methods: We enriched the Theriaque pharmaceutical database with the French national Comorbidities List to identify drugs associated with at least one major comorbid condition and diagnoses associated with a drug indication. Then, we compared the drug indications in the Theriaque database with the ICD-10 billing codes in EHR to detect potentially missing comorbidities based on drug prescriptions. Finally, we improved comorbidity detection by matching drug prescriptions and laboratory test results. We tested the obtained algorithm by using two retrospective datasets extracted from the Rennes University Hospital (RUH) CDW. The first dataset included all adult patients hospitalized in the ear, nose, throat (ENT) surgical ward between October and December 2014 (ENT dataset). The second included all adult patients hospitalized at RUH between January and February 2015 (general dataset). We reviewed medical records to find written evidence of the suggested comorbidities in current or past stays.

Results: Among the 22,132 Common Units of Dispensation (CUD) codes present in the Theriaque database, 19,970 drugs (90.2%) were associated with one or several ICD-10 diagnoses, based on their indication, and 11,162 (50.4%) with at least one of the 4878 comorbidities from the comorbidity list. Among the 122 patients of the ENT dataset, 75.4% had at least one drug prescription without corresponding ICD-10 code. The comorbidity diagnoses suggested by the algorithm were confirmed in 44.6% of the cases. Among the 4312 patients of the general dataset, 68.4% had at least one drug prescription without corresponding ICD-10 code. The comorbidity diagnoses suggested by the algorithm were confirmed in 20.3% of reviewed cases.

Conclusions: This simple algorithm based on combining accessible and immediately reusable data from knowledge databases, drug prescriptions and laboratory test results can detect comorbidities.

Keywords: Databases, Pharmaceutical, Clinical data warehouse, Comorbidity, Billing codes, Drug prescriptions, Laboratory test results

* Correspondence: emmanuelle.sylvestre@chu-martinique.fr
[1]INSERM, U1099, F-35000 Rennes, France
[2]Université de Rennes 1, LTSI, F-35000 Rennes, France
Full list of author information is available at the end of the article

Background

Medical coding [1] is used for a variety of activities, from observational studies to hospital billing [2, 3]. Therefore, medical codes should match as much as possible the information of the patient's medical record [4]. However, clinical coders do not fill in medical records or take care of patients. Several studies demonstrated that the agreement between medical records and medical codes is variable, if not suboptimal [5], and that comorbidities, particularly, tend to be under-reported. In this context, the term comorbidities includes all diagnoses beside the principal diagnosis (i.e., the main reason for the patient's hospitalization) that required specific diagnostic and/or therapeutic interventions during the hospital stay [6]. Yet, codes are used on the basis of the assumption that they contain detailed clinical and outcome data [7, 8]. For this, clinical coders need to have access to all the data contained in the medical record.

With the increasing use of electronic health records (EHR), such data become more easily available, especially through clinical data warehouses (CDW) that are great sources of integrated heterogeneous and exhaustive information [9, 10]. In parallel, knowledge databases, such as pharmaceutical databases, are used to analyze and process clinical data and can also support clinical decision-making [11, 12]. The challenge lies in combining these different sources of information to improve the accuracy and exhaustivity of medical codes.

The aim of this study was to develop an algorithm to detect comorbidities in EHR using a clinical data warehouse and knowledge databases. We focused on two different types of data, drug prescriptions and laboratory tests, to assess how they contribute and complement each other for identifying comorbidities.

Methods

Data sources

We used three data sources: clinical data from the Rennes University Hospital (RUH) CDW, knowledge data from a pharmaceutical database and the French reference list of comorbidities.

The RUH CDW (EHOP)

The EHOP [10, 13] CDW contains most of the EHR, including clinical notes, drug prescriptions, laboratory test records and administrative data. Each patient's EHR includes all information about his/her hospital stay. If the patient was hospitalized several times, all these hospital stays are grouped in a single EHR. Diagnoses are coded using the French version of the international classification of diseases, 10th edition (ICD-10), that incorporates the specific French modifications. Data are de-identified and subdivided in structured (drug prescriptions, laboratory test records...) and unstructured (clinical notes) data. EHOP does not include records from the Anesthesiology Department and the Intensive Care Unit (available only in paper form) and the nursing files.

Theriaque database

The Theriaque database [14] is one of the four drug databases [15] certified by the French Health Authorities (specifically by the Haute Autorité en Santé) and provides exhaustive information on drugs with a marketing authorization. For each drug, this database gives one or more indications (ICD-10 codes, when possible), its Anatomical Therapeutic Chemical (ATC) code [16, 17] and an unique identifier called "Common Unit of Dispensation" (CUD) ("Unité Commune de Dispensation" in French). CUD codes are the French standard for drug identification and are used to process drug data in the Hospital Information System.

The french comorbidity list

The French Comorbidity List ("Liste des Comorbidités et Morbidités Associées") is a reference list from the French Program of Medicalization of the Information Systems (Programme de Médicalisation des Systèmes d'Information) that is based on the Diagnosis-Related-Group (DRG) system. The Program of Medicalization of Information Systems takes comorbidities into account for hospital reimbursement and the major comorbid conditions are identified in this reference list. The aim of this list is to identify comorbidities (ICD-10-coded) with a financial impact on the patient's hospital stay.

Algorithm development

To detect comorbidities, we developed a three-step algorithm that we then tested in a retrospective observational study (Figure 1).

Step one: Enrichment of the theriaque database with the comorbidity list

We paired the Theriaque database with the Comorbidity List to identify drugs associated with at least one major comorbid condition. This step also identified ICD-10 codes associated with a drug indication and eliminated all ICD-10 codes that could not be paired with at least one drug indication. It also excluded drugs with very broad (i.e., more than twenty indications) or only imprecise (e.g., "Pain, unspecified", R52.9) indications, based on their ATC classification (Additional file 1).

Step two: Detection of comorbidities in the EHR by using drug prescriptions

2.Pairing the ICD-10 drug indications with the ICD-10 billing codes The aim of this step was to estimate the proportion of existing ICD-10 codes from the EHR that

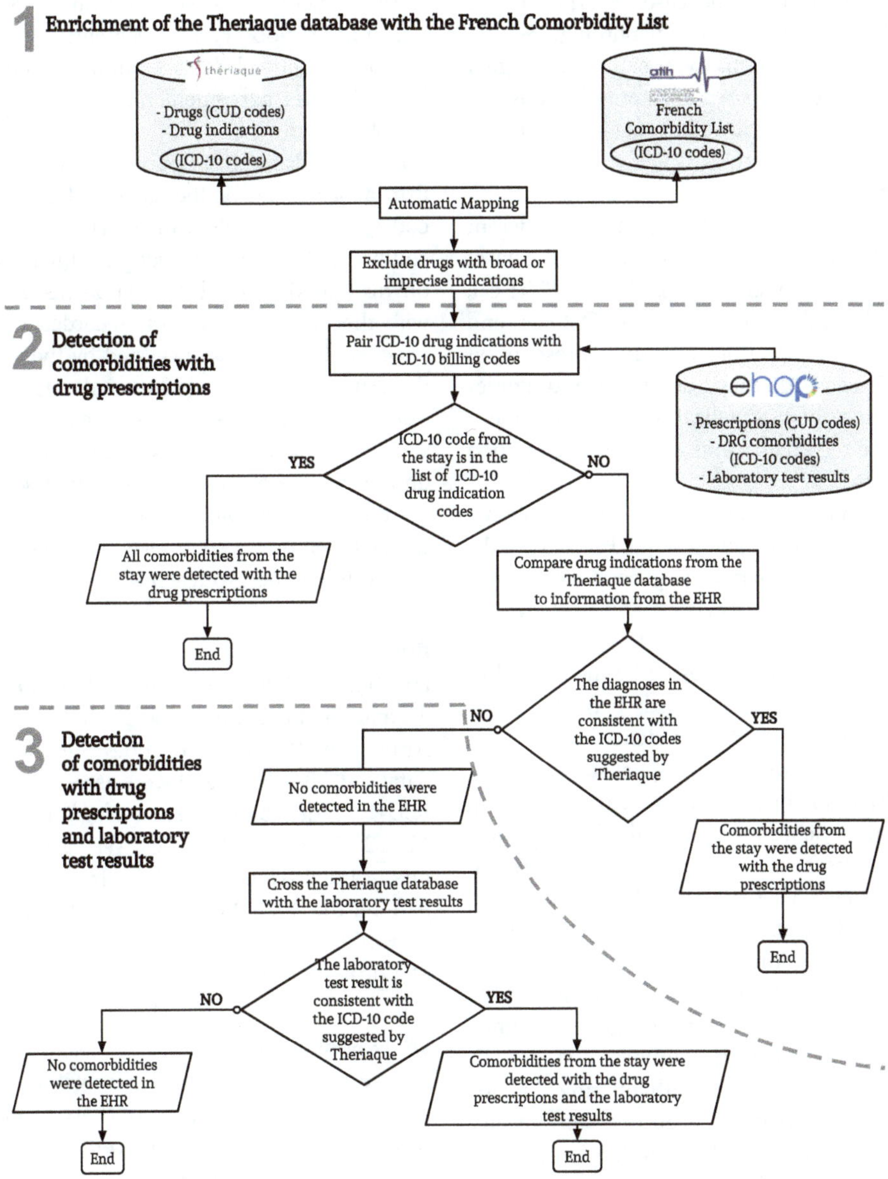

Fig. 1 Three-step algorithm. CUD: Common unit of Dispensation (Drug unique identifier). DRG: Diagnosis-Related-Group. EHR: Electronic Health Record. ICD-10: International Classification of Diseases, 10th revision

can be correctly retrieved by the algorithm. For each hospital stay, we retrieved the names of all the prescribed/administered drugs and all ICD-10 codes originally assigned to that hospital stay by the non-medical coding staff. Then, we compared these ICD-10 codes with those suggested by the Theriaque database for each prescribed/administered drug. This step led to the identification of stays where all ICD-10 codes and drug prescriptions were matched.

3.Comparing the theriaque database drug indications with the EHR information For the stays where not all drug prescriptions were matched with ICD-10 codes, we derived the potentially missing diagnoses using the prescribed drugs. Briefly, each drug prescription without at least one ICD-10 code that matched the drug indications, according to the Theriaque database, was a clue for a possible missing comorbidity. For these drugs, the Theriaque database suggested a list of ICD-10 codes, among which some were included in the Comorbidity List and were thus flagged as possible comorbidities.

Step three: Detection of comorbidities in the EHR using drug prescriptions and laboratory test results

In the last step, we improved comorbidity detection by using another source of structured data. For this study, we focused on sodium polystyrene sulfonate (SPS), because this drug is only prescribed in the case of hyperkalemia (ICD-10 code E87.5). As the French Nephrology Society defines hyperkalemia as a plasma potassium level higher than 5.0 mmol/L [18], we compared drug prescriptions and laboratory test results to detect hyperkalemia in all EHR.

Study populations

We retrospectively tested the algorithm using two different datasets extracted from the EHOP CDW. The first dataset included all stays of adult patients hospitalized at RUH ear, nose, throat (ENT) surgical ward between October and December 2014 and with at least one drug prescription (ENT dataset). We chose this unit because comorbidities unrelated to the cause of hospitalization are rarely mentioned in the surgical record and thus, it represented a good test for our algorithm.

The second dataset included the stays of all adult patients hospitalized at RUH between January and February 2015 and with at least one drug prescription (general dataset).

Algorithm evaluation

We reviewed all the diagnoses suggested by the algorithm using the data from the medical records extracted from the EHOP CDW, to find written evidence about such comorbidities in the current or past hospital stays.

We evaluated the algorithm performance by computing Precision, Recall and F-Score metrics for the ENT dataset. For the general dataset, we did not compute Recall because the value obtained for the ENT dataset suggested that the algorithm could efficiently detect comorbidities based on the drug prescriptions.

Precision is the ratio between the number of stays with confirmed diagnoses and all stays with suggested diagnoses. Recall is the ratio between the number of stays with confirmed diagnoses and all stays with missing diagnoses. The F-Score is the harmonic mean of Precision and Recall. The detailed description of the evaluation process can be found in Additional file 2.

Statistical analysis

We described quantitative variables using means and standard deviation and categorical variables using counts and percentages. We calculated the inter-expert agreement using the Cohen's Kappa (κ) coefficient. We performed all statistical analyses with R 3.3.1 [19].

The suggested diagnoses were confirmed or not by one medical expert for the ENT dataset and by two medical experts for the general dataset. These investigators had a public health background and were familiar with the EHOP CDW and the Program of Medicalization of Information Systems. They also knew well the coding guidelines because they have been involved in coding for a few years before this study. The two experts reviewed all records from the ENT dataset and only a random sample from the general dataset, to estimate the algorithm metrics and inter-observer agreement. We calculated that the size of the general dataset sample required to have a 90% inter-observer agreement rate, with $\beta = 0.80$ and $\alpha = 0.05$, was 285 stays.

For each drug prescription, the two experts had to confirm at least one of the suggested comorbidities (ICD-10 codes) or to reject all of them. To confirm a diagnosis, they compared the title of the suggested ICD-10 code or its synonyms (based on the list of synonyms provided by ICD-10) with the diseases/symptoms recorded in the EHR. If they rejected all diagnoses suggested by the algorithm based on the drug prescriptions (structured data), they examined the discharge notes (unstructured data) to confirm their decision. This was done to ensure that the rejection was based on the absence of data on a given disease/symptom and not on the CDW inability to extract all available data. Any disagreement between experts required a consensus session with a third expert to reach a final decision.

Results

Enrichment of the theriaque database with the comorbidity list and identification of the relevant ICD-10 codes

Among the 22,132 CUD codes presents in the Theriaque database, 19,970 (90.2%) were associated with one or more ICD-10 codes, based on the drug indication(s). Moreover, 11,162 (50.4%) CUD codes were associated with at least one of the 4878 comorbidities from the Comorbidity List. Among the 40,000 codes included in the French ICD-10, only 4407 (11.0%) were present in the Theriaque database as a drug indication.

Study populations

After excluding all hospital stays without at least one drug prescription, or with prescriptions of excluded drugs or without at least one ICD-10 code associated with a drug, the ENT dataset included 122 stays and the general dataset 4312 stays (Figure 2).

Inter-observer agreement

We assessed the inter-expert agreement using a random sample ($n = 285$) from the general dataset (see Materials and Methods). The two medical experts reached an agreement on 280 cases ($\kappa = 0.74$; 95% CI, 0.58–0.90). For the five remaining stays, the experts' disagreement could be explained by the Program of Medicalization of the Information Systems coding rules. For instance, the reimbursement guidelines do not allow coding some diagnoses/symptoms. Accordingly, even if present in the medical record (and, thus, confirming the suggested comorbid conditions), these diagnoses will not be coded in the hospital stay (and, as a consequence, the drug will not be associated with an ICD-10).

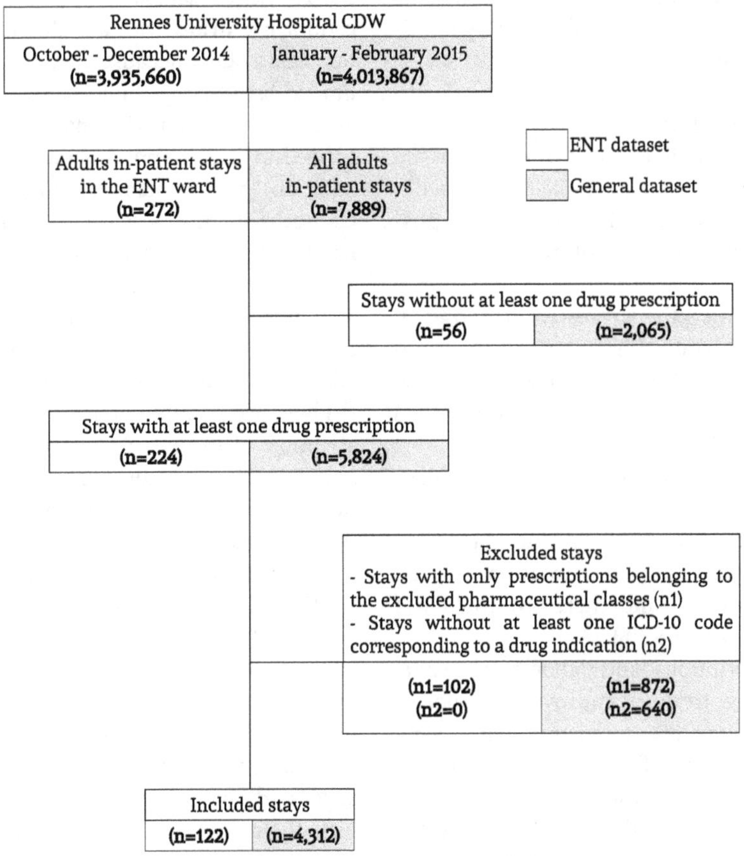

Fig. 2 Study flow chart. CDW: Clinical Data Warehouse; ENT: Ear, Nose, Throat; ICD-10: International Classification of Diseases, 10th revision

Detection of comorbidities in the EHR

Evaluation of the ENT dataset

Among the 730 ICD-10 billing codes present in the 122 stays of the ENT dataset, 339 (46.4%) were detected by the algorithm. The algorithm suggested a possible missing comorbidity in 92 of the 122 stays (75.4%) (Additional file 3).

The expert confirmed the suggested diagnoses in 41 of these 92 stays (44.6%) and added 58 ICD-10 codes to the stay (Additional file 4). Among these 41 stays, 12 (29.2%) had a major comorbidity (i.e., included in the French Comorbidity List) (Table 1) (Additional file 5). Recall was 95.3% and Precision was 44.6%, with an F-Score of 60.7%.

The medical expert did not confirm the suggested diagnoses in 51 of the 92 stays for two main reasons: i) the stays did not contain information concerning the suggested comorbidity ($n = 31$; 60.8%); ii) the drug indication was based on implicit judgments and, therefore, could not be added to the stay ($n = 20$; 39.2%).

Table 1 Number of stays in which comorbidities (ICD-10 codes) were detected by the algorithm using the drug prescriptions

	ENT dataset		General dataset	
	Stays (n = 122)	ICD-10 codes (n = 730)	Stays (n = 4312)	ICD-10 codes (n = 4932)
Comorbidities detected using the drug prescriptions; number (%)	30 (24.5)	339 (46.4)	1362 (31.6)	1271 (25.8)
Missing comorbidities; number (%)	92 (75.4)	–	2950 (68.4)	–
Suggested comorbidities	n = 92		n = 285[b]	
Suggested comorbidities, confirmed; number (%)	41 (44.6)	58 (+7.9 [a])	58 (20.3)	76 (+6.0 [a])
Added major comorbidity; number (%)	12/41 (29.2)	12 (+1.6[a])	18/58 (31.0)	29 (+2.3 [a])

[a]Improvement after code addition. [b]Random sample from the general dataset. ENT: Ear, Nose, Throat; ICD-10: International Classification of Diseases, 10th revision

Drug prescriptions could not be combined with the laboratory test results (step 3) because only one stay in this dataset included a SPS prescription.

Evaluation of the general dataset

Among the 4932 ICD-10 billing codes present in the 4312 stays of the general dataset, 1271 (25.8%) were detected by the algorithm. The algorithm suggested a possible missing comorbidity in 2950 of the 4312 stays (68.4%) (Table 1).

The two experts confirmed the suggested diagnoses in 58 of the 285 reviewed stays (Precision, 20.3%) and added 76 ICD-10 codes (Additional file 4). Among these 58 stays, 18 (31.0%) had a major comorbidity added (Table 1) (Additional file 5).

The two experts could not confirm the suggested diagnoses in 227 reviewed stays for two mains reasons: i) the EHR had no information concerning the suggested comorbidity ($n = 95$; 41.9%); ii) the indication for the drug prescription was implicit and therefore could not be added to the stay ($n = 132$; 58.1%).

Combining SPS prescriptions and laboratory results (plasma potassium concentration) improved the detection of hyperkalemia by 66.8%, compared with using only the laboratory results. Specifically, 1270 stays in the general dataset had laboratory results including blood potassium values and in 152 of them (12%) this value was higher than 5 mmol/L, but without a hyperkalemia ICD-10 billing code. This means that for 12% of stays in this dataset the hyperkalemia ICD-10 code could be added only on the basis of the laboratory test results. Moreover, 299 stays in this dataset included an SPS prescription. Among them, 85 did not have a hyperkalemia ICD-10 billing code and 67 had a potassium concentration value higher than 5 mmol/L, which means that in 78.8% (67/85) of stays, the algorithm could detect a hyperkalemia ICD-10 code by combining the laboratory test result and the SPS prescription.

Discussion

This study demonstrates that an algorithm based on clinical data and knowledge databases can detect comorbidities in EHR. The algorithm suggested missing comorbidities for more than half of the stays and, depending on the dataset, billing codes were improved by 6–8% after expert review. Moreover, by combining drug prescriptions and laboratory test results hyperkalemia detection was improved by 67%.

To develop this algorithm, we applied strategies similar to those used for adverse drug event detection [20–22]. First, we enriched a pharmaceutical database with a comorbidity list. Indeed, 90% of drugs in the Theriaque database have at least one ICD-10 drug indication. However, only 11% of the existing billing codes are present in the Theriaque database. On the other hand, the algorithm cannot use drugs with a wide range of indications (up to hundred codes) because they cannot be associated with a limited list of comorbidities. Moreover, in specialties, such as psychiatry and rheumatology, most drugs are prescribed to treat symptoms rather than specific diseases. In addition, some major comorbidities from the French Comorbidity List are treated surgically (e.g., gastrocolic fistulas [23]) and therefore cannot be detected with this algorithm. Despite these limitations, the algorithm covers 75% of stays with at least one drug prescription and about half of all hospital stays, confirming that drugs are adequate to capture comorbidities.

Then, we combined laboratory test results and prescription of drugs with narrow indications (SPS, in this study) to improve comorbidity detection [24]. This result needs to be confirmed in other similar situations, to further validate the algorithm performance.

We then used data extracted from the EHOP CDW to confirm the diagnoses suggested by the algorithm. The EHOP CDW gives the opportunity to get back to the free text reports (unstructured data) [13]. This allowed us not only to identify relevant information with the help of rules based on structured data, but also to validate and ensure the accuracy of such information. The suggested codes were always manually validated to confirm their accuracy and relevance. Indeed, the objective our system is not to automatically add codes to the EHR, but rather to highlight patient records that could be improved without the need to systematically review all records.

Although the algorithm can identify missing comorbidities, the method has some limitations. First, some drug prescriptions are not covered by the Theriaque database, because it only records indications approved by regulatory agencies for the drug original marketing authorizations, but not "off-label" usage [25]. Yet, doctors do prescribe "off-label" and regulatory agencies recognize this use for patient groups not included in the original approval [26]. As a result, several discrepancies exist between the "official" indication for a drug in the Theriaque database and the actual reasons for its prescription. The algorithm cannot detect these situations because it only relies on official drug indications.

Second, the Cohen's kappa coefficient value (0.74) indicates a substantial agreement between observers, which could be explained by their common background and similar training. This value could have been improved by involving more human experts, but very few were available at the time of the study.

Furthermore, the suggested diagnoses were confirmed only in 20% of cases. The remaining diagnoses could not be confirmed mainly because information was often implicit, a recurring issue in healthcare [27], particularly in the case of preventive treatments. For example, secondary prevention after a cardiac event is an essential part of cardiovascular disease management and is integrated in the everyday practice, as recommended by clinical guidelines [28]. Thus, for patients with cardiovascular diseases, physicians do not explicitly write down the arguments for their prescription in their notes, because they expect other physicians to understand the initial reasoning by (i) reading the patient's medical history, and (ii) by consulting the official guideline practices related to that condition. Here, the algorithm suggested a disease, while the clinical notes mentioned a risk factor rather than a comorbid condition. To improve the algorithm limitations concerning implicit information, the use of natural language processing (NLP) methods could be explored. Indeed, NLP methods can identify implicit information in medical notes [29] using machine learning-based [30], rule-based [31] or both approaches [32, 33]. Although NLP methods yield good results [29, 34], they often target specific diseases, and it would be hard to differentiate between main disease and comorbidities. Future studies should determine whether combining our approach with NLP methods and focusing on the most frequently missing comorbidities might improve the algorithm performance [35].

Nevertheless, our algorithm can improve the patients' characterization using EHR data [36]. This is important because patient phenotyping [37] is now employed to describe patients not only for optimal reimbursement [38], but also for research purposes [36, 39]. EHR-driven phenotyping is efficient only if ICD-10 billing codes are sufficiently exhaustive [40]. Our algorithm adds another level of information to the clinical data by using knowledge databases. It improves the reliability of the ICD-10 billing codes used to describe patients. We think that this could help ensuring accurate reimbursement of patient stays and improve knowledge discovery from studies based on EHR data. The next step in our project is to ask clinical coders to test the algorithm in the daily practice. We think that they could use the algorithm to improve their initial coding from scratch and we would like to fully implement it in the EHOP CDW. In the future, we want to automatically send to the coding software the list of stays with potentially missing comorbidities and the codes suggested by the algorithm. Thus, all clinical coders will benefit from the system for their daily practice.

Conclusions

We developed a fairly simple algorithm based on accessible and immediately reusable data. This study highlights that knowledge databases, drug prescriptions and laboratory test results can be used together to improve comorbidity detection. Combining this approach with NLP methods focused on implicit information should improve the algorithm performance.

Additional files

Additional file 1: List of excluded drugs with broad or imprecise indications according to their Anatomical Therapeutic Chemical (ATC) class. This table lists all drugs that were not included in the first step of the algorithm, with their ATC code and label. (DOCX 12 kb)

Additional file 2: Algorithm Evaluation: Inter-observer agreement process. This file explains in detail inter-observer agreement process: the data used, all the different steps, the formalization, the process in case of disagreement between the experts. (DOCX 19 kb)

Additional file 3: Characteristics of all ICD-10 codes suggested by the Theriaque database. This table describes the aggregated characteristics of all ICD-10 codes suggested by the algorithm for each dataset. The codes are separated between "Match" codes (codes added after expert review) and "Non-match" codes (codes that could not been added after expert review). (DOCX 15 kb)

Additional file 4: Characteristics of the ICD-10 codes added after expert review. This table describes the aggregated characteristics of the ICD-10 codes added to each dataset after the manual review by the two experts. It also count the number of ICD-10 codes that were part of the CMA list. (DOCX 13 kb)

Additional file 5: List of the ICD-10 codes added after expert review. This table lists all ICD-10 codes that were added after expert review, the number of stays were they were added, and specify if these codes are part of the CMA list. (DOCX 17 kb)

Additional file 6: Ethics committee approval. This file (in French) is the official ethics committee approval for the study. (DOC 85 kb)

Abbreviations

ATC: Anatomical therapeutic chemical terminology; CDW: Clinical data warehouse; CMA: French comorbidity list; CUD: Common units of dispensation; DRG: Diagnosis-related groups; EHR: Electronic health records; ENT: Ear; Nose, Throat; ICD-10: International classification of diseases, 10th edition; NLP: Natural language processing; RUH: Rennes university hospital; SPS: Sodium polystyrene sulfonate; κ: Cohen's Kappa coefficient

Acknowledgements

Not applicable.

Funding

This work was supported by a grant from the Brittany Region, through the ID2Santé program (QUALIMED).

Authors' contributions

ES, GB, EC, MC and CR defined the study methodology. ES and GB built the algorithm. ES, and CHM reviewed every patient from the datasets. GB reviewed the cases where ES and CHM could not reach a consensus. ES wrote the manuscript and MC, EC and GB carefully reviewed it. All authors read and approved the final manuscript.

Competing interests

The authors declare that they have no competing interests.

Author details

[1]INSERM, U1099, F-35000 Rennes, France. [2]Université de Rennes 1, LTSI, F-35000 Rennes, France. [3]CHU Rennes, CIC Inserm 1414, F-35000 Rennes, France. [4]CHU Rennes, Centre de Données Cliniques, F-35000 Rennes, France. [5]Département de Santé Publique, Université de Lille EA 2694, CHU Lille, F-59000 Lille, France.

References

1. Slee DA, Slee VN, Joachim Schmidt H. Slee's health care terms 5th edition. 5th ed; 2007.
2. O'Leary KJ, Devisetty VK, Patel AR, Malkenson D, Sama P, Thompson WK, et al. Comparison of traditional trigger tool to data warehouse based screening for identifying hospital adverse events. BMJ Qual Saf. 2013 Feb; 22(2):130–8.
3. Prokosch HU, Ganslandt T. Perspectives for medical informatics. Reusing the electronic medical record for clinical research. Methods Inf Med. 2009;48(1):38–44.
4. Ladha KS, Eikermann M. Codifying healthcare–big data and the issue of misclassification. BMC Anesthesiol. 2015 Dec 15;15:179.
5. Januel J-M, Luthi J-C, Quan H, Borst F, Taffé P, Ghali WA, et al. Improved accuracy of co-morbidity coding over time after the introduction of ICD-10 administrative data. BMC Health Serv Res. 2011 Aug 18;11:194.
6. ATIH: Agence technique de l'information sur l'hospitalisation [Internet]. [cited 2015 Apr 20]. Available from: http://www.atih.sante.fr/
7. Quan H, Parsons GA, Ghali WA. Validity of information on comorbidity derived rom ICD-9-CCM administrative data. Med Care. 2002 Aug;40(8):675–85.
8. Quan H, Sundararajan V, Halfon P, Fong A, Burnand B, Luthi J-C, et al. Coding algorithms for defining comorbidities in ICD-9-CM and ICD-10 administrative data. Med Care. 2005 Nov;43(11):1130–9.
9. Murphy SN, Weber G, Mendis M, Gainer V, Chueh HC, Churchill S, et al. Serving the enterprise and beyond with informatics for integrating biology and the bedside (i2b2). J Am Med Inform Assoc. 2010;17(2):124–30.
10. Cuggia M, Garcelon N, Campillo-Gimenez B, Bernicot T, Laurent J-F, Garin E, et al. Roogle: an information retrieval engine for clinical data warehouse. Stud Health Technol Inform. 2011;169:584–8.
11. Xie M, Weinger MB, Gregg WM, Johnson KB. Presenting multiple drug alerts in an ambulatory electronic prescribing system: a usability study of novel prototypes. Appl Clin Inform. 2014;5(2):334–48.
12. Faustini A, Canova C, Cascini S, Baldo V, Bonora K, De Girolamo G, et al. The reliability of hospital and pharmaceutical data to assess prevalent cases of chronic obstructive pulmonary disease. COPD. 2012 Apr;9(2):184–96.
13. Delamarre D, Bouzille G, Dalleau K, Courtel D, Cuggia M. Semantic integration of medication data into the EHOP clinical data warehouse. Stud Health Technol Inform. 2015;210:702–6.
14. Husson M-C. Theriaque: independent-drug database for good use of drugs by health practitioners. Ann Pharm Fr. 2008 Dec;66(5–6):268–77.
15. Hacin L, Mainar A, Édouard B. Assessment of pharmaceutical databases available in France. Ann Pharm Fr. 2013 Mar;71(2):123–34.
16. WHOCC - Structure and principles [Internet]. [cited 2016 Nov 1]. Available from: http://www.whocc.no/atc/structure_and_principles/
17. Liu Z, Guo F, Gu J, Wang Y, Li Y, Wang D, et al. Similarity-based prediction for anatomical therapeutic chemical classification of drugs by integrating multiple data sources. *Bioinformatics*. 2015 Jun 1;31(11):1788–95.
18. Collège Universitaire des Enseignants de Néphrologie. Néphrologie. 7e édition ed; 2016.
19. R Core Team. R: a language and environment for statistical computing. Vienna, Austria: R Foundation for Statistical Computing; 2016. URL https://www.R-project.org/
20. King WJ, Paice N, Rangrej J, Forestell GJ, Swartz R. The effect of computerized physician order entry on medication errors and adverse drug events in pediatric inpatients. Pediatrics. 2003 Sep 1;112(3):506–9.
21. Mekhjian HS, Kumar RR, Kuehn L, Bentley TD, Teater P, Thomas A, et al. Immediate benefits realized following implementation of physician order entry at an academic medical center. J Am Med Inform Assoc. 2002 Oct; 9(5):529–39.
22. Bonnabry P, Despont-Gros C, Grauser D, Casez P, Despond M, Pugin D, et al. A risk analysis method to evaluate the impact of a computerized provider order entry system on patient safety. J Am Med Inform Assoc. 2008 Aug; 15(4):453–60.
23. Yin J, Zheng Z, Cai J, Song J, Wang J, Zhang J, et al. Current diagnosis and management of malignant gastrocolic fistulas: a single surgical unit's experience. Int J Clin Exp Med. 2014;7(11):4123–30.
24. Ficheur G, Chazard E, Beuscart J-B, Merlin B, Luyckx M, Beuscart R. Adverse drug events with hyperkalaemia during inpatient stays: evaluation of an automated method for retrospective detection in hospital databases. BMC Med Inform Decis Mak. 2014 Sep 12;14:83.
25. Wittich CM, Burkle CM, Lanier WL. Ten common questions (and their answers) about off-label drug use. Mayo Clin Proc. 2012 Oct;87(10):982–90.
26. Elias M, Monique M, Tom W. Regulating pharmaceuticals in Europe: striving for efficiency, equity and quality: striving for efficiency, equity and quality. UK: McGraw-Hill Education; 2004. p. 390.
27. Hanlon JT, Schmader KE. The medication appropriateness index at 20: where it started, where it has been, and where it may be going. Drugs Aging. 2013 Nov;30(11):893–900.
28. Smith SC, Benjamin EJ, Bonow RO, Braun LT, Creager MA, Franklin BA, et al. AHA/ACCF secondary prevention and risk reduction therapy for patients with coronary and other atherosclerotic vascular disease: 2011 update: a guideline from the American Heart Association and American College of Cardiology Foundation. Circulation. 2011 Nov 29;124(22):2458–73.
29. Uzuner O, Goldstein I, Luo Y, Kohane I. Identifying patient smoking status from medical discharge records. J Am Med Inform Assoc. 2008 Feb;15(1):14–24.
30. Wicentowski R, Sydes MR. Using implicit information to identify smoking status in smoke-blind medical discharge summaries. J Am Med Inform Assoc. 2008 Feb;15(1):29–31.
31. Wang Y, Chen ES, Leppik I, Pakhomov S, Sarkar IN, Melton GB. Identifying family history and substance use associations for adult epilepsy from the electronic health record. AMIA Jt Summits Transl Sci Proc. 2016;2016:250–9.
32. Chen Q, Li H, Tang B, Wang X, Liu X, Liu Z, et al. An automatic system to identify heart disease risk factors in clinical texts over time. J Biomed Inform. 2015 Dec;58(Suppl):S158–63.
33. Urbain J. Mining heart disease risk factors in clinical text with named entity recognition and distributional semantic models. J Biomed Inform. 2015 Dec; 58(Suppl):S143–9.
34. Uzuner O. Recognizing obesity and comorbidities in sparse data. J Am Med Inform Assoc. 2009 Aug;16(4):561–70.
35. Ford E, Nicholson A, Koeling R, Tate A, Carroll J, Axelrod L, et al. Optimising the use of electronic health records to estimate the incidence of rheumatoid arthritis in primary care: what information is hidden in free text? BMC Med Res Methodol. 2013 Aug 21;13:105.
36. Peissig PL, Santos Costa V, Caldwell MD, Rottscheit C, Berg RL, Mendonca EA, et al. Relational machine learning for electronic health record-driven phenotyping. J Biomed Inform. 2014 Dec;52:260–70.
37. Wojczynski MK, Tiwari HK. Definition of phenotype. Adv Genet. 2008;60:75–105.
38. Palmer KS, Agoritsas T, Martin D, Scott T, Mulla SM, Miller AP, et al. Activity-based funding of hospitals and its impact on mortality, readmission, discharge destination, severity of illness, and volume of care: a systematic review and meta-analysis. PLoS One. 2014;9(10):e109975.
39. Kho AN, Pacheco JA, Peissig PL, Rasmussen L, Newton KM, Weston N, et al. Electronic medical records for genetic research: results of the eMERGE consortium. Sci Transl Med. 2011 Apr 20;3(79):79re1.
40. Newton KM, Peissig PL, Kho AN, Bielinski SJ, Berg RL, Choudhary V, et al. Validation of electronic medical record-based phenotyping algorithms: results and lessons learned from the eMERGE network. J Am Med Inform Assoc. 2013 Jun;20(e1):e147–54.

2

Identifying direct temporal relations between time and events from clinical notes

Hee-Jin Lee[1], Yaoyun Zhang[1], Min Jiang[2], Jun Xu[1], Cui Tao[1] and Hua Xu[1*]

From The 2nd International Workshop on Semantics-Powered Data Analytics
Kansas City, MO, USA. 13 November 2017

Abstract

Background: Most of the current work on clinical temporal relation identification follows the convention developed in the general domain, aiming to identify a comprehensive set of temporal relations from a document including both explicit and implicit relations. While such a comprehensive set can represent temporal information in a document in a complete manner, some of the temporal relations in the comprehensive set may not be essential depending on the clinical application of interest. Moreover, as the types of evidence that should be used to identify explicit and implicit relations are different, current clinical temporal relation identification systems that target both explicit and implicit relations still show low performances for practical use.

Methods: In this paper, we propose to focus on a sub-task of conventional temporal relation identification task in order to provide insight into building practical temporal relation identification modules for clinical text. We focus on identification of *direct* temporal relations, a subset of temporal relations that is chosen to minimize the amount of inference required to identify the relations. A corpus on direct temporal relations between time expressions and event mentions is constructed, and an automatic system tailored for direct temporal relations is developed.

Results: It is shown that the direct temporal relations constitute a major category of temporal relations that contain important information needed for clinical applications. The system optimized for direct temporal relations achieves better performance than the state-of-the-art system developed with comprehensive set of both explicit and implicit relations in mind.

Conclusions: We expect direct temporal relations to facilitate the development of practical temporal information extraction tools in clinical domain.

Keywords: Temporal relation identification, Direct temporal relation, Information extraction, TLINK, Syntactic structure

Background

Clinical narratives are a rich source of information with details about patients' medical conditions, treatments, and responses that can be utilized for various clinical research projects and applications. Since understanding temporality regarding clinical events conveyed in the narrative text is a crucial prerequisite for the utilization of the narratives, automatic means to identify temporal information from clinical narratives have gained much attention from the community [1–10].

While the task of temporal information identification ranges from identifying time mentions from the text [11, 12] to answering time-related questions [1, 13], this paper focuses on temporal relation identification, which is an essential task in understanding temporality from clinical text. In general, the task of temporal relation identification is formulated as follows: given

* Correspondence: hua.xu@uth.tmc.edu
[1]School of Biomedical Informatics, The University of Texas Health Science Center at Houston, Houston, TX, USA

time expressions and event mentions in clinical narratives, determine what kind of temporal relation does a pair of event mentions and/or time expressions have. Here, a time expression can represent time, date, duration or frequency, such as "7:00 AM", "Sep. 2. 2016", "two weeks", and "daily", and a clinical event mention can refer to problem, treatment, or test, such as "diabetes", "metformin", and "blood glucose test". For instance, the sentence "The patient underwent the surgery on Tuesday." contains an event mention "surgery" and a time expression "Tuesday", and a temporal relation of type "overlap" between the event mention and the time expression.

There are de facto standard corpora on clinical temporal relations that are released through community challenges (i.e., the 2012 Informatics for Integrating Biology and the Bedside (i2b2) challenge [14], the 2013/2014 CLEF/ShARe challenges [4], and the 2015/2016/2017 Clinical TempEval challenges [5–7]). Many systems have been developed based on these corpora [8–10]. Albeit with small differences in the exact annotation guidelines, the corpora are constructed in similar manner. That is, the corpora include implicit temporal relations that are only identifiable through inference, combining multiple pieces of information, as well as temporal relations that are explicitly stated in the text. For instance, temporal relations between mentions across multiple sentences are included. Moreover, since the number of potential temporal relations for a given text is too large (i.e., up to N (N – 1)/2 temporal relations for a document with N mentions [3]), rather than annotating every temporal relation by hand, the notion of transitivity among the temporal relations is introduced. The transitive closure[1] Of a given set of manually annotated temporal relations is calculated and used as the full set of temporal relations identifiable from a text.

While such a comprehensive way of representing temporal relations provides a complete view of temporal relations for a given document, the resulting set of temporal relations often comprises an overly complex network (c.f., Fig. 1). Such a complex network is difficult to comprehend for humans, and some part of the network may be non-essential depending on the clinical application of interest. For instance, if one wants to build a timeline of clinical events for a patient, only the relations between a time expression and an event mention would become essential, and identifying other relations between two events or between two time expressions would become less relevant.

Moreover, evidence that can be used to identify explicit or implicit temporal relations is different. While explicit relations can be identified based on textual clues, implicit relations can be identified based on inference combining multiple pieces of temporal information. Thus, mixing the two types of relations makes automatic systems unable to fully utilize the different types of clues, making it difficult to develop optimized NLP methods. Although much work has been done for temporal relation identification from clinical text, the state-of-the-art performance is still not adequate for wide adoption in practical applications; the best systems' performances for recent challenges have F1-scores of 57.3 [9] and 69.43 [10], respectively. Therefore, it is important to separate the tasks of explicit relation and implicit relation extraction and investigate methods for each type of relations in depth.

In our previous work [15], we proposed to focus on a sub-problem of the standard temporal relation identification task. Instead of targeting all temporal relations identifiable from a text, we focused on a subset of relations between temporal expressions and events. Our subset was chosen to minimize the amount of inference required to identify the relations, so that an automatic method fully utilizing textual evidence can be developed to achieve better performance while maintaining as much of information as possible that is useful in clinical applications. We focused on "direct" temporal relations, which are intra-sentential relations with limited syntactic distance between a temporal expression and an event mention. A small corpus was constructed to perform initial analysis.

In this paper, we extend our previous work to enlarge the corpus of direct temporal relations between time expressions and events by leveraging the 2012 i2b2 challenge corpus. In addition, a Support Vector Machine (SVM)-based system optimized for direct temporal relations is developed. Our analysis shows that the direct temporal relations constitute a major category of temporal relations, and the system tailored to direct temporal relations shows much better performance on direct temporal relations than a state-of-the-art system developed for the complete temporal relation identification task.

Related work

The task of temporal relation identification from clinical narratives has been tackled with various approaches, including machine-learning frameworks such as SVM [8–10], Markov Logic Network (MLN) [16], and structured learning [17]. In many systems, the entire set of temporal relations is often decomposed into several groups based on their characteristics. For instance, the Vanderbilt system [10] divides the temporal relations into six groups (i.e., event-admission time relations, event-discharge time relations, intra-sentential event-event relations, intra-sentential event-time relations, inter-sentential relations across consecutive sentences, and inter-sentential relations with co-references), and trains a separate SVM classifier for each group. Similar approach is adopted by other systems that

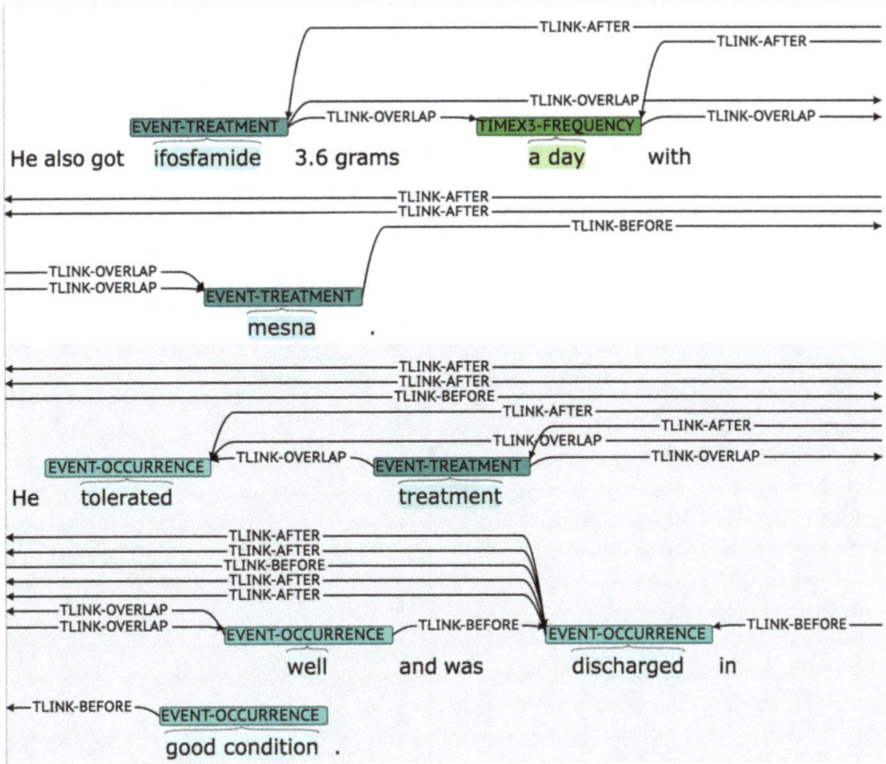

Fig. 1 Visualization of a small partial temporal relation network excerpted from the i2b2 2012 corpora [14]. Two sentences contain 8 temporal mentions and 26 temporal relations. For clarity, when there are more than one relations for a pair of temporal mentions, only one of the relations is shown

use SVM [8, 9]. These systems differentiate intra-sentential relations from inter-sentential relations, but do not differentiate implicit relation within a sentence from explicitly stated relations.

Some focus on identifying implicit relations. Xu et al. [16] train 10 separate SVM classifiers to identify both explicit and implicit relations, and then apply MLN to further infer implicit relations based on the results produced by the SVM classifiers. Leeuwenberg and Moens [17] use structured perceptron model that jointly learns the relations between events and the document-creation time and the relations between events and time expressions in the text. The model training and prediction is done at a document level using global features that can exploit local evidences. While these systems report increased performance with enhanced identification of implicit relations, the systems do not include any specialized method for explicit relations.

The rest of this paper is organized as follows: in the METHODS Section, we first introduce direct temporal relation and describe the procedure to construct a corpus of direct temporal relations (Section Direct Temporal Relations). And then, we introduce an automatic relation identification system tailored to the direct relations (Section Automatic Identification System). After that, we detail the experiments done in this paper (Section Experimental Setup). The results of the experiments are reported in Section RESULTS, followed by Section DISCUSSION and Section CONCLUSION.

Methods

Direct temporal relations

In this section, we define direct temporal relation in Section *Definition*, and detail the procedure to construct the direct temporal relation corpus in Section *Corpus construction*. Examples of direct and non-direct temporal relations are shown in Fig. 2 and Fig. 3, respectively. In the examples, a constituency parse tree of the target sentence is shown as our definition of direct temporal relation is based on constituency-based syntax, and the target time expression and the target event mention are marked with square brackets and subscripts 't' and 'e', respectively. Note that non-direct temporal relations refer to the temporal relations that are not direct.

Definition

We define a direct temporal relation as either 1) a temporal relation whose time expression modifies the event mention (or vice versa), or 2) a temporal relation whose time expression and event mention are arguments or adjuncts of the same predicate. Here, a temporal relation is an ordered relation between a time expression and an

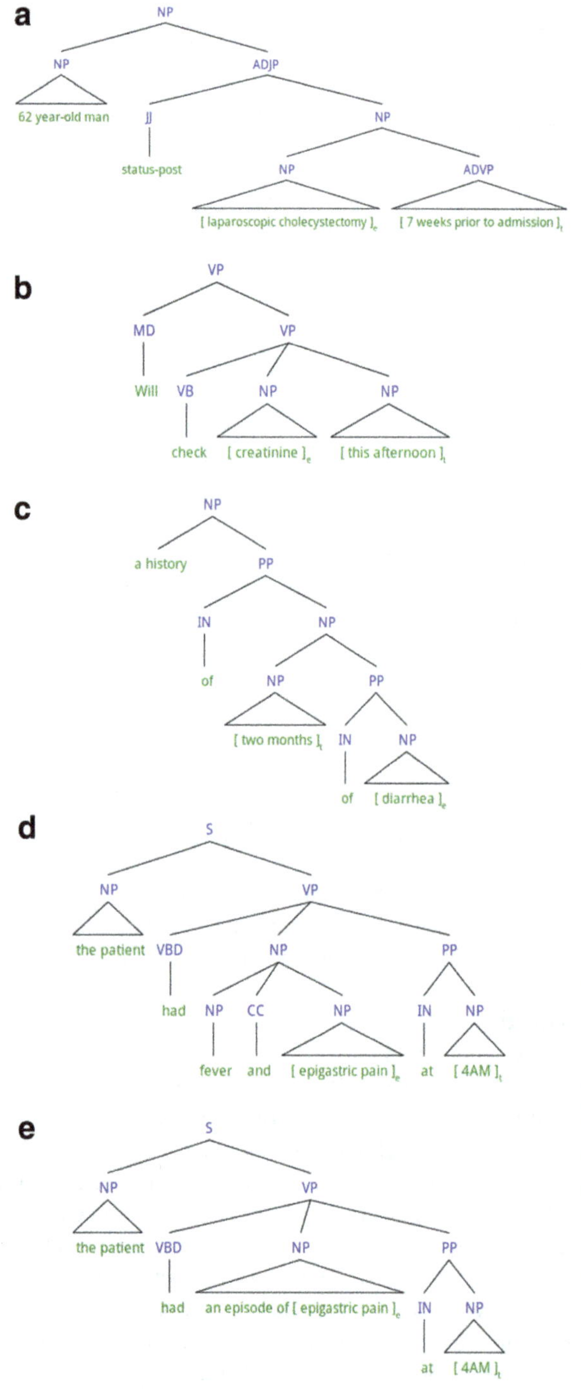

Fig. 2 Examples of direct temporal relations. Five examples with labels, **a**, **b**, **c**, **d**, **e**, are illustrated

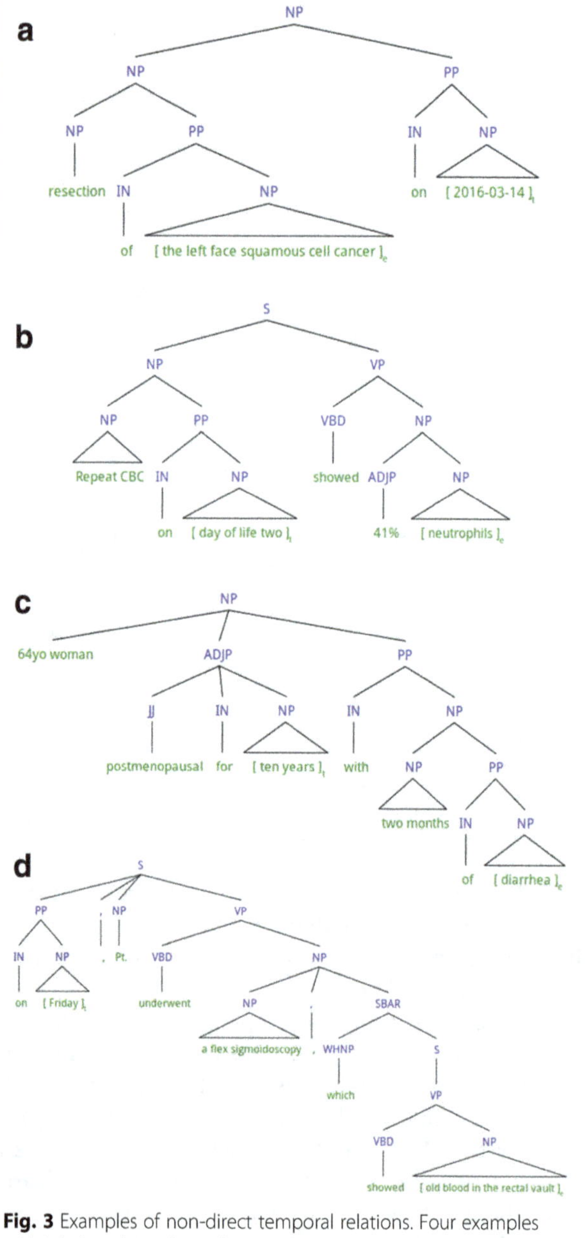

Fig. 3 Examples of non-direct temporal relations. Four examples with labels, **a**, **b**, **c**, **d**, are illustrated

event mention, which can have one of the following three types: "before", "after", or "overlap". The types of the temporal relations follow the types used in the 2012 i2b2 challenge. While conventional temporal relation work covers temporal relations between two event mentions as well, our direct temporal relations focus on temporal relations between a time expression and an event mention.

Modification of an event mention by a time expression refers to a syntactic construction that the event mention is accompanied (or modified) by the time expression to form a bigger grammatical element. For instance, for the example in Fig. 2(a), the target time expression "7 weeks prior to admission" forms an adverbial phrase (ADVP), and the target event mention "laparoscopic cholecystectomy" forms a noun phrase (NP). The ADVP containing the time expression is modifying the NP containing the event mention, forming a bigger NP "laparoscopic cholecystectomy 7 weeks prior to admission". Thus, by the first rule of the definition of direct temporal relations, the time expression "7 weeks prior to admission" and the event mention "laparoscopic cholecystectomy" form a direct temporal relation.

Usually, a verb or a noun is considered as a predicate in linguistics. A predicate needs one or more arguments acting in different syntactic/semantic roles to complete its meaning. Adjuncts are another type of grammatical elements used to modify and complete the meaning of predicates. Different from arguments, adjuncts can be removed from a sentence without making it grammatically wrong. Taking Fig. 2(b) as an example, the NP formed by the mention of a lab test event "creatinine" serves as an object of the verb "check". Meanwhile, the NP formed by the time expression "this afternoon" modifies the same verb "check" as an adjunct, providing additional information on when the event of "check creatinine" will happen. Thus, according to the second rule of the definition of direct temporal relations, the time expression and the event mention in Fig. 2(b) form a direct temporal relation.

Note that the time expression and the event mention should be the head of the phrase that modifies the other phrase (or being modified by the other phrase), or the phrase serving as an argument or an adjunct of the predicate. Head of a phrase is a sub-phrase that determines the syntactic type of the phrase. Every event mention and time expression shown in Fig. 2(a) and (b) constitutes a NP by itself, thus all of them are heads of the respective NPs. By contrast, in the example shown in Fig. 3(a), the time expression "2016–03-14" is part of a prepositional phrase (PP) "on 2016–03-13", and the event mention "the left face squamous cell cancer" is part of a NP "resection of the left face squamous cell cancer". The PP modifies the NP, but the event mention is not the head of the NP ("resection" is the head), thus, the time expression and the event mention in this example cannot form a direct temporal relation. Similarly, in Fig. 3(b), the time expression "day of life two" is contained in a NP "repeat CBC on day of life two", and the even mention "neutrophils" is contained in a NP "41% neutrophils". The two NPs are both arguments of the same verb "showed". However, the time expression is not the head of the NP ("repeat CBC" is the head), thus, the time expression and the event mention cannot form a direct temporal relation. Examples of non-direct temporal relations with more complex sentence structures are shown in Fig. 3(c) and (d).

However, there are cases where even when the time expression or the event mention is not the head of the respective phrase, it is rather straightforward to identify the temporal relation (i.e., not requiring inference that combines multiple pieces of information). Since our initial goal was to identify a subset of temporal relations that requires less number of inferences to identify but still contains as much important information as possible, we make exceptions to the above "head-of-the-phrase" rule.[2] There are three cases in which the pairs are allowed to form direct temporal relations even when the time expressions and the event mentions are not the heads of the phrases:

- Case 1: The time expression or the event mention is contained inside a PP, which can be decomposed into a preposition (which is the head of the PP) and a NP. If the time expression or the event mention is the head of the NP, then the time expression or the event mention is allowed to form a direct temporal relation.
- Case 2: The time expression or the event mention is contained inside a coordinated NP, which contains multiple smaller NPs (coordinates) and conjunction words (e.g., "and", "or", ","). If the time expression or the event mention is the head of one of the coordinates (smaller NPs), then the time expression or the event mention is allowed to form a direct temporal relation.
- Case 3: The time expression or the event mention is the head of a phrase P, and P is contained in a bigger phrase which is one of the type-preserving phrases (c.f. Table 1).

The example in Fig. 2(c) shows a pair with case 1. The time expression "two months" itself is a NP, which is modified by a PP "of diarrhea". Although the event mention "diarrhea" is not the head of the PP (the preposition "of" is the head), by exception case 1, this pair can form a direct temporal relation. An example pertinent to case 2 is shown in Fig. 2(d). The verb "had" has the NP "fever and epigastric pain" as an argument and the PP "at 4 AM" as an adjunct. Although the event mention "epigastric pain" is not the head of the NP "fever and epigastric pain", it can form a direct temporal relation, since the NP "fever and epigastric pain" is coordinated and the event mention "epigastric pain" is one of the coordinates.

Table 1 Examples of type-preserving phrases

Template[a]	Examples[b]
the first course of [Event-Treatment]	the first course of *Velban*
episodes of [Event-Problem]	episodes of *gastric pain*
the time of [Time-Date]	the time of *3/21*
period of [Time-Duration]	period of *14 days*

[a]In the templates, squared parentheses mark the placeholder for a time expression or an event mention
[b]In the examples, italicized letters mark a time expression or an event mention

A "type-preserving phrase", as mentioned in case 3, is a phrase whose semantic type can be regarded as time (i.e., time, date, duration, or frequency) or clinical event (i.e., problem, treatment, or test), even though its head is not a time expression or an event mention. For instance, for the NP "an episode of diarrhea", "an episode" is the head of the phrase, but the phrase can be regarded as conveying the meaning of a problem type clinical event, "diarrhea". Thus, the phrase can be a type-preserving phrase. In order to avoid confusion during annotation, a pre-compiled list of type-preserving phrases is added to the annotation guideline. Table 1 shows some of the type-preserving phrases. During annotation, type-preserving phrases are manually identified given types of time expressions and event mentions (i.e., "time", "date", "duration", or "frequency" for time expressions and "problem", "test", or "treatment" for event mentions). In Fig. 2(e), the problem type event mention, "epigastric pain", is contained inside a type-preserving phrase "an episode of epigastric pain", which serves as an argument of the verb "had". Although the even mention is not the head of this phrase, by exception case 3, the pair shown in Fig. 2(e) can form a direct temporal relation.

Corpus construction

A corpus of direct temporal relations is constructed by leveraging the 2012 i2b2 corpus. The corpus construction process is shown in Fig. 4. First, the transitive closure of the 2012 i2b2 corpus is calculated to produce the set of all inferable temporal relations from the 2012 i2b2 corpus. The rules for transitive closure calculation are shown in Table 2. Second, only the intra-sentential temporal relations between a time expression and an event mention is selected. Finally, each intra-sentential time-event temporal relation is reviewed by domain experts to be decided whether it is a direct temporal relation or not. The experts followed the definitions in Section *Definition* and the annotation guidelines[3] that were developed through the pilot annotation phase with small number of documents. The whole 2012 i2b2 corpus (310 discharge summaries, including both training and test set) is reviewed by an expert. Randomly selected 16 discharge summaries containing 383 pairs of time expressions and event mentions are reviewed by another expert, to measure the inter-annotator agreement rate. After manual review, only the direct temporal relations are collected. As a result, a new corpus of direct temporal relations is constructed. Note that the direct temporal relations preserve the temporal relation type (i.e., "after", "before", or "overlap") from the original 2012 i2b2 corpus.

Automatic direct temporal relation identification system

In this section, we introduce a SVM-based system tailored to direct temporal relations. The system takes as input a document with annotations of time expressions and event mentions, and outputs direct temporal relations found in the document. The system is composed of three parts: a pre-processing module, a SVM classifier, and a post-processing module. Fig. 5 shows the structure of the system. We chose to use SVM as the classification algorithm since it has shown good performances in many temporal relation identification systems [8–10].

The pre-processing module includes tokenization and section identification by the CLAMP tool [18], POS (Part Of Speech) tagging by OpenNLP [19], dependency parsing by ClearTK [20], and semantic role labeling by SENNA [21].

The SVM classifier determines if a candidate intra-sentential pair of a time expression and an event

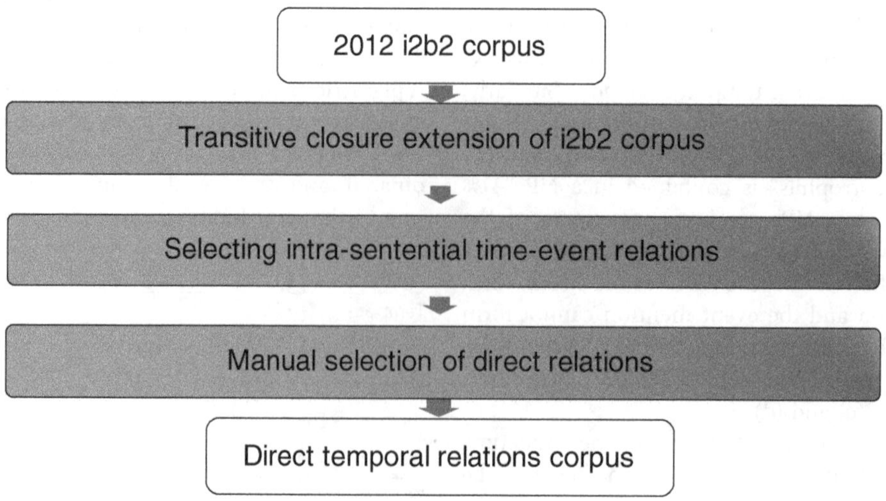

Fig. 4 The process of direct temporal relations corpus construction

Table 2 Rules for transitive closure calculation[a]

- If A overlap B, then B overlap A
- If A before B, then B after A
- If A after B, then B before A
- If A overlap B, and B overlap C, then A overlap C
- If A before B, and B before C, then A before C
- If A before B, and B overlap C, then A before C
- If A overlap B, and B before C, then A before C

[a]It is possible that the rules may produce false positive or false negative temporal relations. For instance, A and C may not overlap even when A overlap B and B overlap C. The false positive relations are removed and missing relations are added during the manual annotation process by the domain experts

mention forms a direct temporal relation or not, and classifies the pair into "overlap", "before", or "after" (when the pair forms a direct temporal relation), or "no-relation" (when the pair does not form a direct temporal relation). Since direct temporal relations are defined based on syntactic structure and predicate-argument structure, features derived from parse trees and semantic role labels are included in addition to the features that have shown to be effective for clinical temporal relation identification [9, 10]. The features are listed below:

1) Time expression type: one of "date", "time", "duration", and "frequency", as given in the original i2b2 corpus
2) Event mention attributes: "type", "polarity", "modality" of the event mention, as given in the original i2b2 corpus
3) Tokens of the mentions and the context: bag of tokens of the time expression and the event mention, preceding and following three tokens of the mentions, bag of tokens in-between the mentions, number of tokens in-between the mentions
4) POS tags: POS tags of the tokens of the mentions
5) Punctuations: number of punctuations in-between the mentions
6) Verb tense: tense and position of the verbs in the sentence
7) Section type: type of the section in which the target mentions are found, e.g., "History of present illness", "Brief hospital course"
8) Sentence type: if the sentence starts with an enumeration mark such as "2.", and "a)", or if the sentence ends with a colon
9) Dependency features: common ancestor of the time expression and the event mention on the dependency parse tree of the sentence, whether a noun exists or not in the dependency path from the event mention to the time expression
10) Semantic roles: predicates of the time expression and the event mention, whether the time expression and the event mentions are arguments/adjuncts of the same predicate or not

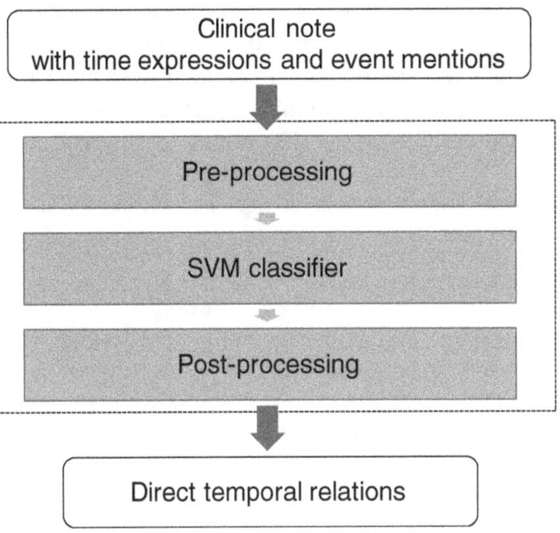

Fig. 5 Structure of the direct temporal relation identification system

Since the type distribution of the direct temporal relations is imbalanced (c.f. Table 3), cost-sensitive learning is applied by assigning weights to each type that are inversely proportional to the type frequency. LibSVM [22] implementation of SVM is used.

Lastly, the post-processing step consists of deterministic rules to fix common errors observed during the development period. For instance, a direct temporal relation is regarded as a false positive and removed from the final output when the relation is between a problem type event mention and a frequency type time expression, and the time expression represents frequency of medication (e.g., "bid", "prn", or "q2h"). Similarly, a direct temporal relation is regarded as a false positive if there's a word "where" in-between the time expression and the event mention of the direct temporal relation.

Experimental setup

In order to examine the extent of coverage of direct temporal relations in the 2012 i2b2, we compare the direct temporal relation corpus to the 2012 i2b2 corpus. Similar to the evaluation method in the i2b2 challenge [14], the set of direct relations is first extended to its transitive closure, and then the extended set is compared to the i2b2 annotations.

Table 3 Type distribution of direct temporal relations

Temporal relation type	Training set	Test set	Overall
Before	387 (17%)	355 (20%)	742 (18%)
After	345 (15%)	299 (16%)	644 (16%)
Overlap	1518 (68%)	1173 (64%)	2690 (66%)
total	2249 (100%)	1827 (100%)	4076 (100%)

The performance of the SVM-based system that is developed specifically for the direct temporal relations is reported. The performance is also compared to other baseline systems. We employ three baseline systems: 1) the Vanderbilt system [10], which is the best-performing system in the 2012 i2b2 challenge, 2) a syntactic graph kernel based system [23], and 3) a Conditional Random Fields (CRF)-based system [24]. The Vanderbilt system is the state-of-the-art system that is developed for the complete set of temporal relations (i.e., including both explicit and implicit relations). We re-implement the system and re-train it with direct temporal relations corpus. Such an evaluation provides insight on how effective the Vanderbilt systems features (i.e., features for machine learning and other gazetteers/rules) are for identification of direct temporal relations. In addition, we also evaluate the results produced by the Vanderbilt system for the 2012 i2b2 challenge (i.e., the submission by the Vanderbilt system to the TLINK-only track) against direct temporal relations. This second evaluation of the Vanderbilt system provides a view on how accurately the direct temporal relations are handled among the complete set of temporal relations in the standard task of temporal relation identification. Since the submission contains non-direct temporal relations as well as direct temporal relations, a procedure similar to that of temporal relations corpus construction is adopted: 1) the transitive closure of the Vanderbilt systems output is calculated, 2) only the relations between direct pairs of a time expression and an event mention are kept (i.e., temporal relations between pairs that do not conform to the rules for direct temporal relations are excluded), and 3) the resulting set of temporal relations is compared to the direct temporal relations corpus for evaluation. Syntactic graph kernel based methods [23, 25] are shown to achieve high performance for relation extraction tasks when the target relations are highly dependent on syntactic structure. Thus, the method is expected to perform well for direct temporal relations. CRF-based methods [24, 26] are shown to achieve good performance when the surface distance between the two entities of relation is short, thus selected as another strong baseline.

Results

In this section, we report the results of our experiments and discuss the results.

Statistics on the direct temporal relation corpus

The direct temporal relation corpus contains 310 discharge summaries. The discharge summaries are split into a training set of 190 documents and a test set of 120 documents following data split in the original 2012 i2b2 corpus (i.e., the documents in the training and test sets of direct temporal relation corpus are the same as the documents in the training and test sets of the original 2012 i2b2 corpus, respectively). Table 3 shows the type distribution of direct temporal relations in the corpus. The type distribution is similar to the type distribution of the 2012 i2b2 corpus (71.1% of the temporal relations have type "overlap", and the rest "before" or "after").

The inter-annotator agreement rate between the two experts is shown to be 80.10 (Cohens kappa [27]), which represents a good agreement.

Comparison to the standard temporal relation identification task

The direct temporal relations in our corpus constitutes 88.75% of all intra-sentential temporal relations between a time expression and an event mention in the 2012 i2b2 corpus. The direct relations also constitute 73.37% of all the temporal relations between a time expression and an event mention in the 2012 i2b2 corpus. This indicates that the direct temporal relations constitute a major category of temporal relations.

The performance of the Vanderbilt system (using submission to the 2012 i2b2 challenge) on direct temporal relations is precision 43.53, recall 76.99, and F1-score 55.61, indicating the need for the development of methods specialized for direct temporal relations.

Automatic identification performance

The performance of the SVM-based direct temporal relation identification system is shown in Table 4, along with the performances of other systems. The F1-score of the SVM-based system is shown to be 63.77, the best among all the systems. Specifically, the performance is much higher than the F1-score of the original Vanderbilt system (55.61) or the re-implemented Vanderbilt system (55.66). This shows that a system specialized for the direct temporal relations can achieve much better performance than the state-of-the-art system developed for the standard temporal relation identification task. The original Vanderbilt system shows best recall, probably due

Table 4 Performances of automatic direct temporal relation identification systems

System	P	R	F_1
SVM-based system	63.93	63.62	**63.77**
Original Vanderbilt system (submission to 2012 i2b2 challenge)	43.53	**76.99**	55.61
Re-trained Vanderbilt system (re-impremented, re-trained on direct temporal relation corpus)	64.16	49.15	55.66
Syntactic graph kernel based system	**64.46**	54.27	58.92
CRF-based system	48.51	39.52	43.56

Best scores for precision, recall and F_1-score are marked bold

to the fact that the system is developed for the entire set of temporal relations. Syntactic graph kernel shows second-best F_1-score and best precision, showing that syntactic information is indeed important in identifying direct temporal relations. On the other hand, the CRF-based system performs poorer than the other systems. We conjecture that such a poor performance is due to the fact that the CRF-based system does not utilize any syntactic-level information.

Table 5 shows example outputs of the SVM-based system. The table shows both correctly identified direct temporal relations and erroneous outputs.

Discussion

In this paper, we focused on direct temporal relations, instead of targeting the entire set of inferable temporal relations from a document as done in the standard temporal relation identification tasks. We defined direct temporal relation based on the syntactic structures and shallow semantic structures of the sentences, and our goal was to limit the amount of inference required to identify the temporal relations. A corpus of direct temporal relations was constructed by leveraging an existing corpus. An automatic system optimized for the direct temporal relations was developed using the new corpus. We showed that the direct temporal relations constitute a major category of temporal relations, and the automatic identification system optimized for direct temporal relations achieved much better performance than the state-of-the-art system that is developed for the complete temporal relation identification task.

The performance of the original Vanderbilt system (using the submission to the i2b2 challenge) on direct temporal relations is reported to be F_1-score 55.61 (Table 4). Interestingly, the performance of the system on the entire set of temporal relations (i.e., the official TLINK-only track record of the system) is shown to be F_1-score 69.32 [10], which is much higher than the system's performance on direct temporal relations. In fact, the entire set of temporal relations provided by the 2012 i2b2 challenge corpus contains relations between clinical event mentions and section times (i.e., admission time and discharge time as the 2012 i2b2 corpus is composed of discharge summaries). Such relations to section times constitute almost half of the entire temporal relations (45.87%), and are shown to be much easier to identify than other types of temporal relations [14]. This demonstrates the complexity of the complete temporal relation extraction task and the need to separate the entire task into different sub-tasks and develop optimized methods for each of the sub-tasks.

The SVM-based direct temporal relation identification system shows much better performance than other baseline systems, but the performance is still not ideal for practical use (F_1-score 63.77). During the development of the system, we identified three major obstacles hindering accurate identification of direct temporal relations. The first is difficulty in identifying the correct syntactic structures of the sentences, particularly, of ambiguous sentences such as the followings:

1) On [post-op day #3]$_t$, the patient's pacing wires were removed, and his [17opressor]$_e$ was started.
2) The patient presents with a [four day]$_t$ prodrome of dry cough, rhinorrhea, chills, loose bowel movements with diarrhea and no blood, [decreased urine output]$_e$, no sick contacts.

For the first sentence, it is ambiguous whether the PP "On post-op day #3" is an adjunct of both of the verbs "removed" and "started", or of only the first verb "removed". For the second sentence, it is ambiguous how many of the symptoms listed in this sentence are included in the "four day prodrome" (i.e., is it four day prodrome of dry cough only? Or of dry cough and all other symptoms mentioned in the sentence?). Such

Table 5 Example outputs of svm-based system

Sentence	Predicted	Gold standard
Subsequently [his creatinine]$_e$ rose for [three days]$_t$ and then stabilized at 10.	overlap	overlap
[Cardiac catheterization]$_e$ was performed without complication from the right neck and right groin on [the day]$_t$ of admission.	overlap	overlap
3. On [the morning of 12–01]$_t$, the patient had some transient episodes of hypotension with [SBP s]$_e$ in the 70 s.	overlap	N/A
Initially on [Vanc]$_e$ and Cipro on [Friday]$_t$ but then seen by ID who recommended no abx but a bone biopsy, blood cx.	N/A	overlap
Anti-coagulation was started with Warfarin 5 mg with a goal of 2–3 and a plan for [cardioversion]$_e$ in [6 weeks]$_t$.	overlap	after
[POD# 15/6]$_t$, she resumed [TF]$_e$'s and TPN was tapered again.	overlap	after

In the "sentences", the target time expression and the target event mention are marked with square brackets and subscripts 't' and 'e', respectively. "Predicted" is the type of direct temporal relation predicted by the SVM-based system. "Gold standard" is the gold standard type of direct temporal relation. When the temporal relation is non-direct, it is represented as "N/A"

ambiguity was in fact a major source of disagreement among the human annotators.

In addition, long sentences with complex syntactic structures often produced errors, probably due to the false parse trees produced by the automatic parser. For example, for the pair of a time expression and an event mention shown in the following sentence, the system missed a direct temporal relation of type "overlap".

1) On 9–28-92, the patient will return for chemotherapy and she will follow up with her primary doctor, Dr. Jescspald, for $[\text{repeat PT}]_e$ and Coumadin dosing on $[\text{Monday, 9–14-02}]_t$.

The second difficulty in accurately identifying direct temporal relations is the required use of common/domain knowledge in assigning appropriate types to direct temporal relations. The direct temporal relations are defined in a syntactically motivated way. Thus, the classification of a temporal relation into a direct or non-direct one can be done based on the constituency parse tree or the predicate-argument structure of the sentence. However, assigning type (i.e., "after", "before", "overlap") to the direct temporal relations still often requires inference based on common and domain knowledge. For instance, consider the three sentences following:

1) On $[\text{post-op day\#2}]_t$, $[\text{chest tubes}]_e$ were removed.
2) $[\text{The next day}]_t$, he developed $[\text{orthostasis}]_e$.
3) $[\text{Friday}]_t$, the patient underwent $[\text{a flex sigmoidoscopy}]_e$.

The three sentences above have similar predicate-argument structure to one another; both the time expression and the event mention are arguments/adjuncts of the main verb of the sentence. Thus, all three pairs of time expression and event mention form direct temporal relations. However, the type of the temporal relation differs from one another depending on the meaning of the sentence. For the first sentence, the type of the temporal relation between the treatment event "chest tube" and the time expression "post-op day #2" should be "before", since one can infer that "chest tubes" was applied before "post day #2". For the second sentence, the type of the temporal relation should be "after", since "orthostasis" will remain until being treated starting from "The next day". Finally, for the third sentence, the type of the temporal relation should be "overlap", since "sigmoidoscopy" will start and end on "Friday". In fact, the performance of the SVM-based system on detecting direct temporal relations not considering type assignment is shown to be much higher (precision 78.80, recall 84.33, and F1-score 81.47) than the performance of identifying direct temporal relations considering types. This indicates that type assignment is indeed a major source of error in direct temporal relation identification. We plan to devise methods that can incorporate common/domain knowledge into the direct temporal relation identification process.

Note that the inference here that uses common and domain knowledge is different from the kind of inference that is required to identify non-direct implicit relations such as inter-sentential relations. In order to identify non-direct implicit relations, one needs first to identify multiple direct temporal relations and then perform inference combining the direct relations. In this way, the direct temporal relations can be viewed as the basic building blocks that can be used to infer the complete set of all inferable temporal relations.

The last difficulty in accurately identifying direct temporal relations is the imbalanced nature of the direct temporal relations corpus (c.f., Table 3). Although cost-sensitive learning is applied to counter-balance the imbalance in the dataset, the performance of the minor relation types, "after" and "before", is much lower than the major type, "overlap" (Table 6). We plan to incorporate synthetic data generation techniques such as SMOTE algorithm [28], in order to improve the performance on minor types.

Lastly, we discuss on some real example outputs produced by the SVM-based system. See Table 5 of the Automatic identification performance Section for the examples. The first and second examples of Table 5 show direct temporal relations of type "overlap" that are correctly identified by the SVM-based system. Interestingly, all other baseline systems failed to identify the "overlap" type direct temporal relations for these two examples. One possible reason for such difference is that the SVM-based system is the only system that utilizes predicate-argument structure as feature; all other baseline systems do not utilize predicate-argument structure information. Note that in both examples, the event mention and the time expression are arguments or adjuncts of the same predicates (i.e., in the first example, the event mention "his creatinine" and the time expression "three days" are argument and adjunct of the verb predicate "rose"; in the second example, the event mention "Cardiac catheterization" and the time expression "the day" are argument and adjunct of the verb predicate "performed".).

Table 6 Performance of svm-based system for each relation type

Temporal relation type	P	R	F_1
After	53.44	33.78	31.39
Before	56.87	42.21	48.46
Overlap	66.74	77.66	71.79

In the third example of Table 5, the system wrongly classified a non-direct temporal relation between the event mention "SBP s" and the time expression "the morning of 12-10" as a direct temporal relation of type "overlap". We conjecture that such an error is produced by the failure in correctly identifying the syntactic tree structure of the sentence (i.e., attachment of the PP "with SBPs in the 70s" to the verb "had" instead of the noun "hypotension"). In the fourth example, the system failed to identify an "overlap" type direct temporal relation between the event mention "Vanc" and the time expression "Friday". Again, this error seems to be due to the failure in correctly identifying syntactic structure of the sentence (i.e., attachment of the PP "on Friday" to the NP "Cipro" instead of the NP "Vanc and Cipro").

For the last two examples, the system incorrectly identified direct temporal relations of type "after" as direct temporal relations of type "overlap". For the fifth example, while the preposition "in" usually signals temporal relation of type "overlap", in this context it conveys the meaning that "cardioversion" would be performed after a time period of "6 weeks". The system failed to identify such information. For the last example, the verb "resume" conveys the information that "TF" started on "POD# 15/6" and continued for some time after "POD# 15/6". However, the system failed to identify this information. In fact, all other baseline systems also failed to identify correct direct temporal relations for these two examples.

As future work, we plan to investigate different ways to improve the performance of automatic direct temporal relation identification. We plan to investigate how different features contribute to the performance, and to test diverse types of machine learning algorithms including deep learning. We are also considering using a rule-based system instead of machine-learning based systems as our definition of direct temporal relations describes a deterministic process of direct temporal relation identification based on syntactic structures of the sentences.

Conclusion

In this paper, we proposed to focus on direct temporal relations instead of targeting all inferable relations from a document. A corpus of direct temporal relations is constructed, and an automatic system that is tailored to the direct temporal relations is developed. It is shown that the direct temporal relations constitute a major category of temporal relations, and that a system optimized for direct temporal relations can achieve much better performance than a state-of-the-art system targeting all inferable temporal relations. We expect methods for direct temporal relations to advance wide adoption of automatic temporal information extraction tools in practical medical applications.

Endnotes

[1]Transitive closure of a set of temporal relations is the minimal set of minimal transitive relations that contains the original set of temporal relations.

[2]Based on our annotation, about 26% of direct temporal relations strictly follow the "head-of-the-phrase" rule, and the rest of direct temporal relations are identified based on the exception cases.

[3]The annotation guideline is available at https://sbmi.uth.edu/ccb/resources/temporal.htm.

Funding

This work is supported in part by NIGMS R01GM103859, NLM R01LM010681, NLM R01LM011829, NCI U24CA194215, and NIAID R01AI130460. Publication of this article was supported by National Institutes of Health under Award Number R01 GM103859.

Authors' contributions

HX conceived the idea of direct temporal relations. HX and HL developed the definition of direct temporal relations. HL, YZ, and MJ participated in the annotation process. HX, HL, YZ and CT wrote the manuscript. All authors read and approved the final manuscript.

Competing interests

The authors declare that they have no competing interests.

Author details

[1]School of Biomedical Informatics, The University of Texas Health Science Center at Houston, Houston, TX, USA. [2]Pieces Technologies, Dallas, TX, USA.

References

1. L. Zhou, C. Friedman, S. Parsons, and G. Hripcsak, "System Architecture for Temporal Information Extraction, Representation and Reasoning in Clinical Narrative Reports," presented at the AMIA Symposium, 2005, pp. 869–874.
2. L. Zhou, S. Parsons, and G. Hripcsak, "Handling implicit and uncertain temporal information in medical text," presented at the AMIA Symposium, 2006, p. 1158.
3. Sun W, Rumshisky A, Uzuner O. Annotating temporal information in clinical narratives. J Biomed Inform. 2013;46(S):S5–S12.
4. D. L. Mowery, S. Velupillai, B. R. South, L. Christensen, D. Martinez, L. Kelly, L. Goeuriot, N. Elhadad, S. Pradhan, G. Savova, and W. Chapman, "Task 2: ShARe/CLEF eHealth Evaluation Lab 2014," presented at the Proceedings of CLEF 2014, Sheffield, 2014.
5. S. Bethard, L. Derczynski, G. Savova, J. Pustejovsky, and M. Verhagen, "SemEval-2015 Task 6: Clinical TempEval," presented at the the 9th International Workshop on Semantic Evaluation, Stroudsburg, PA, USA, 2015, pp. 806–814.
6. S. Bethard, G. Savova, W.-T. Chen, L. Derczynski, J. Pustejovsky, and M. Verhagen, "SemEval-2016 Task 12 - Clinical TempEval.," presented at the Proceedings of the 10th International Workshop on Semantic Evaluations, 2016, pp. 565–572.
7. S. Bethard, G. Savova, M. Palmer, and J. Pustejovsky, "SemEval-2017 Task 12: Clinical TempEval," presented at the Proceedings of the 10th International Workshop on Semantic Evaluations, 2017, pp. 565–572.
8. Lin C, Dligach D, Miller TA, Bethard S, Savova GK. Multilayered temporal modeling for the clinical domain. J Am Med Inform Assoc. 2015;23(2): ocv113–9.
9. H. J. Lee, Y. Zhang, J. Xu, S. Moon, J. Wang, Y. Wu, and H. Xu, "UTHealth at SemEval-2016 task 12: an end-to-end system for temporal information extraction from clinical notes," presented at the SemEval 2016, 2016.
10. Tang B, Wu Y, Jiang M, Chen Y, Denny JC, Xu H. A hybrid system for temporal information extraction from clinical text. J Am Med Inform Assoc. 2013;20(5): 828–35.

11. A. X. Chang and C. D. Manning, "SUTIME: a library for recognizing and normalizing time expressions," Presented at the 8th international conference on language resources and evaluation LREC, 2012.
12. J. Strötgen and M Gertz, "HeidelTime - High Quality Rule-Based Extraction and Normalization of Temporal Expressions," presented at the Proceedings of the 5th International Workshop on Semantic Evaluation, 2010, pp. 321–324.
13. Zhou L, Parsons S, Hripcsak G. The evaluation of a temporal reasoning system in processing clinical discharge summaries. J Am Med Inform Assoc. 2008;15(1): 99–106.
14. Sun W, Rumshisky A, Uzuner O. Evaluating temporal relations in clinical text: 2012 i2b2 challenge. J Am Med Inform Assoc. 2013;20(5):806–13.
15. H.-J. Lee, Y. Zhang, J. Xu, C. Tao, M. Jiang, and H. Xu, "Towards practical temporal relation extraction from clinical notes: an analysis of direct temporal relations," presented at the SEPDA-BIBM, 2017, pp. 1–4.
16. Xu Y, Wang Y, Liu T, Tsujii J, Chang EI-C. An end-to-end system to identify temporal relation in discharge summaries: 2012 i2b2 challenge. J Am Med Inform Assoc. 2013;20(5):849–58.
17. A. Leeuwenberg and M.-F. Moens, "Structured learning for temporal relation extraction from clinical records," presented at the the th Conference of the European Chapter of the Association for Computational Linguistics, 2017, pp. 1150–1158.
18. Soysal E, Wang J, Jiang M, Wu Y, Pakhomov S, Liu H, Xu H. CLAMP – a toolkit for efficiently building customized clinical natural language processing pipelines. J Am Med Inform Assoc. 2017; https://doi.org/10.1093/jamia/ocx132.
19. J. Baldridge, "The opennlp project," 2005. [Online]. Available: http://opennlp.apache.org/index.html. [Accessed: 13-Mar-2017].
20. S. Bethard, P. V. Ogren, and L. Becker, "ClearTK 2.0 - Design Patterns for Mach Learn in UIMA.," presented at the LREC, 2014, pp. 3289–3293.
21. Collobert R, Weston J, Bottou L, Karlen M, Kavukcuoglu K, Kuksa P. Natural Language Processing (Almost) from Scratch. JMLR. 2011;12(Aug):2493–537.
22. Chang C-C, Lin C-J. LIBSVM: a library for support vector machines. ACM Trans Intell Syst Technol. 2011;2(3):27.
23. Zhang Y, Wu H-Y, Xu J, Wang J, Soysal E, Li L, Xu H. Leveraging syntactic and semantic graph kernels to extract pharmacokinetic drug drug interactions from biomedical literature. BMC Syst Biol. 2016;10(3):67.
24. J. Xu, Y. Zhang, J. Wang, Y. Wu, M. Jiang, E. Soysal, and H. Xu, "UTH-CCB: The Participation of the SemEval 2015 Challenge – Task 14," presented at the the 9th International Workshop on Semantic Evaluation, Stroudsburg, PA, USA, 2015, pp. 311–314.
25. Airola A, Pyysalo S, Björne J, Pahikkala T, Ginter F, Salakoski T. All-paths graph kernel for protein-protein interaction extraction with evaluation of cross-corpus learning. BMC Bioinformatics. 2008;9(11):S2.
26. Bundschus M, Dejori M, Stetter M, Tresp V, Kriegel H-P. Extraction of semantic biomedical relations from text using conditional random fields. BMC Bioinformatics. 2008;9:207.
27. Cohen J. A coefficient of agreement for nominal scales. Educ Psychol Meas. 1960;20(1):37–46.
28. Chawla NV, Bowyer KW, Hall LO, Kegelmeyer WP. SMOTE - synthetic minority over-sampling technique. J Artif Intell Res. 2002;16(1):321–57.

3

A mathematical modelling tool for unravelling the antibody-mediated effects on CTLA-4 interactions

Aravindhan Ganesan[1†], Theinmozhi Arulraj[1,2†], Tahir Choulli[3] and Khaled H. Barakat[1,4*]

Abstract

Background: Monoclonal antibodies blocking the Cytotoxic T-lymphocyte antigen 4 (CTLA-4) receptor have revolutionized the field of anti-cancer therapy for the last few years. The human T-cell-based immune responses are modulated by two contradicting signals. CTLA-4 provides a T cell inhibitory signal through its interaction with B7 ligands (B7–1 and B7–2), while CD28 provides a stimulatory signal when interacting with the same ligands. A previous theoretical model has focused on understanding the processes of costimulatory and inhibitory complex formations at the synapse. Nevertheless, the effects of monoclonal antibody (mAb)-mediation on these complexes are relatively unexplored. In this work, we expand on the previous model to develop a new mathematical framework for studying the effects of anti-CTLA-4 mAbs on the co-stimulatory (CD28/B7 ligands) and the co-inhibitory (CTLA-4/B7 ligands) complex formation at the immunological synapse. In particular, we focus on two promising anti-CTLA-4 mAbs, tremelimumab (from AstraZeneca) and ipilimumab (from Bristol-Myers Squibb), which are currently in clinical trials and the market, respectively, for targeting multiple tumors.

Methods: The mathematical model in this work has been constructed based on ordinary differential equations and available experimental binding kinetics data for the anti-CTLA-4 antibodies from literature.

Results: The numerical simulations from the current model are in agreement with a number of experimental data. Especially, the dose-curves for blocking the B7 ligand binding to CTLA-4 by ipilimumab are comparable with the results from a previous competitive binding assay by flow cytometry and ELISA. Our simulations predict the dose response and the relative efficacies of the two mAbs in blocking the inhibitory CTLA-4/B7 complexes.

Conclusions: The results show that different factors, such as multivalent interactions, mobility of molecules and competition effects, could impact the effects of antibody-mediation. The results, in particular, describe that the competitive effects could impact the dose-dependent inhibition by the mAbs very significantly. We present this model as a useful tool that can easily be translated to study the effects of any anti-CTLA-4 antibodies on immunological synaptic complex formation, provided reliable biophysical data for mAbs are available.

Keywords: CTLA-4, Immune checkpoints, Ipilimumab, Tremelimumab, Antibody, Mathematical modeling

* Correspondence: kbarakat@ualberta.ca
[†]Aravindhan Ganesan and Theinmozhi Arulraj contributed equally to this work.
[†]Equal contributors
[1]Faculty of Pharmacy and Pharmaceutical Sciences, University of Alberta, Edmonton, Canada
[4]Li Ka Shing Institute of Virology, University of Alberta, Edmonton, Canada
Full list of author information is available at the end of the article

Background

Blockade of immune checkpoints has recently been proven as a revolutionary strategy in the fight against cancers [1–6]. T-cells play a pivotal role in modulating the immune response against pathogens [7] and also in the prevention of autoimmunity [6]. According to the classic 'two-signal' model in immunology [8, 9], T-cell-mediated immune responses are activated by two different protein-protein interactions taking place at the immunological synapse [1–5, 10–12] (Fig. 1). The first signal is triggered when the T-cell receptors (TCRs) recognize the major histocompatibility complex (MHC) on the surface of antigen-presenting cells (APCs). A second signal comes from the binding of CD28, a co-receptor expressed on the T-cell surface, with its' complementary B7 ligands, known as B7–1 (or CD80) and B7–2 (or CD86), on the surface of APCs. This second signal is required to activate and sustain the activity of T-cells [3, 5, 13, 14]; hence it is known as a co-stimulatory signal and CD28 is dubbed as a co-stimulatory receptor (Fig. 1). On the other hand, there are a number of negative signal stimuli (known as the inhibitory receptors) that act to inactivate the T-cells, including cytotoxic T-lymphocyte-associated protein-4 (CTLA-4 or CD152) and programmed death 1 (PD1 or CD279) [3]. Particularly, CTLA-4, a CD28 homologue (with ~ 30% sequence identity) expressed on the T-cell surface, binds with the same set of B7-ligands of CD28; albeit with higher affinity towards B7–1 and B7–2. Both CD28 and CTLA-4 are transmembrane proteins of the immunoglobulin superfamily that exist as homodimers [15] .Nevertheless, CD28 is known to bind the ligands monovalently; whereas, CTLA-4 is bivalent in nature that, infact, allows it to bind the B7 ligands with high avidity [15, 16]. Given such differences, under competitive environments, CTLA-4 would be able to out-compete CD28 for ligand-binding [17]. The functionalities of CD28 and CTLA-4 are interlinked and both co-stimulatory and co-inhibitory signals are required for maintaining the immunological balance between self-tolerance and defending against foreign entities and pathogens under normal conditions [4–6, 18, 19].

Cancer cells are able to escape the immunological surveillance of T-cells, by overexpressing the inhibitory receptors that attenuate anti-tumor immune response [4, 5]. As a result, in principal, blocking the co-inhibitory receptor-ligand interactions (schematically shown in Fig. 1) should be able to facilitate the re-activation of T-cells, which in-turn will recognize and eliminate cancers. Monoclonal antibodies (mAbs) blocking inhibitory immune checkpoints have demonstrated exceptional therapeutic benefits in clinical trials [20–22], which is transforming human cancer treatment. Ipilimumab, a completely human IgG1 antibody from Bristol-Myers Squibb, became the first-in-class anti-CTLA-4 mAb to be approved by the US Food and Drug Administration (FDA) in 2011 for the treatment of metastatic melanoma [23, 24]. Several clinical trials showed

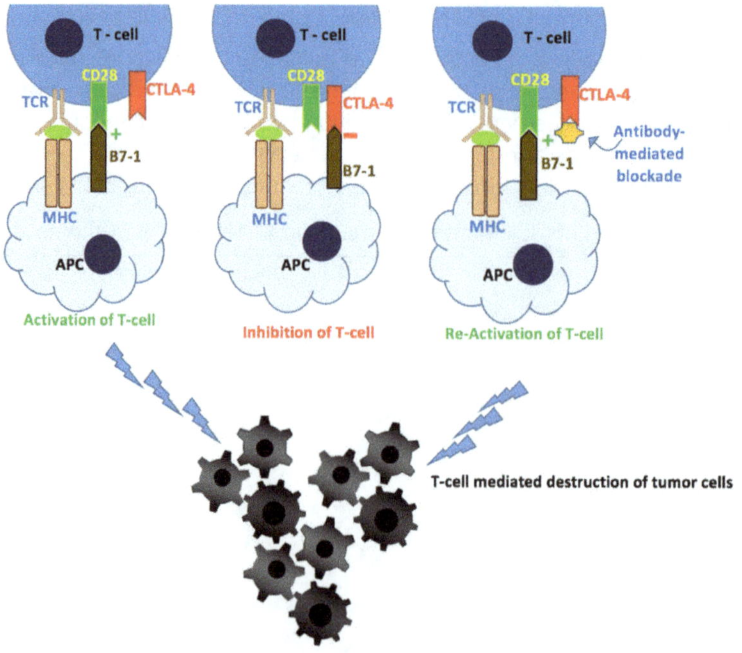

Fig. 1 Schematic representation of T-cell activation and inhibition by the interactions of CD28 and CTLA-4 with the B7 ligands, B7–1 and B7–2, respectively

that monotherapy with ipilimumab in metastasis melanoma patients increased the overall responsive rate by 10–20% [1, 25]. When combined with other immune checkpoint therapies, ipilimumab is able to offer much enhanced benefits [26, 27]. Another IgG2 anti-CTLA-4 mAb, Tremelimumab from AstraZeneca, is currently in phase III clinical trials [1, 5]. Similar to Ipilimumab, AstraZeneca's tremelimumab binds specifically to CTLA-4 and blocks its interaction with the B7 ligands. Tremelimumab is also being tested in combination with other immune checkpoint mAbs for targeting multiple tumors [28, 29], including melanoma, colon cancer, and mesothelioma [28, 29]. The progress made by these two antibodies, from bench to final clinical trial phases or to the market, has boosted the interests towards developing more promising immune-checkpoint blocking inhibitors (both mAbs and, lately, small molecules).

Very recently, He et al. [1] investigated the binding profiles of both mAbs against CTLA-4 using surface plasmon resonance (SPR) experiments and reported their K_D values as 18.2 nM for ipilimumab/CTLA-4 complex and 5.89 nM for tremelimumab/CTLA-4 complex. These binding affinity values are higher than (or, in some cases, comparable to) those reported for B7–1 ligands with CTLA-4 [1]. However, it is important to note that different range of affinity values have been reported for the CTLA-4/B7–1 complexes. For example, an earlier study reported that a soluble B7–1 Ig fusion protein bound to CTLA-4 with a dissociation constant of ~ 12 nM [30]. However, this value was argued to be higher when compared with other protein-protein interactions occurring between T-cell surface and APCs [31]. The authors of this work [30] had described that the CTLA-4Ig in their experiments was not monomeric in solution, and possibly formed higher aggregates that might have possibly resulted in the high apparent K_D values for the interactions of CTLA-4Ig/B7Ig fusion protein. Another study [31] based on SPR experiments reported that, at 37 °C, soluble recombinant B7–1 bound to CTLA-4 with a K_D value of 0.42 μM. This indicates that affinity between B7–1 and CTLA-4 is relatively lower than that of ipilimumab/CTLA-4 and tremelimumab/CTLA-4 complexes. The association rate constant (k_a) of ipilimumab (3.83×10^5/Ms) and tremelimumab (3.08×10^5/Ms) are almost close to each other, however, their dissociation rate constants (k_d) were significantly different [1]. The k_d value for ipilimumab was 6.96×10^{-3}/s, whereas for tremelimumab it was 1.8×10^{-3}/s [1]. This clearly indicates that the tremelimumab is able to form much stable complex with CTLA-4 when compared to that of ipilimumab. Thus, understanding the effects of these two potent anti-CTLA-4 antibodies on the co-stimulatory and the co-inhibitory complex formation at the synapse will be useful to develop effective next-generation anti-CTLA-4 therapeutics. The ultimate objective of this work is to precisely study these effects using mathematical modelling and simulations.

Mathematical modelling and simulation remains a powerful tool to gain quantitative insights into the dynamics of complicated systems [32–40]. Especially, mathematical modelling is gaining more popularity in the field of cancer immunotherapy. For example, Kirschner et al. [38] developed a mathematical model, based on ordinary differential equations (ODEs) to simulate the dynamics between tumor cells, immune-effector cells and cytokine interleukin-2. This model was useful to explore the effects of adoptive cellular immunotherapy (ACI) on the model and found that a combination therapy with ACI and IL-2 could boost the immune system sufficiently to clear the tumor [38]. Krnoik et al. [37] developed an expanded mathematical model, from a previously published model, in order to simulate cellular immunotherapy in melanoma. This model was useful to understand the findings from clinical trials suggesting that patients with the smallest tumor load respond better for this kind treatment [37]. Mathematical models have also been useful to understand tumor growth, response to therapy and the interactions of immune cells with the cancer cell [39–42]. Bidot et al. [43] developed a mathematical model for studying the kinetics of monoclonal T-cell-specific activation. This model attempted to account for the sequence of events starting from the TCR-MHC binding to T-cell activation and response [43]. Mathematical modelling has also been employed to study the complex formation between PD-1 receptor and its ligands [44]. Jansson et al. [33] developed a theoretical model for simulating the synaptic accumulation of the molecules involved in co-stimulation and inhibition of T-cells. This model, which was developed based on the Ordinary Differential Equations (ODEs) and rigorous biophysical and expression data from literature, explained the interactions of CTLA-4 and CD-28 with their B7-ligands in the context of a potentially dynamic synaptic microenvironment [33]. However, until now, there is no model that could predict the response to CTLA-4 blocking antibodies and the consequent effects on complex formation at immunological synapse.

In this work, we expand the model of Jansson et al. [33] by including the effect of an anti-CTLA-4 antibody. Our model is based on ODEs and additional biophysical data for antibody-CTLA-4 complexes [1]. Using this new model, we studied how the binding of mAbs (with different affinities) to CTLA-4 dynamically changed the interactions among co-inhibitory complexes (CTLA-4/B7–1 and CTLA-4/B7–2) and co-stimulatory complexes

(CD28/B7–1 and CD28/B7–2) at the immunological synapse. The numerical simulations from the model have been validated by different experimental data reported earlier. This model should be a useful tool to predict the dose response of any anti-CTLA-4 antibodies and their impacts on synaptic complex formation processes.

Methods

Mathematical modelling assumptions

As mentioned above, the mathematical model in this work is based on the previous two-compartment model by Jansson et al. [33], which was constructed to simulate the CD28 and CTLA-4 complex formation with the B7-ligands at immunological synapses. In this study, we developed an expanded model to assess the changes in the co-stimulatory (CD28/B7 ligands) and the co-inhibitory (CTLA-4/B7 ligands) interactions upon binding of the antibody to the free CTLA-4 receptor sites. This model, as in Jansson's model [33], involves two components that includes the synapse and the region outside of the synapse. It is assumed that CD28, B7–1 and B7–2 are primarily unbound and distributed uniformly over the surface. CTLA-4, on the other hand, is present intracellularly and gets injected into the synapse upon activation [45, 46]. The 'free-diffusion' model has been applied to control the mobility of the molecules, such that only the mobile molecules are able to diffuse into the synapse, while the immobile species outside of the synapse are ignored. It is understandable that the immobile species outside of the synapse are, anyway, not able to participate in any complex formation. On the other hand, the immobile molecules inside the synapse stay there and are involved in the protein-protein interactions. The model also assumes that the CTLA-4 receptors, once injected from the intracellular environment, stay within the synapse. In the case of antibody, unlike the membrane-bound ligands, it is in the free solution and is assumed to bind to free CTLA-4 monovalently. The model assumes that the binding site of B7–1, B7–2 and the antibody molecules on CTLA-4 overlap considerably [2], and, therefore, only one of them (B7–1 or B7–2 or the antibody) is able to bind with a CTLA-4 molecule. Moreover, in our model, the antibody is allowed to bind an unbound CTLA-4 monomer that is part of a dimer, where the other monomer can be bound with a B7 ligand. Due to the lack of parameters for the association and dissociation of complexes in the model, rate constants from similar complexes are used and reactions are modelled as parallel mass action reactions. Bivalent association and dissociation rate constants are employed for the binding/unbinding of B7 ligands to a CTLA-4 monomer that is part of a dimer, where the other monomer is bound to an antibody.

Parameters

The parameters for the interactions of CTLA-4 and CD28 with the B7 ligands in the current model are almost similar to those in Jansson's model [33], which are given in the supplementary information (Additional file 1: Table S1). However, the association and dissociation rate constants for the interactions of antibodies, tremelimumab and ipilimumab, with CTLA-4 receptor are collected from the literature [1] and employed in the current model. The reported SPR experiments [1] measured the association rate constants of ipilimumab and tremelimumab with CTLA-4 to be 3.83×10^5/Ms. and 3.08×10^5/Ms., respectively. Whereas, their dissociation rate constants were observed to be 6. 96×10^{-3}/s (ipilimumab) and 1.8×10^{-3}/s [1] (tremelimumab). It is important to note that the rate constants for the interactions of antibodies are not converted to 2-D rates, as the antibodies are present in the solution. This approximation is reasonable, when the binding site is accessible [47].

Antibody complex formation

The equations related to the modelling of rates of change for the complex formation between different species, such as CD28, CTLA-4, B7–1 and B7–2, are all similar to those of Jansson et al. [33]. However, a number of additional terms are employed in the current model in order to account for the increase or decrease in density of these species in response to the association and dissociation of antibodies to that of CTLA-4 monomers. Please note that the rate of change of the density of complexes for the newly added terms in the model are also written using the mass-action law.

Rate of change of density of antibody/CTLA-4 complex

The antibody associates with a CTLA-4 dimer at the rate of k_{on}, in order to form the antibody/(CTLA-4)$_2$ complex (referred as Ac complex in the equation). The rate for dissociation of antibody from the Ac complex is k_{off}. An unbound B7–1 associates with the Ac complex at the rate of $\alpha_{44}$to form a complex of Ac/B7–1 (or EAb_1), whereas, an unbound B7–2 associates with the Ac complex at the rate of α_{33} to form Ac/B7–2 (or Ab/CTLA4/B72). An antibody binds to the Ac complex at the rate of Kon to form the resultant Ab/Ac (or AcA) complex. The association of either of the B7–1 ligands or antibody to the Ac complex reduces the density of the latter. On the other hand, dissociation of B7–1 (rate = δ_{44}), B7–2 (rate = δ_{33}) and antibody (rate = k_{off}) from the EAb1, Ab/CTLA4/B72, AcA complexes, respectively, increases the density. Hence, the rate of change in the density of the Ac complex can be written as follows,

$$\frac{dAc}{dt} = -\alpha_{44}{}^*Ac^*B71 + \delta_{44}{}^*EAb_1 - k_{on}{}^*Ac^*Ab + k_{off}{}^*AcA + k_{on}{}^*CTLA4^*Ab - k_{off}{}^*Ac - \alpha_{33}{}^*Ac^*B72 + \delta_{33}{}^*Ab/CTLA4/B72 \quad (1)$$

The rate of change of density for the other antibody-mediated complexes are given in supplementary information, Additional file 2: Table S2. The numbers of free antibody molecules is increased by the dissociation of mAb from any of the antibody-included complexes (such as, Ac, AcA, Ab/CTLA-4/B72, EAb, CAb, DAb). On the other hand, association of free antibody to form any of the above complexes decreases the total number of free antibody molecules,and this rate of change in the antibody can be written as,

$$\frac{dAb}{dt} = -k_{on}{}^*CTLA4^*Ab + k_{off}{}^*Ac - k_{on}{}^*Ac^*Ab + k_{off}{}^*AcA - k_{on}{}^*Ab^*\sum_{k=1}^{\infty}E_k + k_{off}{}^*\sum_{k=1}^{\infty}EAb_k - k_{on}{}^*Ab^*\sum_{k=1}^{\infty}C_k + k_{off}{}^*\sum_{k=1}^{\infty}CAb_k - k_{on}{}^*Ab^*\sum_{k=1}^{\infty}CAb_k + k_{off}{}^*\sum_{k=1}^{\infty}DAb_k - k_{on}{}^*CTLA4/B72^*Ab + k_{off}{}^*Ab/CTLA4/B72 \quad (2)$$

Density of mobile CD28, B71 and B72 molecules, present outside synapse is estimated by subtracting the total number of mobile molecules of CD28, B71,B72 that are part of complexes formed at synapse.

$$CD28out = t_{CD28,tot}{}^*m_{CD28} - (CD28 + CD28/B71 + 2^*(CD28)_2/B71 + CD28/B72 - i_{CD28}) * a_{syn} \quad (3)$$

$$B71out = t_{B71,tot}{}^*m_{B71} - (B71 + CD28/B71 + (CD28)_2/B71 + \sum_{k=1}^{\infty}B_k(k+1) + \sum_{k=1}^{\infty}C_k k + \sum_{k=1}^{\infty}E_k k + \sum_{k=1}^{\infty}EAb_k k + \sum_{k=1}^{\infty}CAb_k k + \sum_{k=1}^{\infty}DAb_k k - i_{B71}) * a_{syn} \quad (4)$$

$$B72out = t_{B72,tot}{}^*m_{B72} - (B72 + CD28/B72 + CTLA4/B72 + 2^*CTLA4/(B72)_2 + Ab/CTLA4/B72 - i_{B72}) * a_{syn} \quad (5)$$

Similarly, the number of CTLA4 molecules present inside the cell is calculated by subtracting it from total number of CTLA4 molecules.

$$CTLA4int = t_{CTLA4,tot}{}^*m_{CTLA4} - (CTLA4 + CTLA4/B72 + CTLA4/(B72)_2 + \sum_{k=1}^{\infty}B_k k + \sum_{k=1}^{\infty}C_k(k+1) + \sum_{k=1}^{\infty}E_k k + \sum_{k=1}^{\infty}EAb_k k + \sum_{k=1}^{\infty}CAb_k(k+1) + \sum_{k=1}^{\infty}DAb_k(k+1) + Ab/CTLA4/B72 + Ac + AcA) * a_{syn} \quad (6)$$

Modelling and simulations

Mathematical modelling and simulation procedures in this study were programmed using MATLAB software from MathWorks (https://www.mathworks.com/products/matlab.html). A stiff ordinary differential equation solver, ode15s, was used for solving the equations in the current model. The different components included in the model and their abbreviations are provided in the supplementary information (Additional file 3: Table S3). Each simulation was performed for 7 h (i.e., 25,200 s) unless otherwise stated. Initially, the simulations are performed with '0' concentration of antibody, in order to reproduce the results from Jansson's model [33]. Later, the simulations were performed with different concentrations of tremelimumab and ipilimumab and the effects on CTLA-4 and CD28 complex formation were analyzed.

Results

Simulation of antibody-free complex formation

Initially, the simulation based on the free-diffusion model (Fig. 2a) was performed for ~ 7 h, without the inclusion of any antibody (i.e., 0 μM antibody concentration).This situation is ideally to reproduce the simulation from Jansson et al. [33].This simulation mimics an activated T-cell environment, where both CD28 and CTLA-4 are present at the synapse and are competing for ligand-binding. During the initial hours (~ 15 min), the expression levels of B7–2 at synapse is much higher and hence, it remained the leading ligand for CTLA-4 and CD28. Particularly, at about 6 min, the CTLA-4/B72 interactions reached a peak with ~ 600 CTLA-4 monomers were bound to B7–2, against ~ 140 CTLA-4/B7–1 and 108 CD28/B7–2 complexes. The domination of CTLA-4/B7–2 remained until ~ 17 min, however, this number (of CTLA-4/B7–2 complex) dropped significantly to < 50 at ~ 1 h of simulation. Gradually, as more CTLA-4 moved from the intracellular region to the synapse (see in Fig. 2b), the CTLA-4/B7–1 complex replaced CTLA-4/B7–2 and became the most populated complex after ~ 20 min. After reaching the steady state, it can be seen (in Fig. 2a) that the majority of the B7–1 was bound to CTLA-4 (resulting ~ 790 CTLA-4/B7–1 complexes), while only small numbers of B7–1 (~ 50)

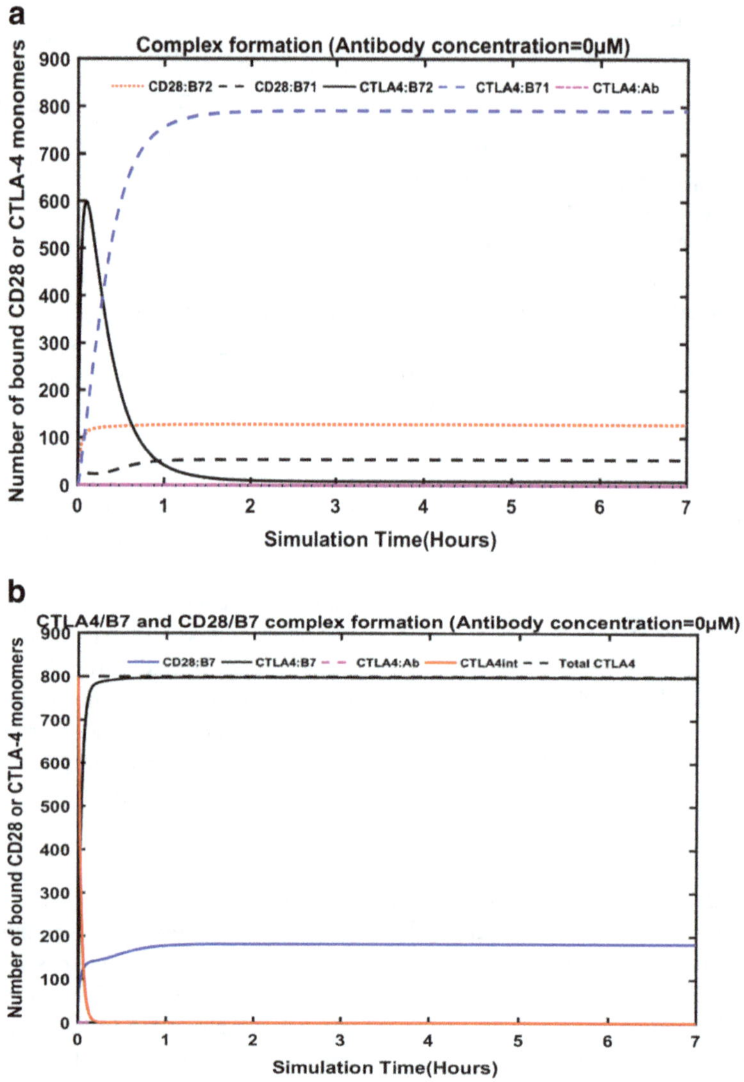

Fig. 2 Complex formation in the free-diffusion model from the antibody-free simulations. The number of CD28 and CTLA-4 molecules bound to B7–1 and B7–2 at the immunological synapse, during the antibody-free simulations (**a**). The dynamic changes in the total numbers of CTLA-4/B7 complex, CD28/B7 complex, amount of CTLA-4 at the intra-cellular environment and the total number of CTLA-4 monomers are provided (**b**)

were engaged with the CD28 receptor. On the other hand, the amount of CD28/B7–2 complexes (~ 127) outnumbers the complexes formed by CTLA-4 monomers and B7–2(~ 8). As Jansson et al. [33] noted, these behaviors in the simulation are in good agreement with previous findings that B7–1 is the preferred ligand for CTLA-4 and B7–2 preferentially recruits CD28 at the synapse [48, 49]. Hence, 99% of CTLA-4 are complexed with B7–1, while only 1% of the receptor is engaged with the B7–2 ligand. Overall, however, the percentage of CTLA-4 complexed with the B7 ligands is much higher than that of CD28/B7 complexes (Fig. 2b). This trend is expected as CTLA-4 has a higher affinity towards B7 ligands than that of CD28.

Binding of the antibodies to CTLA-4

Initially, we performed two simulations with an in silico knockout model, where CD28 and the B7 ligands (both B7–1 and B7–2) were muted and only CTLA-4 was allowed to bind with the antibodies, ipilimumab and tremelimumab, at different concentrations (0.002 μM to 0.018 μM). These simulations were carried out in order to confirm that, in a non-competitive setting, 50% of CTLA-4 had formed complex with the antibodies when the concentration of the antibodies equaled their respective K_D values. As shown in Figs. 3, 50% of the CTLA-4 monomers were bound to antibody at the concentrations of 0.018 μM and 0.0058 μM of ipilimumab (Fig. 3a) and tremelimumab (Fig. 3b),

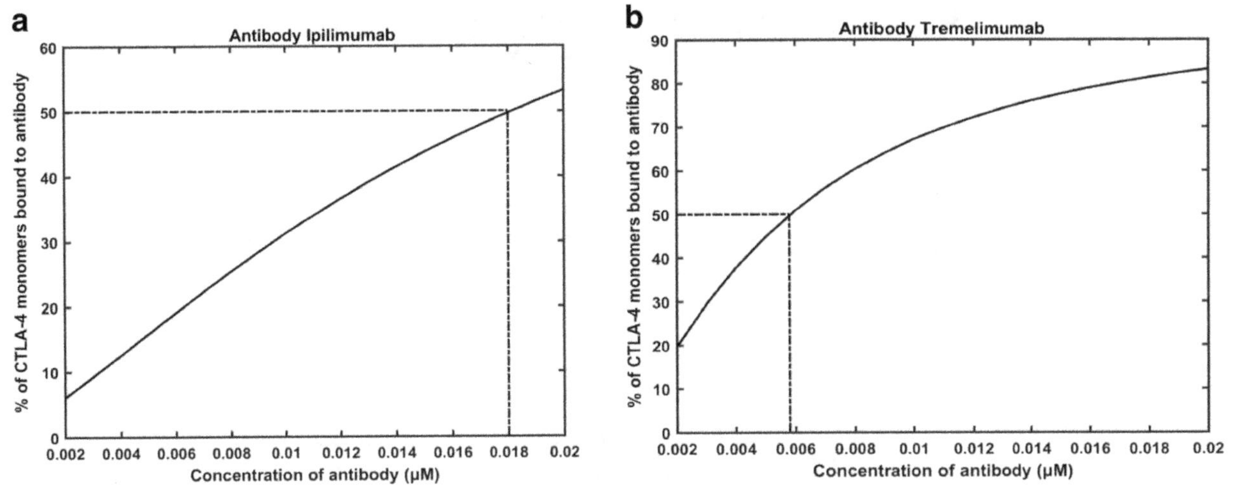

Fig. 3 The reproduction of the experimental K_D values for the binding of CTLA-4 to ipilimumab (**a**) and tremelimumab (**b**)

respectively. These concentrations are approximately close to the K_D values for these antibodies (ipilimumab – 18.2 nM; Tremelimumab – 5.89 nM), as reported by He et al. [1] based on their SPR experiments. Nevertheless, since the association and dissociation rate constants of the antibodies for the current model was obtained from the work of He et al. [1], it is expected that the model is able to achieve 50% complex formation at the concentration of the K_D values of mAbs. Hence, this confirms that the model simulates the complex formation correctly.

Competitive binding of the antibodies to CTLA-4 and model validation

Next, we performed the simulations to study how the antibodies, in the absence of CD-28, competed with either B7–1 or B7–2 for binding to CTLA-4. In order to perform these simulations, CD-28 and either of the B7 ligands were muted in the model. The resulting dose response curves for the percent inhibition of B7–1 binding and B7–2 binding with CTLA-4 at different concentrations of the antibodies, as predicted by the model, are shown in Fig. 4a and b, respectively. As shown in Fig. 4a and b, the model was able to simulate the dose-dependent inhibition of CTLA-4/B7 interactions by the competitive binding of ipilimumab and tremelimumab.

The dose-curves for blocking B7–1 and B7–2 binding by ipilimumab (Fig. 4a) is comparable with the experimental dose curves reported by Keler et al. [50] for the same antibody. It is important to note that no values from this experimental work have been used in our simulations or in the construction of our model. In this previous work [50], the scientists at Medarex performed competitive binding assay by flow cytometry and ELISA to demonstrate the ability of ipilimumab (dubbed as 10D1 in the paper) [50] to block the interactions of CTLA-4 with B7–1 and B7–2, separately. The simulations based on our model was also carried out by having only one of the B7 ligands active at a time, so as to mimic the experimental set-up [50]. Although the overall trends in the dose-response curves for ipilimumab obtained from our model and the previous experiment [50] are in agreement, the percent inhibition predicted for each dose of the antibody by our model are higher than those observed in the experiments [50]. For example, our model predicts that, at 10 μM concentration of ipilimumab, ~ 89% of B7–1 and ~ 92% of B7–2 are blocked; the experiments, on the other hand, reported ~ 70% and ~ 90% inhibition of B7–1 and B7–2 binding [50], respectively. Nevertheless, it should be noted that the previous experiments [50] were carried out with a human CTLA-4 (hCTLA-4) expressing cell, which was constructed by a hCTLA-4/murineCD3 chimeric gene. Thus, taking into account this difference and other experimental conditions, in general, the predictions from our model and the experiments are in reasonable agreement. Particularly, Keler et al. [50] reported an IC_{50} value of ~ 1–3 μM for ipilimumab (or 10D1 as named in the paper) to block the B7 ligands, which is in excellent agreement with the values predicted by our model (IC_{50} = 1.11 μM for B7–2 blocking; and 3.5 μM for B7–1 blocking). This validates the ability of our model to simulate the competitive binding between antibodies and the B7 ligands reasonably well.

By comparing the dose-response curves for the two antibodies as predicted from our simulations, it is

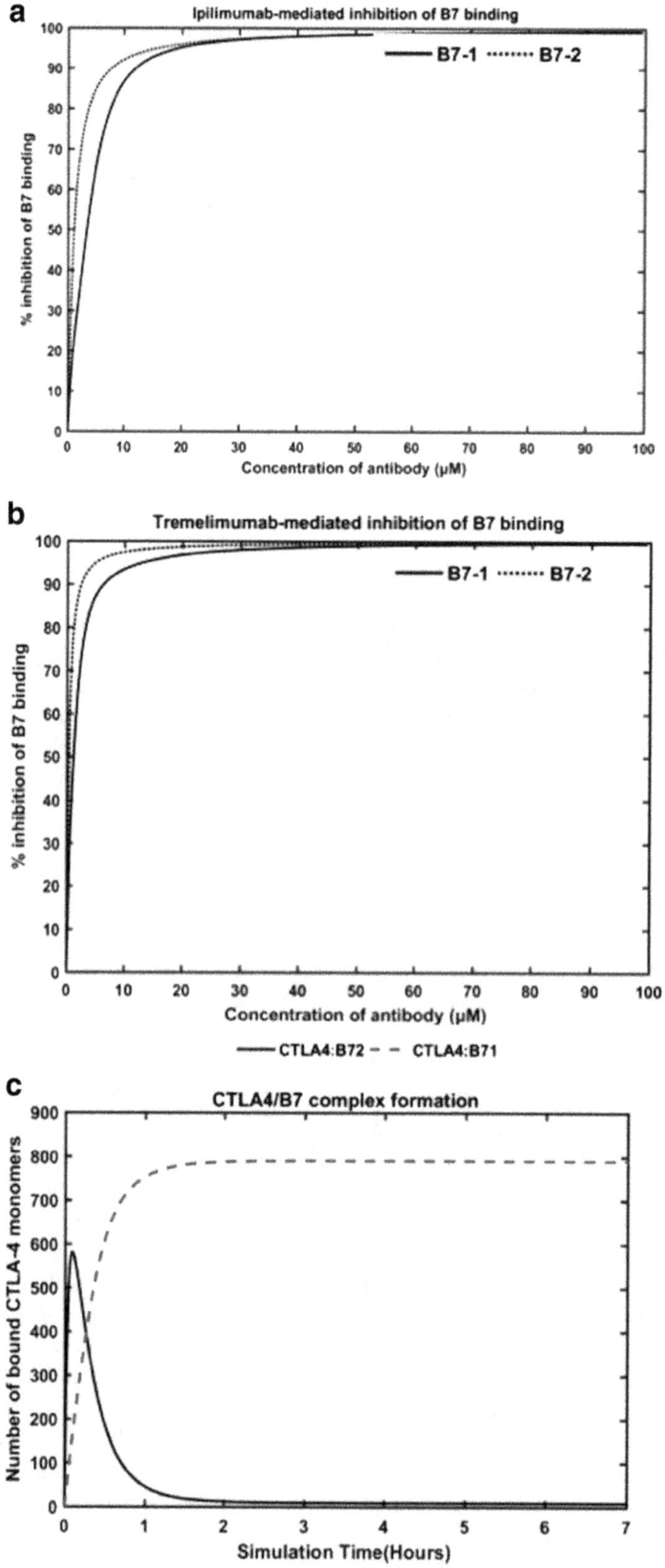

Fig. 4 The dose-curves for the blocking of B7 ligands to CTLA-4 by ipilimumab (**a**) and tremelimumab (**b**) in the simulations performed in either of the B7 -knock-out model, where either of the B7 ligands and CD28 were removed. The complex formation of CTLA-4/B7–1 and CTLA-4/B7–2 in the absence of CD28 and antibody is also simulated (**c**)

apparent that, at any given dose concentration, tremelimumab (Fig. 4b) is able to inhibit higher percentage of B7–1 and B7–2, when compared to that of ipilimumab (Fig. 4a). For instance, 1 μM of tremelimumab was found to inhibit ~ 54% of B7–1 binding and ~ 76% of B7–2 binding, which are much higher % inhibition than those obtained from 1 μM of ipilimumab (~ 25% of B7–1 inhibition; ~ 47% inhibition of B7–2) in our simulations. Such trends are in line with the affinity of these antibodies against CTLA-4 as reported by He et al [1]. It has been reported that both the antibodies have comparable association rate constants, however, the dissociation rate constants of ipilimumab is much higher than that of tremelimumab [1]. Hence, tremelimumab is able to block much higher amounts of B7 ligands from binding to CTLA-4, when matched with ipilimumab. In addition, it can be noted that higher percent inhibition of CTLA-4/B7–2 interactions than CTLA-4/B71 interactions can be achieved with low concentrations (≤ 10 μM) of the antibodies. This again accords with previous observation that the affinity of CTLA-4 to B7–1 is higher than its affinity to B7–2 [51]. In order to test this statement, we performed a simulation with our model, where only B7–1 and B7–2 were allowed to competitively bind with CTLA-4. To model this scenario, we again left the total initial concentrations of the antibodies and the CD28 receptor to 0, such that they do not have any effects on CTLA-4 binding to the B7 ligands. The result from this simulation is shown in Fig. 4c. Except for the first few minutes of the simulations, when the synapse was dominated by B7–2, the predominant amount of CTLA-4 remained in complex with B7–1 and the proportion of CTLA-4/B7–2 complex was meager.

Effects of antibody-mediation on the overall complex formation

Subsequently, we tested the effects of antibody-mediation on the co-stimulatory (CD28/B7 ligands) and the co-inhibitory (CTLA-4/B7 ligands) complex formation at the synapse. Simulations were performed with a restraint-free competitive environment facilitated by the model, where all the species (such as CTLA-4, B7–1, B7–2 and CD28) were present and a specific concentration of either of the antibodies was added. Initially, 10 μM concentration of ipilimumab (Fig. 5a) and tremelimumab (Fig. 5b) were added in the simulations to study their effects. The results are comparable to Fig. 2a, where the simulation performed without the antibodies (concentration = 0 μM) is provided. As expected, upon addition of 10 μM concentration of antibodies, the antibody-bound CTLA-4 complex out-numbered the other complex formations. Particularly, in the antibody-free simulations, the B7–2-bound CTLA-4 complex (~ 600) was dominant during the initial hours; however, the presence of the antibody reduced the initial dominance of this complex (CTLA-4/B7–2) by at least 75%.

In the case of simulation with ipilimumab (concentration = 10 μM), it can be seen that both the B7 ligands and ipilimumab contested for CTLA-4 binding during the early hours. However, the antibody out-competed the B7 ligands to form complexes with CTLA-4. It can be seen in Fig. 5a that, at the end of the simulations, there were ~ 630 CTLA-4/ipilimumab complexes against ~ 129 CTLA-4/B7–1 complexes. This is, particularly, a significant reduction in the sheer dominance of CTLA-4/B7–1 complexes (790 numbers) seen in the antibody-free simulations. On the other hand, 10 μM concentration of tremelimumab was able to bind more effectively with CTLA-4, thus remaining the most populated complex (~ 760 CTLA-4/tremelimumab complexes) at the steady state of the simulations, as shown in Fig. 5b. As a result, there were only 20 complexes of CTLA-4 and B7–1 at the end of simulations with tremelimumab (10 μM). In summary, the antibody-mediation has significantly impacted the CTLA-4/B7 ligand complex formation, which reduced from ~ 800 numbers (in antibody-free simulations) to ~ 168 and ~ 42 in the simulations with 10 μM of ipilimumab and tremelimumab, respectively. Later, we increased the dose of the antibodies to 15 μM and performed simulations (Fig. 5c-d). The higher dose of antibodies naturally increased the effects on CTLA-4 binding and B7-ligand blockade. In fact, predominant CTLA-4 monomers were engaged in complexes with the antibodies, ipilimumab (~ 707) and tremelimumab (~ 780). And as a result, the inhibitory complex formation between CTLA-4 and the B7-ligands had significantly diminished (~ 23 with 15 μM of tremelimumab; ~ 92 with 15 μM of ipilimumab). However, the addition of antibody did not significantly impact the interactions of CD28 with the B7 ligands. While the amount of CD28/B7–2 complexes remained almost the same in antibody-free and antibody-included simulations, the number of CD28/B71 complexes increased only slightly. The total numbers of different complexes (such as CTLA-4/mAb, CTLA-4/B7 and CD28/B7) at the end of simulations performed with different concentrations of ipilimumab and tremelimumab are summarized in Table 1.

Next, we simulated full dose-response curves for the two antibodies (Fig. 6), ipilimumab and tremelimumab. The inhibition percentage of the B7 ligands (i.e., B7–1 and B7–2) at each concentration of the antibodies in this figure was calculated as follows,

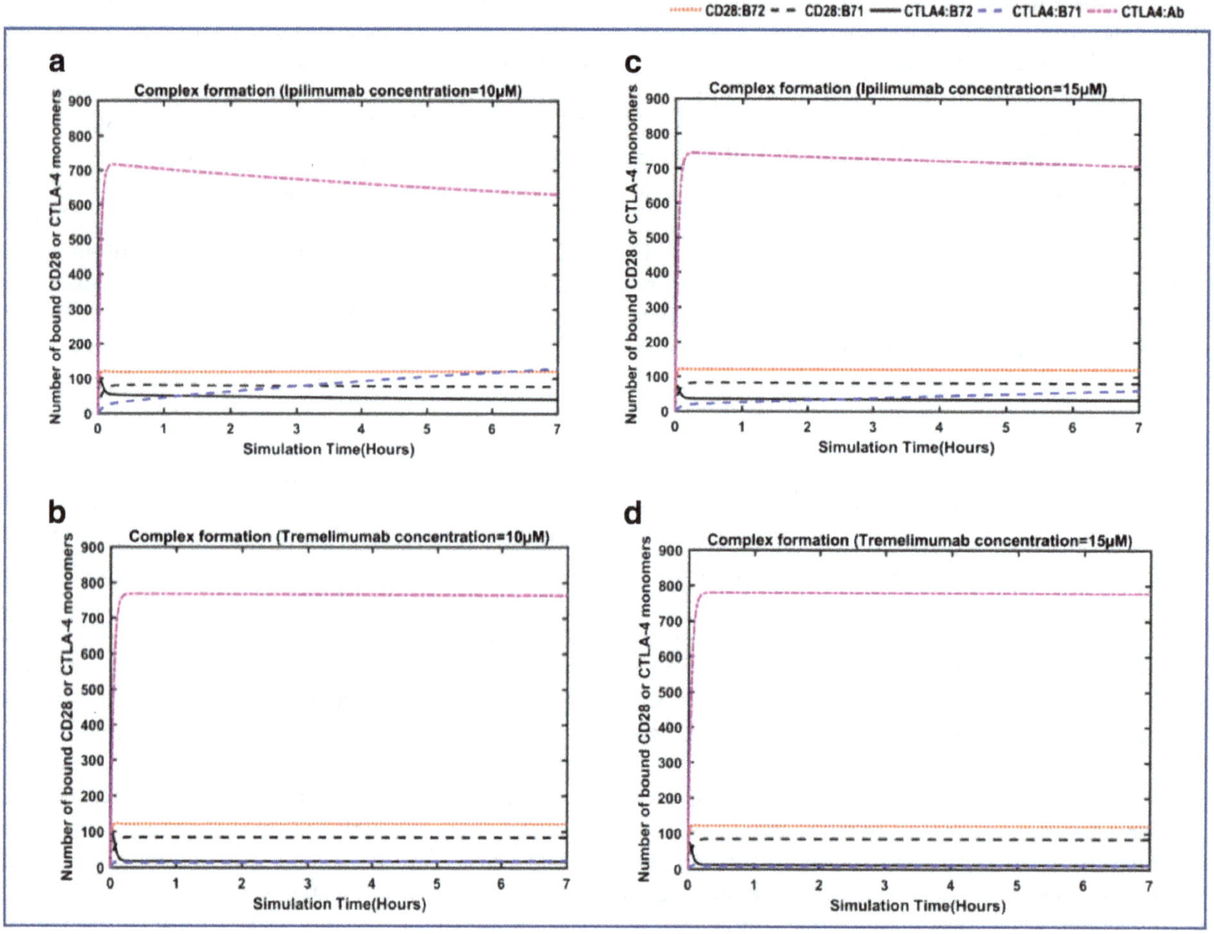

Fig. 5 Antibody-mediated changes in the complex formation at the synapse in the free-diffusion model: The dynamic changes in the different complexes, such as CTLA-4/antibody, CTLA-4/B7 ligands and CD28/B7 ligands, at the synapse are simulated at 10 μM and 15 μM of antibodies, ipilimumab (**a**, **c**) and tremelimumab (**b**, **d**)

$$\%B7\ inibition@x\ \mu M\ of\ mAb = \left(1 - \frac{(No.of\ CTLA{-}4/B7\ complex)@x\ \mu M\ of\ mAb}{(No.of\ CTLA{-}4/B7\ complex)@0\ \mu M\ of\ mAb}\right) \times 100 \quad (7)$$

Table 1 Comparison of the total numbers of CTLA-4/mAb, CTLA-4/B7 and CD28/B7 complexes formed at the end of simulations performed with the different concentrations (= 0 μM, 10 μM and 15 μM) of ipilimumab and tremelimumab

Interactions	Number of interacting CTLA-4/CD28 monomers					
	Initial	Antibody =0 μM	Tremelimumab		Ipilimumab	
			(10 μM)	(15 μM)	(10 μM)	(15 μM)
CD28/B7–2	0	127	121	121	121	120
CD28/B7–1	0	54	83	84	77	81
CTLA-4/B7–2	0	8	17	12	40	32
CTLA-4/B7–1	0	790	20	11	129	60
CTLA-4/mAb	0	0	763	778	631	707

From the dose curves, it is clear that both the antibodies have effectively inhibited the bivalent interactions of CTLA-4 and B7–1 even at very small concentrations. In fact, 50% of the B7–1 interactions with CTLA-4 were inhibited at concentrations < 5 μM in the case of both the antibodies. As much as 10 μM of either of the antibodies was sufficient to achieve ~ 90% (or more) inhibition of CTLA-4/B7–1 interactions (Fig. 6a). These percentage inhibition values for CTLA-4/B7–1 interactions shown by the antibodies in the fully competitive simulations are almost similar to those observed for B7–2 knockout-simulations (where B7–2 and CD28 were absent, in Fig. 4). Nevertheless, the inhibition of B7–2 interactions (with CTLA-4), in the full model simulations, required really very high dose of the antibodies. In fact, it can be seen that the CTLA-4/B7–2 inhibition was seen only at concentrations ≥20 μM for Tremelimumab and > 60 μM for ipilimumab (Fig. 6b). This indicates that at lower concentrations of the antibodies,

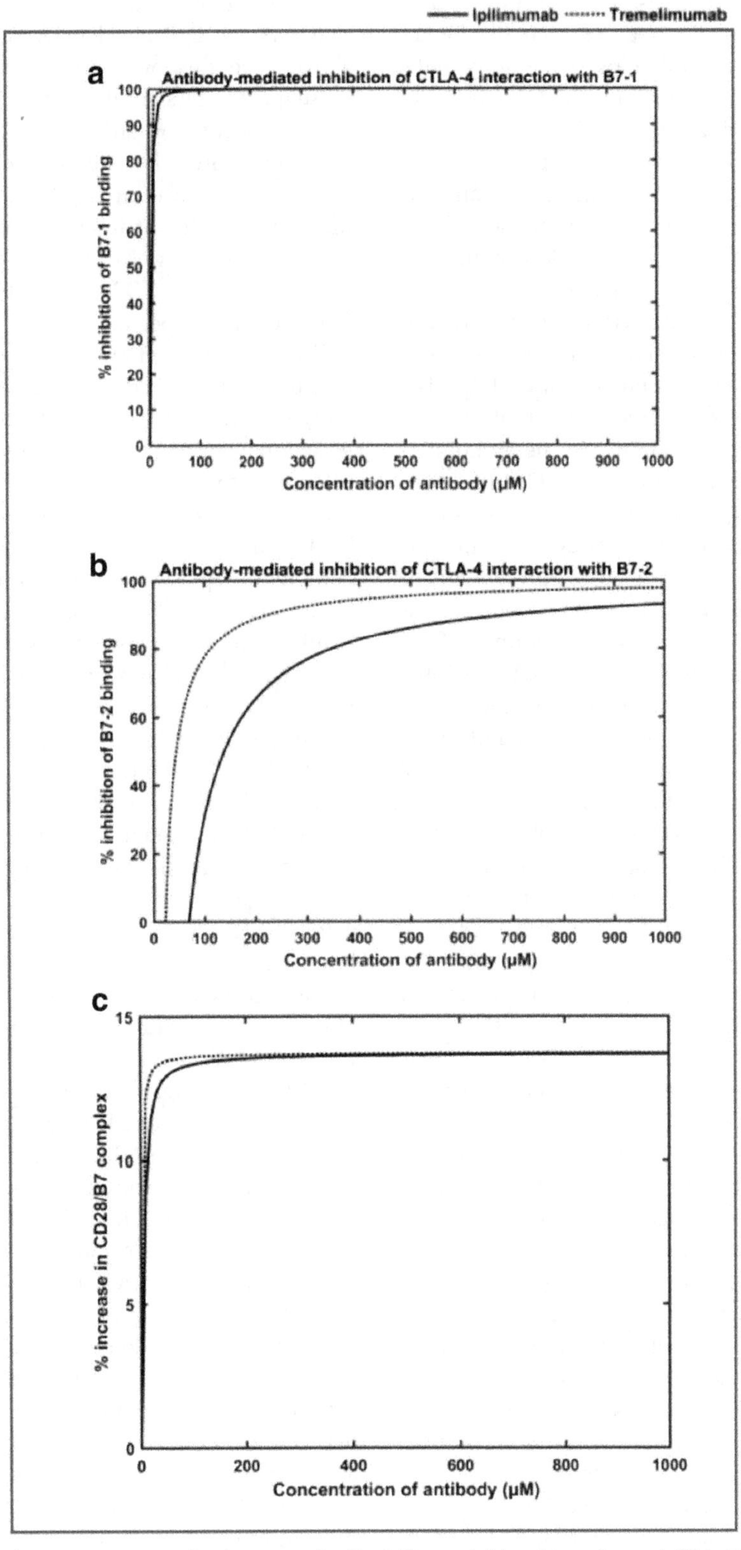

Fig. 6 The simulation of full dose-response curves for the two antibodies, ipilimumab (**a**) and tremelimumab (**b**) in the free-diffusion model. The % increase in the CD28/B7 complex during the full-dose response simulations with ipilimumab and tremelimumab are also plotted (**c**)

there were actually some increase in the CTLA-4/B7–2 complexes, when compared to those seen in the untreated (or antibody-free) simulations. It should be noted that, in the antibody-free simulations, the CTLA-4/B7–2 complex dominated during the initial stages until the bivalent CTLA-4/B7–1 complex suppressed the monovalent CTLA-4/B7–2 interactions to become the dominant complex (see in Fig. 2). Whereas, in the antibody-mediated simulations, at low dose concentrations, the antibodies are more proactive in blocking the multivalent CTLA-4/B7–1 interactions, which relieves the suppression on the monovalent CTLA-4/B7–2 interactions. In addition, the actual numbers of CTLA-4/B7–2 complexes are in general much less than that of CTLA-4/B7–1 complex. For example, at the end of antibody-free simulations, there were only 8 CTLA-4/B7–2 complexes, when compared to 790 CTLA-4/B7–1 complexes. Nevertheless, higher antibody concentrations effectively blocked the CTLA-4/B7–2 interactions as well. This contradicts with the B7–1 knockout simulations (Fig. 4), where even the lower amounts of the antibodies inhibited predominant CTLA-4/B7–2 interactions. This suggests that the competitive effects could implicate the dose response predictions significantly. Finally, as indicated earlier, inhibition of CTLA-4/B7 interactions did not essentially translate to the more proportional increase in the CD28/B7 complex formation. Figure 6c compares the percentage of increase in the CD28/B7 complex seen at each dose concentration (from 0 μM to 1000 μM) of ipilimumab and tremelimumab. It can be seen that there were only a maximum of ~14% gain in the CD28/B7 complexes following the inhibition of CTLA-4/B7 interactions by the mAbs in this study.

Effects of antibody-mediation on the overall complex formation

It is important to acknowledge that any mathematical model is mainly dependent on the parameters employed to build it. Particularly, the sensitivity is much higher in the models that rely on biological parameters. For example, Jansson et al. [33] tested the dependence of their model on the affinity, mobility and expression levels of various species, by reducing each of these parameters by 10-fold, and found that some of the simulated interactions are sensitive to these changes [33]. However, it is true even in the case of measured data, as the experimental conditions, such as stoichiometry and temperature, have been shown to affect the results. For instance, an earlier experimental study reported that the affinity between CTLA-4 and B7–1 was 12 nM [30]; while another experimental study reported the affinity for the same complex to be 0.4 μM [31]. In the current study, we tested the sensitivity of our model towards the changes in the rate constants for association and dissociation of different species in the model (the parameters, P2-P20 listed in Additional file 1: Table S1). To achieve this, we perturbed the values for each of these parameters in the range of −50 to +50% from their respective original values used in the model. Figure 7 compares the effects of changing the association (k_{on}) and dissociation (k_{off}) rate constants for tremelimumab on different interactions, such as CTLA-4/antibody complex (Fig. 7a), CTLA-4/B7–1 (Fig. 7b), CTLA-4/B7–2 (Fig. 7c), CD28/B7–1 (Fig. 7d) and CD28/B7–2 (Fig. 7e). As expected, the CTLA-4/antibody and the CTLA-4/B7 interactions were the most affected by these perturbations; indeed, the effects seen for CTLA-4/antibody complex were inverse to those of CTLA-4/B7 interactions. For example, the 50-fold reduction in the k_{on} value led to the drop of ~60 numbers of monomer CTLA-4/antibody complexes, which was compensated by the increase in the total numbers of CTLA-4/B7 complexes (approximately +48 for CTLA-4/B7–1 complex; +12 for CTLA-4/B7–2 complex). On the other hand, 50-fold increase in the k_{on} value resulted in a small gain of CTLA-4/antibody complexes, which again led to the drop in the total numbers of CTLA-4/B7 complexes (refer to Fig. 7a-c). Similar inverse effects in the CTLA-4/antibody and CTLA-4/B7 complexes were also seen for the changes in the k_{off} values. Nevertheless, the CD28/B7 interactions were mostly insensitive to these perturbations. This highlights the fact that CD28 is not able to compete with the high-affinity and high-avidity interactions of CTLA-4/B7 and CTLA-4/antibody interactions.

The effects of varying the rate constants for association and dissociations for monovalent CD28/B7 complexes, monovalent CTLA-4/B7 complexes, bivalent CD28/B7–1 complex, and multivalent CTLA-4/B7 complexes were also tested (results provided in supplementary information, Additional file 4: Figure S1 and Additional file 5: Figure S2). These manipulated simulations described that the CTLA-4/antibody and CTLA-4/B7–1 interactions are mostly sensitive to the rate constant values for multivalent association and dissociation of CTLA-4/B7–1 complex; whereas, the CTLA-4/B7–2 interactions are predominantly affected by the rate constants for association and dissociation of bivalent CTLA-4/B7–2 interactions. The perturbations in the latter parameters also exhibited small effects on CTLA-4/antibody interactions. Nevertheless, none of the changes corresponding to CTLA-4/B7 interactions made any significant impacts on the CD28/B7 complexes, which were only sensitive to the rate constant values corresponding to their own association/dissociation. Although the model is sensitive to upto 50% variations in the selected kinetics parameters, the qualitative inference based on the original values remain the same.

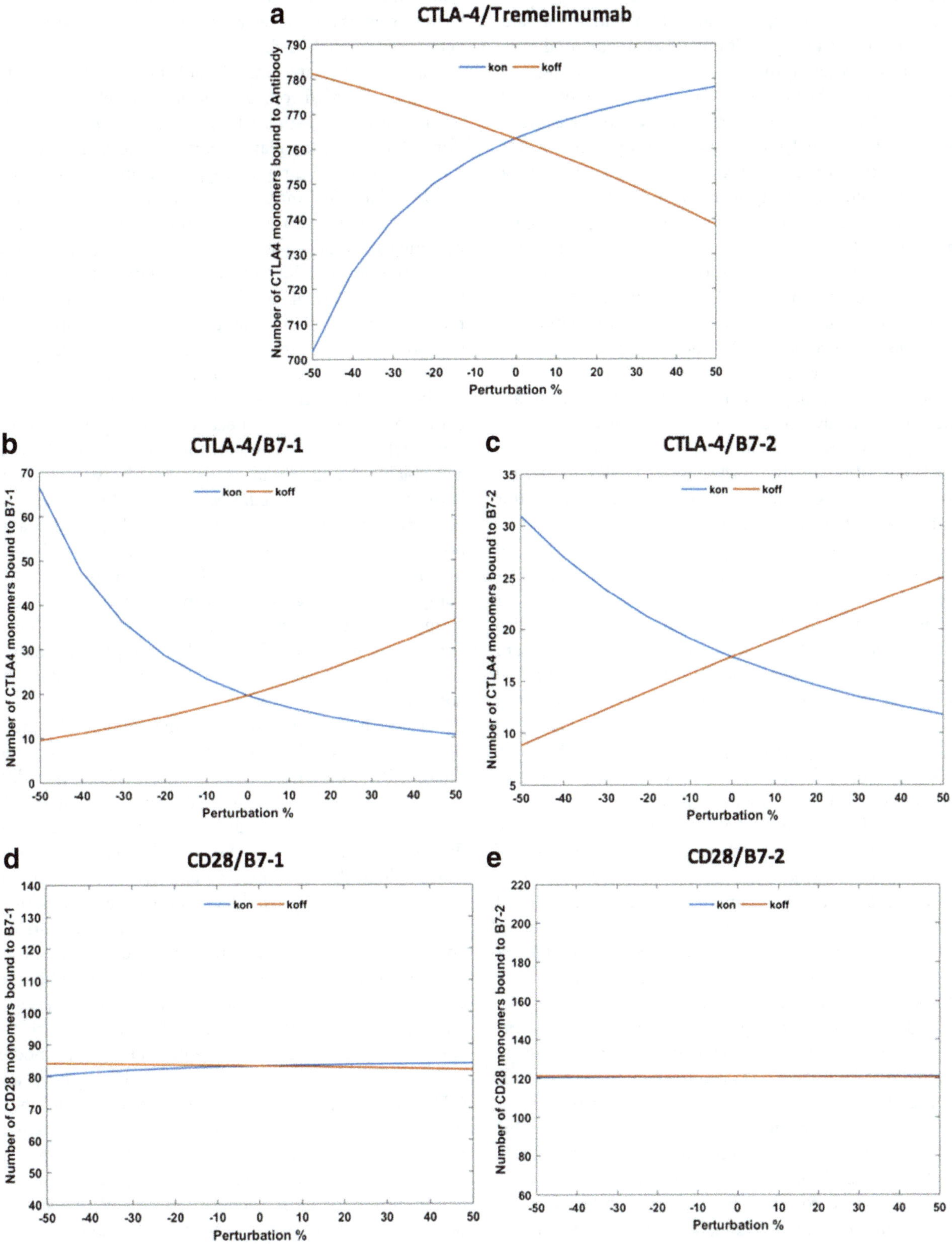

Fig. 7 Sensitivity of the interactions towards the perturbations in the association (k_{on}) and dissociation (k_{off}) rate constants for CTLA-4/Tremelimumab complex. The changes in the numbers of CTLA-4/Tremelimumab complex (**a**), CTLA-4/B7–1 complex (**b**), CTLA-4/B7–2 complex (**c**), CD28/B7–1 complex (**d**), and CD28/B7–2 complex (**e**) in response to the perturbations are shown

Discussions

Mathematical modeling and simulation remains a valuable tool to develop quantitative insights about the dynamic changes taking place within complex systems. It has particularly been employed in the field of cancer immunotherapy. Jansson et al. [33] developed a model for quantitative analysis of costimulatory complex formation, between CTLA4, CD28 and the B7- ligands, at the immunological synapse. However, there have been no study that modelled the effects of antibody-mediation on the complex formation at the synapse. In this study, we have taken one baby-step forward towards analyzing the effects of adding anti-CTLA-4 antibodies on the immunological balance between the co-stimulatory interactions (formed by CD28 and B7 ligands) and the co-inhibitory interactions (formed by CTLA-4 and B7 ligands) at the synapse, using a free-diffusion model. The study mainly focused on two promising CTLA-4 blocking antibodies, ipilimumab and tremelimumab, which are either in the market or in clinical trials, respectively. As acknowledged throughout the paper, this study is an extension of the Jansson's model [33], where we included several new equations and parameters to account for the effects of antibody-mediation at the synapse. The model is able to reproduce the K_D values for the inhibition of CTLA-4 by the two antibodies. We also validated our model by showing a reasonable agreement between the dose-curves, for blocking the binding of B7–1 and B7–2 to CTLA-4 by ipilimumab, from our simulations against a previous experimental data from competitive binding assays by Keler et al. [50]. The study also helped to understand the relative efficacy of the two antibodies in CTLA-4 blockade. Although both tremelimumab and ipilimumab have similar K_D values, the former tends to show more effective inhibition of CTLA-4/B7 interactions, due to its much lower dissociation rate that that of ipilimumab. The modelling and simulations in this work have shown that different factors, such as multivalent interactions, mobility of molecules and competition effects, could impact the effects of antibody-mediation. The results, in particular, highlighted that the competitive effects played an important role in the dose-dependent inhibition of the B7 ligand interactions with CTLA-4 receptor by the antibodies. However, it is important to concede that, as in any case of mathematical modelling, the model in this work is also mainly dependent on the parameters employed to build it. However, it is known that the K_D values measured for the same systems under different experimental conditions could vary significantly. For example, different k_{on} and k_{off} rates for ipilimumab/CTLA-4 complex have been reported in the literature. Hence, in order to minimize the impacts from such variabilities, we have used the k_{on} and k_{off} rates for both ipilimumab/CTLA-4 and tremelimumab/CTLA-4 complexes from the same work of He et al. [1], which was very recently published.

Another important limitation of this model is that it is constructed based on the normal T-cell conditions, where both the co-stimulatory and co-inhibitory interactions at the synapse play important role in maintaining the much-needed immunological balance. However, a CTLA-4 blocking antibody (or any immune-checkpoint drug for that matter) is only administered in an abnormal micro-tumor environment, where the expression of the receptors and ligands will be different than those seen in the normal T-cells, thus shifting the balance more towards inhibitory interactions. But, unfortunately, comprehensive parameter data for simulating cancerous cells in the context of immunological synapse is not available in the literature. Hence, we made an informed choice of simulating the effects of antibody mediation in a normal T-cell environment, for which parameters are available and a preliminary model [33] (without antibody) was also published. Precisely, for this reason, we did not perform simulations by introducing the antibodies at various timescale (after reaching steady-state for instance). Instead, we only focused on simulating the competitive binding aspects of the antibodies to CTLA-4 and how it changes the co-stimulatory (CD28/B7) and the co-inhibitory (CTLA-4/B7) complex formations at the synapse, when compared to untreated (or antibody-free) simulation.

Despite the stated limitations, the numerical simulations performed with the current model are in agreement with different experiments, such as the dose curve for ipilimumab-mediated inhibition of B7 ligands. The model is able to predict the dose-dependent inhibition of CTLA-4/B7 interactions in an immunologically-relevant competitive environment, where both the B7-ligands and antibodies compete to bind with CTLA-4. In general, it is difficult (and not always practical) to measure the specific inhibition percentage of either B7–1 or B7–2 by the antibodies under such fully immunologically-relevant competitive binding environment. Most experiments measure the competitive binding of the anti-CTLA-4 antibodies only in the presence of either of the ligands and CTLA-4. Thus, this mathematical model could be a useful tool to gain some insights about the potencies of the antibodies to compete with both B7–1 and B7–2 to bind with the CTLA-4 receptor, at the dynamic immunological synapse. Although the simulations in this work were performed for only the two known antibodies, the model itself could serve as an easily transferable tool to study the effects of any anti-CTLA-4 antibodies on the co-stimulation by the CD28 pathway, provided the binding kinetics data for the query antibodies and CTLA-4 are available. Therefore, the results presented and the mathematical model will be useful for the research activity in the field of immune-checkpoints-targeted cancer therapy.

Conclusion

In this work, we have developed an expanded mathematical modeling framework to quantitatively analyze the effects of anti-CTLA-4 antibody-mediation on the co-stimulatory and co-inhibitory complex formation at the immunological synapse. The numerical simulations performed using this model have been validated by different experimental data. The model predicted the dose curve for the B7-ligand blockade by ipilimumab, which was in a reasonable agreement with the experimental data obtained from competitive binding assays. Further, the model was also able to reproduce the K_D values for the binding of the antibodies against the CTLA-4 receptor. Our findings show that a number of significant factors, such as multivalent interactions, mobility of moleculesand competition effects contribute to the antibody-mediated interactions at the synapse. In particular, the competitive effects play a more predominant role. The simulations from our model show that in a less-competitive setting, the CTLA-4/B7–2 interactions are inhibited with much lower concentrations of antibodies, while the inhibition of B7–1 interactions required comparatively higher dose of antibodies. This is in concurrent with the previous findings that B7–1 is a preferred ligand for CTLA-4 and also has a higher affinity to CTLA-4 compared with B7–2. Nevertheless, our simulations show that the trend is reversed within a fully competitive and dynamic immunological synapse. In fact, the antibodies are more proactive in inhibiting the divalent CTLA-4/B7–1 interactions, which in turn relieves the suppression of CTLA-4/B7–2 complexes. As a result, the inhibition of CTLA-4/B7–2 in the full model required much higher concentrations of antibodies. Further, the inhibition of the CTLA-4/B7 interactions does not essentially lead to significant increase in the costimulatory CD28/B7 complexes. It is important to acknowledge that the model suffers from some of the important limitations, which are mainly caused due to lack of several parameters required to model a tumor microenvironment. Nevertheless, the current work represents an important first step towards understanding the antibody-mediated effects on synaptic complex formation. The model could also serve as an easily transferable predictive tool to study the effects of any anti-CTLA-4 antibodies on the co-stimulation by the CD28 pathway, provided the binding kinetics data for the query antibodies and CTLA-4 are available. Our natural next step will be expanding the current model by integrating it with the simulation of the main first signal (from TCR-MHC interactions) and also connecting to some downstream signaling processes, such as interleukin-2 activation pathway. Such an integrated mathematical model will be an excellent tool to guide immune-checkpoints research towards complete elimination of cancers.

Additional files

Additional file 1: Table S1. Parameters used in the model. The parameters related to the interactions of CTLA-4 and CD28 with the B7 ligands in the current model are provided in this file. (DOCX 26 kb)

Additional file 2: Table S2. Equations related to the rate of change of density for the antibody included in different complexes. The rate of change of density for the different antibody-mediated complexes are given in this file. Equations related to the rate of change of density for the antibody included in different complexes. The rate of change of density for the different antibody-mediated complexes are given in this file. (DOCX 144 kb)

Additional file 3: Table S3. Different components/species included in the model and their respective abbreviation used in the text. The different components included in our mathematical model, along with their corresponding abbreviations, are provided in this file. Different components/species included in the model and their respective abbreviation used in the text. The different components included in our mathematical model, along with their corresponding abbreviations, are provided in this file. (DOCX 13 kb)

Additional file 4: Figure S1. Sensitivity of the CTLA-4/antibody (a, d) and CTLA-4/B7 (b-c, e-f) interactions towards the perturbations in the association and dissociation for the CTLA-4/B7 and the CD28/B7 complexes. This file includes various figures corresponding to the sensitivity analyses performed to study the impacts of perturbations in the association and dissociation rates for the CTLA-4/B7 and the CD28/B7 complexes. (DOCX 5236 kb)

Additional file 5: Figure S2. Sensitivity of the CD28/B7–1 and CD28/B7–2 interactions towards the perturbations in the association and dissociation for the CTLA-4/B7 and the CD28/B7 complexes. This file includes various figures corresponding to the sensitivity analyses performed to study the impacts of perturbations in the association and dissociation rates for the CTLA-4/B7 and the CD28/B7 complexes. (DOCX 181 kb)

Abbreviations

APCs: Antigen-presenting cells; CTLA-4: Cytotoxic T-lymphocyte antigen 4; FDA: Food and drug administration; mAbs: Monoclonal antibodies; MHC: Major histocompatibility complex; ODEs: Ordinary differential equations; TCRs: T-cell receptors

Funding

The authors would like to acknowledge the funding support from Alberta Cancer Foundation (RES0025662) and Li Ka Shing Applied Virology Institute (Project ID:RES0028141) at the University of Alberta. The funding bodies had no role in this study in any way, including the study design, data collection and analysis, decision to publish and preparation of the manuscript.

Authors' contributions

AG and KB conceived and supervised the project. AG and TA contributed equally in relevant data collection, development of the model, testing and performing simulations. AG, TA , TC and KB analysed of the results and presentation. AG and TA wrote the manuscript. All authors read and approved the final manuscript.

Competing interests

The author declared that they have no competing interests.

Author details

[1]Faculty of Pharmacy and Pharmaceutical Sciences, University of Alberta, Edmonton, Canada. [2]School of Life Sciences, University of Hyderabad, Hyderabad, India. [3]Department of Mathematical and Statistical Sciences, Faculty of Science, University of Alberta, Edmonton, Canada. [4]Li Ka Shing Institute of Virology, University of Alberta, Edmonton, Canada.

References

1. He M, Chai Y, Qi J, Zhang CWH, Tong Z, Shi Y, Yan J, Tan S, Gao GF. Remarkably similar CTLA-4 binding properties of therapeutic ipilimumab and tremelimumab antibodies. Oncotarget. 2017.
2. Ramagopal UA, Liu W, Garrett-Thomson SC, Bonanno JB, Yan Q, Srinivasan M, Wong SC, Bell A, Mankikar S, Rangan VS, et al. Structural basis for cancer immunotherapy by the first-in-class checkpoint inhibitor ipilimumab. Proc Natl Acad Sci. 2017;114(21):E4223–32.
3. Cogdill AP, Andrews MC, Wargo JA. Hallmarks of response to immune checkpoint blockade. Br J Cancer. 2017;117(1):1–7.
4. Tsai H-F, Hsu P-N. Cancer immunotherapy by targeting immune checkpoints: mechanism of T cell dysfunction in cancer immunity and new therapeutic targets. J Biomed Sci. 2017;24(1):35.
5. Lee JY, Lee HT, Shin W, Chae J, Choi J, Kim SH, Lim H, Won Heo T, Park KY, Lee YJ, et al. Structural basis of checkpoint blockade by monoclonal antibodies in cancer immunotherapy. Nat Commun. 2016;7:13354.
6. Pardoll DM. The blockade of immune checkpoints in cancer immunotherapy. Nat Rev Cancer. 2012;12(4):252–64.
7. Strutt TM, McKinstry KK, Swain SL. Control of innate immunity by memory CD4 T cells. Adv Exp Med Biol. 2011;780:57–68.
8. Sharpe AH, Freeman GJ. The B7-CD28 superfamily. Nat Rev Immunol. 2002; 2(2):116–26.
9. Bretscher PA. A two-step, two-signal model for the primary activation of precursor helper T cells. Proc Natl Acad Sci. 1999;96(1):185–90.
10. Bretscher P, Cohn M. A theory of self-nonself discrimination. Science (New York, NY). 1970;169(3950):1042–9.
11. Gao GF, Jakobsen BK. Molecular interactions of coreceptor CD8 and MHC class I: the molecular basis for functional coordination with the T-cell receptor. Immunol Today. 2000;21(12):630–6.
12. Gao GF, Rao Z, Bell JI. Molecular coordination of αβ T-cell receptors and coreceptors CD8 and CD4 in their recognition of peptide-MHC ligands. Trends Immunol. 2002;23(8):408–13.
13. Postow MA, Callahan MK, Wolchok JD. Immune checkpoint blockade in Cancer therapy. Journal of clinical oncology : official journal of the American Society of Clinical Oncology. 2015;33(17):1974–82.
14. Grosso JF, Jure-Kunkel MN. CTLA-4 blockade in tumor models: an overview of preclinical and translational research. Cancer Immun. 2013;13:5.
15. Linsley PS, Nadler SG, Bajorath J, Peach R, Leung HT, Rogers J, Bradshaw J, Stebbins M, Leytze G, Brady W, et al. Binding stoichiometry of the cytotoxic T lymphocyte-associated Molecule-4 (CTLA-4): a DISULFIDE-LINKED HOMODIMER BINDS TWO CD86 MOLECULES. J Biol Chem. 1995;270(25): 15417–24.
16. Stamper CC, Zhang Y, Tobin JF, Erbe DV, Ikemizu S, Davis SJ, Stahl ML, Seehra J, Somers WS, Mosyak L. Crystal structure of the B7-1/CTLA-4 complex that inhibits human immune responses. Nature. 2001;410(6828):608–11.
17. Sansom DM. CD28, CTLA-4 and their ligands: who does what and to whom? Immunology. 2000;101(2):169–77.
18. Merelli B, Massi D, Cattaneo L, Mandalà M. Targeting the PD1/PD-L1 axis in melanoma: biological rationale, clinical challenges and opportunities. Crit Rev Oncol Hematol. 2014;89(1):140–65.
19. Intlekofer AM, Thompson CB. At the bench: preclinical rationale for CTLA-4 and PD-1 blockade as cancer immunotherapy. J Leukoc Biol. 2013;94(1):25–39.
20. Roh W, Chen P-L, Reuben A, Spencer CN, Prieto PA, Miller JP, Gopalakrishnan V, Wang F, Cooper ZA, Reddy SM, et al. Integrated molecular analysis of tumor biopsies on sequential CTLA-4 and PD-1 blockade reveals markers of response and resistance. Sci Transl Med. 2017;9:379.
21. Pitt Jonathan M, Vétizou M, Daillère R, Roberti María P, Yamazaki T, Routy B, Lepage P, Boneca Ivo G, Chamaillard M, Kroemer G, et al. Resistance mechanisms to immune-checkpoint blockade in Cancer: tumor-intrinsic and -extrinsic factors. Immunity. 44(6):1255–69.
22. Zaretsky JM, Garcia-Diaz A, Shin DS, Escuin-Ordinas H, Hugo W, Hu-Lieskovan S, Torrejon DY, Abril-Rodriguez G, Sandoval S, Barthly L, et al. Mutations associated with acquired resistance to PD-1 blockade in melanoma. N Engl J Med. 2016;375(9):819–29.
23. Hodi FS, O'Day SJ, McDermott DF, Weber RW, Sosman JA, Haanen JB, Gonzalez R, Robert C, Schadendorf D, Hassel JC, et al. Improved survival with Ipilimumab in patients with metastatic melanoma. N Engl J Med. 2010; 363(8):711–23.
24. Robert C, Schachter J, Long GV, Arance A, Grob JJ, Mortier L, Daud A, Carlino MS, McNeil C, Lotem M, et al. Pembrolizumab versus Ipilimumab in advanced melanoma. N Engl J Med. 2015;372(26):2521–32.
25. Larkin J, Chiarion-Sileni V, Gonzalez R, Grob JJ, Cowey CL, Lao CD, Schadendorf D, Dummer R, Smylie M, Rutkowski P, et al. Combined Nivolumab and Ipilimumab or monotherapy in untreated melanoma. N Engl J Med. 2015;373(1):23–34.
26. Wolchok JD, Kluger H, Callahan MK, Postow MA, Rizvi NA, Lesokhin AM, Segal NH, Ariyan CE, Gordon R-A, Reed K, et al. Nivolumab plus Ipilimumab in advanced melanoma. N Engl J Med. 2013;369(2):122–33.
27. Postow MA, Chesney J, Pavlick AC, Robert C, Grossmann K, McDermott D, Linette GP, Meyer N, Giguere JK, Agarwala SS, et al. Nivolumab and Ipilimumab versus Ipilimumab in untreated melanoma. N Engl J Med. 2015; 372(21):2006–17.
28. Comin-Anduix B, Escuin-Ordinas H, Ibarrondo FJ. Tremelimumab: research and clinical development. OncoTargets and therapy. 2016;9:1767–76.
29. Kaplon A, Reichert JM. Antibodies to watch in 2018. mAbs. 2018;10(2): 183–203.
30. Linsley PS, Brady W, Urnes M, Grosmaire LS, Damle NK, Ledbetter JA. CTLA-4 is a second receptor for the B cell activation antigen B7. J Exp Med. 1991; 174(3):561–9.
31. van der Merwe PA, Bodian DL, Daenke S, Linsley P, Davis SJ. CD80 (B7-1) binds both CD28 and CTLA-4 with a low affinity and very fast kinetics. J Exp Med. 1997;185(3):393–404.
32. Sengers BG, McGinty S, Nouri FZ, Argungu M, Hawkins E, Hadji A, Weber A, Taylor A, Sepp A. Modeling bispecific monoclonal antibody interaction with two cell membrane targets indicates the importance of surface diffusion. MAbs. 2016;8(5):905–15.
33. Jansson A, Barnes E, Klenerman P, Harlén M, Sørensen P, Davis SJ, Nilsson P. A theoretical framework for quantitative analysis of the molecular basis of Costimulation. J Immunol. 2005;175(3):1575.
34. Aravindhan G, Kumar GR, Kumar RS, Subha K. AJAX Interface: a breakthrough in bioinformatics web applications. Proteomics Insights. 2009; 2(PRI-2-Ganesan-et-al):1–7.
35. Aravindhan G, Kumar RS, Subha K, Subazini TK, Dey A, Kant K, Kumar GR. AIM-BLAST-AJAX interfaced multisequence Blast. Proteomics Insights. 2009; 2(PRI-2-Ganesan-et-al-2):9–13.
36. Subha K, Kumar GR, Rajalakshmi R, Aravindhan G. A novel strategy for mechanism based computational drug discovery. Biomarkers in Cancer. 2010;2:35–42.
37. Kronik N, Kogan Y, Schlegel PG, Wölfl M. Improving T-cell immunotherapy for melanoma through a mathematically motivated strategy: efficacy in numbers? J Immunother. 2012;35(2):116–24.
38. Kirschner D, Panetta JC. Modeling immunotherapy of the tumor – immune interaction. J Math Biol. 1998;37(3):235–52.
39. Sanga S, Sinek JP, Frieboes HB, Ferrari M, Fruehauf JP, Cristini V. Mathematical modeling of cancer progression and response to chemotherapy. Expert Rev Anticancer Ther. 2006;6(10):1361–76.
40. Allison E, Colton AD, Gorman AD, Kurt R, Shainheit M. A mathematical model of the effector cell response to cancer. Math Comput Model. 2004; 39(11):1313–27.
41. Robertson-Tessi M, El-Kareh A, Goriely A. A mathematical model of tumor–immune interactions. J Theor Biol. 2012;294:56–73.
42. de Pillis LG, Radunskaya AE, Wiseman CL. A validated mathematical model of cell-mediated immune response to tumor growth. Cancer Res. 2005; 65(17):7950.

43. Bidot C, Gruy F, Haudin CS, El Hentati F, Guy B, Lambert C. Mathematical modeling of T-cell activation kinetic. J Comput Biol: a journal of computational molecular cell biology. 2008;15(1):105–28.
44. Cheng X, Veverka V, Radhakrishnan A, Waters LC, Muskett FW, Morgan S, Huo J, Yu C, Evans EJ, Leslie AJ, et al. Structure and interactions of the human programmed cell death 1 receptor. J Biol Chem. 2013;288(17): 11771–85.
45. Egen JG, Allison JP. Cytotoxic T lymphocyte Antigen-4 accumulation in the immunological synapse is regulated by TCR signal strength. Immunity. 2002;16(1):23–35.
46. Chikuma S. CTLA-4, an essential immune-checkpoint for T-cell activation. In: Yoshimura A. (eds) Emerging concepts targeting immune checkpoints in cancer and autoimmunity. Current Topics in Microbiology and Immunology. Cham:. Sprinter. 2017;410.
47. Bell GI. Models for the specific adhesion of cells to cells. Science (New York, NY). 1978;200(4342):618.
48. Collins AV, Brodie DW, Gilbert RJC, Iaboni A, Manso-Sancho R, Walse B, Stuart DI, van der Merwe PA, Davis SJ. The interaction properties of costimulatory molecules revisited. Immunity. 2002;17(2):201–10.
49. Pentcheva-Hoang T, Egen JG, Wojnoonski K, Allison JP. B7-1 and B7-2 selectively recruit CTLA-4 and CD28 to the immunological synapse. Immunity. 2004;21(3):401–13.
50. Keler T, Halk E, Vitale L, O'Neill T, Blanset D, Lee S, Srinivasan M, Graziano RF, Davis T, Lonberg N, et al. Activity and safety of CTLA-4 blockade combined with vaccines in Cynomolgus macaques. J Immunol. 2003;171(11):6251–9.
51. Greene JL, Leytze GM, Emswiler J, Peach R, Bajorath J, Cosand W, Linsley PS. Covalent dimerization of CD28/CTLA-4 and oligomerization of CD80/CD86 regulate T cell costimulatory interactions. J Biol Chem. 1996;271(43):26762–71.

4

Informing evaluation of a smartphone application for people with acquired brain injury

Jade Kettlewell[1*], Julie Phillips[2], Kate Radford[3] and Roshan dasNair[4]

Abstract

Background: Brain in Hand is a smartphone application (app) that allows users to create structured diaries with problems and solutions, attach reminders, record task completion and has a symptom monitoring system. Brain in Hand was designed to support people with psychological problems, and encourage behaviour monitoring and change. The aim of this paper is to describe the process of exploring the barriers and enablers for the uptake and use of Brain in Hand in clinical practice, identify potential adaptations of the app for use with people with acquired brain injury (ABI), and determine whether the behaviour change wheel can be used as a model for engagement.

Methods: We identified stakeholders: ABI survivors and carers, National Health Service and private healthcare professionals, and engaged with them via focus groups, conference presentations, small group discussions, and through questionnaires. The results were evaluated using the behaviour change wheel and descriptive statistics of questionnaire responses.

Results: We engaged with 20 ABI survivors, 5 carers, 25 professionals, 41 questionnaires were completed by stakeholders. Comments made during group discussions were supported by questionnaire results. Enablers included smartphone competency (capability), personalisation of app (opportunity), and identifying perceived need (motivation). Barriers included a physical and cognitive inability to use smartphone (capability), potential cost and reliability of technology (opportunity), and no desire to use technology or change from existing strategies (motivation). The stakeholders identified potential uses and changes to the app, which were not easily mapped onto the behaviour change wheel, e.g. monitoring fatigue levels, method of logging task completion, and editing the diary on their smartphone.

Conclusions: The study identified that both ABI survivors and therapists could see a use for Brain in Hand, but wanted users to be able to personalise it themselves to address individual user needs, e.g. monitoring activity levels. The behaviour change wheel is a useful tool when designing and evaluating engagement activities as it addresses most aspects of implementation, however additional categories may be needed to explore the specific features of assistive technology interventions, e.g. technical functions.

Keywords: Brain injuries, Technology, Smartphone application, mHealth, Self-monitoring, Engagement study, Behaviour change

* Correspondence: Jade.Kettlewell@nottingham.ac.uk
[1]Division of Rehabilitation and Ageing, School of Medicine, University of Nottingham, D1409, Medical School, Queens Medical Centre, Nottingham NG7 2UH, UK
Full list of author information is available at the end of the article

Background

Acquired brain injury

Acquired brain injury (ABI) is defined as damage to the brain that has sudden onset and occurs after birth [1]. It includes both traumatic head injures (e.g. road accidents, falls) and non-traumatic causes such as vascular incidents (e.g. stroke), infections (e.g. meningitis), brain tumours hypoxic injuries and other non-generative neurological conditions [1]. Approximately 956 people were admitted to hospital every day due to ABI in 2013–14, which has increased by 10% since 2005–06 [2]. Approximately 1.3 million people in the UK are living with a traumatic brain injury [3], so the number of people with ABI will be even larger. ABI results in a myriad of persistent deficits in cognition (difficulties with memory, problem solving, planning, slower information processing, etc.), psychological and behavioural problems (e.g. increased anxiety, irritability), physical problems (epilepsy, fatigue, etc.), and social problems (e.g. isolation, reliance on family members). The main objective of rehabilitation with people with ABI is to help them recognise their problems, and find strategies to help them achieve the highest quality of life.

Assistive technology

Assistive technology (AT) is an umbrella term that refers to devices developed for people with disabilities, which can be assistive, adaptive, and rehabilitative. AT aims to compensate for loss of function and promotes greater independence, by providing individuals with the support they need to carry out tasks and move towards leading more fulfilling lives. In this study, we focus on ATs for cognition, which refers to technologies that may enhance, enable or extend cognitive function when used. This type of AT does not aim to restore cognitive function, but is used as a compensatory device to support these functions, for example, memory, executive function, language, and attention. Although ATs exist to support rehabilitation, there is limited technology available to support self-management and functional outcomes specifically for people with ABI [4, 5]. With such a large section of the population recovering from ABI, many in their youth, there is a need for ATs that can support all aspects of rehabilitation.

We identified several ATs in the literature available for ABI survivors and a recognised benefit of reminders to improve prospective memory and promote independence [4, 6–10]. 'Neuropage' is a well-established paging device that provides scheduled reminders for people with cognitive problems [9, 11–13]. Multiple studies have corroborated the value of reminder devices like Neuropage, electronic calendars, and personal digital assistants (PDAs) for ABI survivors, in improving performance of everyday tasks [10, 14–17].

Mobile health (mHealth) is becoming increasingly popular and applicable to healthcare. The World Health Organisation (WHO) defines mHealth as, medical or public health practice supported by mobile devices, such as mobile phones, PDAs, pagers and tablets [18]. With smartphone ownership in the UK at an estimated 76% of the adult population, mobile technology is becoming an integral part of everyday living [18, 19]. Smartphone applications (apps) for people with ABI (e.g. Evernote, Google Calendar, Family Tracker, etc.) usually have a calendar or reminder function. However, few apps have been systematically tested in this population, with the majority evaluating the efficacy of such technologies with studies with small sample sizes [7, 15, 20, 21]. One study explored the barriers to technology use, with a smartphone app called 'ForgetMeNot', which incorporates unsolicited prompts to encourage users to input more reminders [22]. Another study explored the use of a mHealth app (PEAT), designed as a scheduling assistant, but was found to be only as effective as paper-based methods [8].

Given the ubiquity of mobile phones and an increasing availability of mHealth apps, we expect that these technologies will be adopted more within healthcare services [23, 24]. Despite a growing awareness of mHealth, there is, however, limited research exploring the benefit of these technologies on executive function such as self-monitoring, problem solving, social interaction, initiation of tasks, and volition [4, 5, 25]. Other common co-morbidities of ABI such as fatigue, depression, anger, anxiety, and lack of confidence, also affect independence and social participation. These sequalae or 'invisible' symptoms are among the greatest unmet rehabilitation needs for this population [26–29]. There is an urgent need for mHealth apps to support people carry out these functions following ABI, and to promote independence and autonomy.

Problems with implementation

Many studies focus on the effectiveness of mHealth interventions, specifically reminding technologies [7, 9, 30, 31], however few address the barriers to use - essential to the development and implementation of these technologies [5, 22, 32–34]. It is important to consider the potential use of the technology in clinical practice when designing and evaluating mHealth interventions. Implementation studies attempt to identify the key features of an intervention and consider its applicability in practice, to better inform necessary developments and meet the needs of the target population [22, 34]. A report by the Voluntary Organisations Disability Group (VODG) identified problem areas associated with implementing smart technologies, such as a lack of care pathway commissioning, a lack of public awareness of mobile technology, and the unchangeable (and sometimes unhelpful) mind-set of healthcare professionals (HCPs) [35]. Some healthcare providers who regard themselves as traditional 'caregivers' might have concerns that physical care and social care may be lost to the increasing use of technology [35, 36]. There may be a certain level of reluctance to change, especially if intervention uptake has the potential to result in the loss of (their) jobs and reduced clinical support. Potential barriers to the uptake of mHealth may be commissioning of clinical services, technical issues (e.g. poor internet connection), fear of change, lack of leadership, and risk of investment [36]. However, increasing staff efficiency, ability to provide information faster, potential cost savings, and increased patient dignity, control and independence may be potential enablers to the uptake of technology [36].

Brain in Hand

A new mHealth app called 'Brain in Hand' (BiH) is currently being implemented in various settings for autism and mental health. BiH is a web-based software that synchronises with a smartphone app. It is readily available and simple to use. The software helps users create a structured daily routine for difficult to remember tasks or problem situations. The smartphone app gives patients instant solutions, which can be easily accessed in real time, thus allowing them to manage their distress levels and improve independence. BiH has a reminder function that enables patients to set alarms for important appointments and tasks, with the ability to record task completion. BiH also has an online portal, which comprises a diary and timeline. The portal acts as a monitoring system whereby a user, carer, mentor or HCP can track app usage. The timeline can record functions selected on the app, whether it be a solution or completion of task.

App data are recorded in real time and stored in the 'cloud', allowing users and HCPs to monitor and better understand issues that cause distress. A traffic light alarm system, prompts users to record their anxiety levels at a specific time: red (I am not coping), amber (I am struggling, but I am coping) and green (I am coping). There is also the option to use this function to access telephone support if needed i.e., when the red button is pressed.

Behaviour change wheel

We chose the Behaviour Change Wheel (BCW) to inform the method of this study, as the technology (BiH) being evaluated aims to encourage changes in behaviour [37]. The BCW model suggests that changing behaviour is based on three components: capability, opportunity and motivation (COM-B). Capability refers to an individual's psychological and physical capability to engage in an activity, opportunity refers to factors not directly linked to the individual that make that behaviour possible (e.g. having access to a smartphone), and motivation refers to reflexive and emotional responses that make the behaviour possible (e.g. knowing something will work) (see Fig. 1). [37, 38].

Examples of anticipated behaviours when using BiH include: activity and medication reminders, fatigue and anxiety monitoring, reminder of strategies to use when a problem occurs. The BCW was appropriate for this

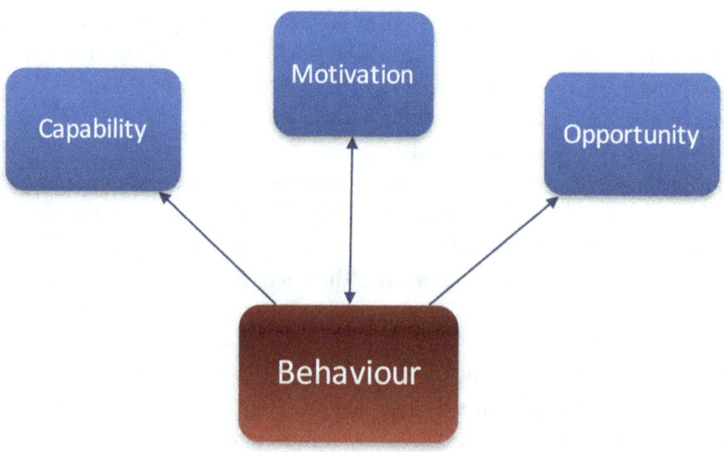

Fig. 1 Model of Behaviour Change (COM-B) [38, 45]. The relationship between capability, opportunity, motivation and behaviour, forming the basis of the BCW. The arrows demonstrate how each part in the COM-B model interacts within the behaviour system. Capability influences motivation, opportunity also influences motivation, which then impacts on behaviour. Motivation tends to drive behaviour, however behaviour can influence motivation. Capability moderates the link between behaviour and motivation, as does opportunity. The behaviour system exists as a cycle and is an important model to consider when designing and evaluating interventions that aim to change behaviour

study because it considers other factors that might influence use, such as the need for training to use the technology. Although the BCW model considers factors such as environmental restructuring (i.e., changing the physical context and enablement), increasing or reducing barriers to use the app, discussions with experts in the use of BiH felt this did not fully explore the usability and acceptability of the actual technology. Therefore, we identified studies that had evaluated technology and used feedback questionnaires to inform potential views of the app.

Rationale

A literature review suggested there is a need to better understand the use of technology in health, and various studies have identified potential problems with the uptake of mobile technologies, such as adaptability, cost, compatibility with existing systems and complexity [35, 36, 39]. The research literature highlights the importance of identifying barriers through consultation with key stakeholders and collaboration, early in the implementation process [39–41]. The rationale for this study was therefore to evaluate the usability and acceptability of the smart technology, and explore its potential use in ABI rehabilitation, through early stakeholder consultation.

Aims

The aim of this paper is to describe the process undertaken to:

- Explore the barriers and enablers, and the potential use of BiH technology in clinical practice with ABI survivors.
- Identify possible adaptations of the technology to meet the needs of the ABI population.
- Determine if the BCW could be used as model for stakeholder engagement.

Method

As the aim of BiH technology is to help users change their behaviour, the method of engagement was informed by the BCW model [37]. Engagement was defined as consulting with patients, carers and HCPs to obtain their views about the technology through different activities. This consisted of verbal engagement with the research team, focus groups, meetings with users and professional groups at their workplace, conferences and completion of questionnaires. We considered a mixed method approach appropriate for this type of study. We followed Johnson, Onwuegbuzie and Turner's view [42] of taking a broad interpretation of the word 'methods' here, in that it incorporates a variety of data collection methods, research approaches, and philosophies. We felt that this approach would enable us to identify various perspectives on the potential uses, enablers and barriers of the technology, and enable us to evaluate the potential use of the BCW as a tool for engagement, by using both quantitative and qualitative methods. We also felt that a mixed methods approach would increase the breadth of the research, by providing a fuller picture of people's experiences, attitudes and feelings about the technology. The data collection process was divided into three stages, with an ongoing iterative approach (Fig. 2). We followed the UK Health Research Authority (HRA) guidance regarding ethics approval via an online assessment tool, and were advised that it specific ethical approval was not required, as this project was viewed as stakeholder consultation. Participants were identified through voluntary organisations, special interest groups and conferences that had a focus on ABI/technology, and at organised events for the lay public.

Stage 1: Identify stakeholders and develop a format for engagement

The study management group consisted of academics and clinicians. They identified the stakeholder groups as: ABI survivors who would use the technology, carers or support workers who would mentor people with ABI and support them to use BiH, and HCPs who would potentially recommend using BiH as part of a treatment programme. We took a pragmatic approach to accessing the identified user groups, and incorporated engagement activities within meetings held by stakeholders. Additionally, focus groups were held to specifically engage both ABI survivors and carers.

As BiH is a novel mHealth app and currently unused with the ABI population, we provided potential stakeholders with information about the system during small groups or presentations, during which we explained the functions of BiH, its potential uses in daily life and in clinical practice. In addition, we gave people the opportunity to explore and experience the app themselves using a smartphone or iPad.

Our academic advisory panel suggested using existing technology questionnaires such as the Mobile Application Rating Scale (MARS) [43] and the System Usability Scale (SUS) [44] to capture stakeholders' opinions about similar technologies. These scales were evaluated by the researchers and the most appropriate elements incorporated into a questionnaire. The study management group agreed that a questionnaire would provide further in-depth quantitative data (particularly relating to the technical aspects of the app), and give people the opportunity to provide feedback outside of a group setting. A questionnaire was designed to be piloted with all stakeholders.

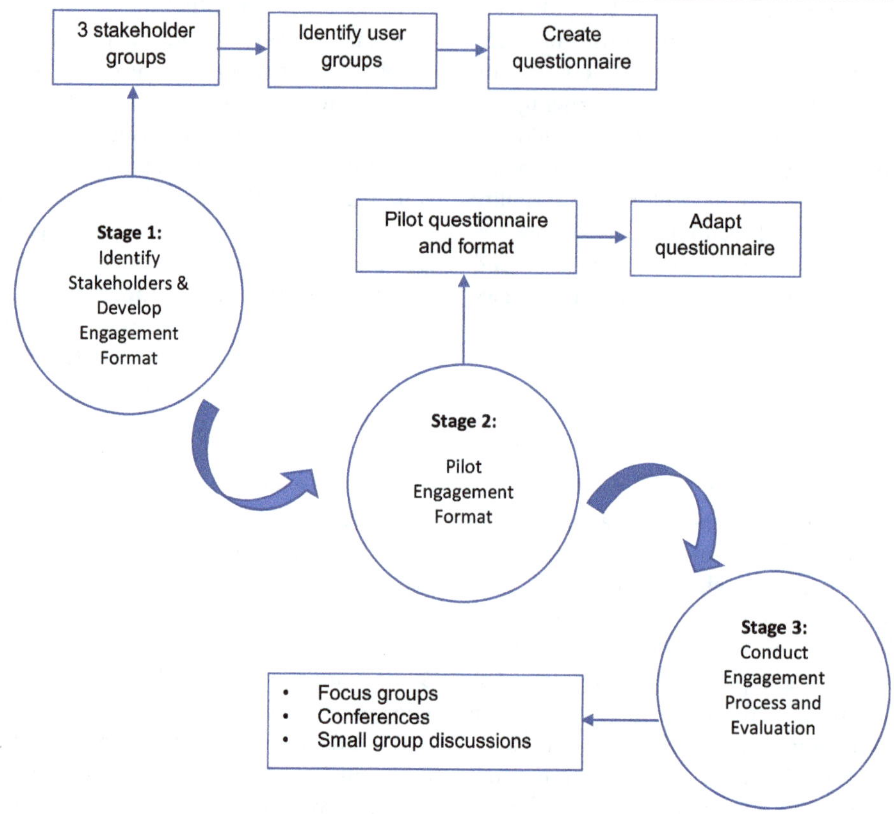

Fig. 2 Summary of engagement method. The iterative method used to identify stakeholders and carry out engagement activities

Stage 2: Piloting the engagement format

To determine if our methods of engagement were appropriate, and would obtain the relevant feedback, we piloted the format of discussion and questionnaire with a small group (ABI survivors, carers and HCPs) that had an interest and familiarity with smart technology. Feedback obtained from this activity informed necessary changes to the engagement approach and questionnaire. We contacted the local technology special interest group known to the researchers and a meeting was arranged. Participants were recruited during the group session and questionnaires completed following discussion. The group is run by a local therapist involving people with an ABI who have an interest in and review technology for, and on behalf of people with ABIs. Group members are former service users/carers themselves and interested in helping other people with an ABI. The group was chosen because of its focus on technology. Participants were not current UK health department service users.

Stage 3: The engagement process

The final stage involved identifying opportunities to engage with the stakeholders. We identified conferences and meetings where we could present and discuss the technology with professionals. We were invited to present our study and demonstrate the technology at a head injury conference organised by the local brain injury community service, where most of these participants were recruited. This was held in close proximity to the university and comprised a range of professionals (therapists, solicitors, case managers and business owners). We informed the professionals that we were soliciting feedback from them as stakeholders to help us identify the potential for the technology to help people with ABIs achieve their rehabilitation goals (and inform outcome measurement for a subsequent study). Professionals were invited to complete questionnaires following discussion if they wished (Additional file 1). Further participants were recruited at meetings identified by the authors (JK and JP) through their existing professional contacts, which all had a focus on ABI and/or technology. These groups exist to share information about specific aspects of their areas of interest, and to offer support, guidance, and feedback for various projects or cases. As before, stakeholders were invited to complete questionnaires following the meeting.

To ensure ABI survivors and carers were fully involved, we organised focus groups. The APEASE criteria [38, 45] along with the BCW was used to create a topic guide for the focus groups. The focus groups were facilitated by two people (JK, a PhD researcher, and JP, a research/clinical occupational therapist). The group discussions were audio recorded, analysed by the groups facilitators, and the findings discussed with the study management group. Views generated in the focus groups and from other engagement activities were mapped onto the BCW behaviour components.

The two focus groups comprised 8–10 service users and carers in each group. ABI participants and carers were recruited from various sources. Some participants were identified using a database of people with ABIs (who had previously expressed an interest in taking part in brain injury research) at the University of Nottingham. These people had previously consented to being contacted by researchers in our department regarding future studies and being involved in patient and public involvement (PPI) activities. This database is stored securely within the University and accessible only to members of our research team (long term conditions). It was accessed by author JP and potential participants were invited to take part in a focus group by email, giving them the opportunity to respond in their own time. Other ABI participants and carers were identified via social media posts by Headway and the Stroke Association (two UK charities), from an existing stroke specific PPI group (University of Nottingham Stroke Partnership Research Group (UNSPRG)), and local Headway and stroke groups. We used purposive sampling to ensure a heterogeneous sample, including people who did and did not use technologies.

Results

Stage 1: Identify stakeholders and develop a format for engagement

We engaged with 50 stakeholders: 20 ABI survivors (16 completed the questionnaire), 5 carers (4 completed the questionnaire), and 25 professionals (21 completed the questionnaire) who worked with people with ABI including therapists from NHS and private sector, and solicitors. Demographic characteristics of the stakeholders are presented in Table 1.

Table 1 Demographic information of stakeholders

Total = 50		Age			Gender	
		18–30	31–50	51+	Male	Female
ABI survivors (n = 20)	n	3	9	8	15	5
	% total	*6%*	*18%*	*16%*	*30%*	*10%*
Carers (n = 5)	n	1	0	4	2	3
	% total	*2%*	*0%*	*8%*	*4%*	*6%*
Professionals (n = 25)	n	2	12	11	4	21
	% total	*4%*	*24%*	*22%*	*8%*	*42%*
Overall	n	6	21	23	21	29
	% total	*12%*	*42%*	*46%*	*42%*	*58%*

Stage 2: Piloting the engagement format

We piloted our engagement format with an ABI user group (n = 6) that had a special interest in smartphone apps and were familiar with technology like BiH. Feedback from this stakeholder group suggested ideas for technological development and identified barriers to uptake, thus indicating that the format did facilitate informed discussion of the smartphone app. Based on their feedback, we adapted the questionnaire to make it more accessible and easier to complete by creating two versions: one for ABI survivors and carers (Additional file 2) and one for professionals (Additional file 1). We also removed the frequently unanswered and irrelevant questions that did not provide useful information about BiH.

Stage 3: The engagement process

We took a pragmatic and opportunistic approach to consult with the stakeholders. All were asked to complete a questionnaire. The engagement activities included:

- A formal presentation followed by a discussion with 30 professionals (therapists, case managers, solicitors) at an ABI meeting.
- Three informal presentations, to discuss and demonstrate BiH to two groups of therapists treating neurological patients (six per group), an ABI technology user group, and at a day centre (Headway) specifically for people with brain injury.
- An exhibition stand at a lay stroke conference where information was provided to delegates (stroke survivors, carers and professionals) on a 1:1 basis. The environment was not suitable for questionnaire completion. Some delegates took questionnaires home, but none were returned. Suggestions for improvement and any comments about the technology were noted on the day.

Results from discussion and questionnaires

The main points identified by the focus groups and other discussions complemented the questionnaire responses. However, the questionnaire approach limited responses, and did not allow individuals to elaborate on their views. For example, during one focus group, a suggestion was to change the word 'problems' to 'issues' on the app, as the ABI survivor felt the language was negative. Another person suggested linking the app to activity monitoring. This information would not have been captured with questionnaires alone. However, the questionnaire enabled us to quantify some responses such as potential uses and reporting on the technical aspects of the app (e.g. appearance of BiH). Over half of stakeholders stated that seeing the app made them want to use it (65%, 17/25). This suggests that the app is visually appealing.

Capability

Participants felt they would be confident using the app if they were existing technology users (22/24, 95%), but only a quarter of people felt it was completely appropriate for the ABI population (6/25, 24%). This finding is reflected by comments from professionals who felt that users needed an awareness of their problems and an ability to use strategies for the app to be effective (Table 2). Most stakeholders identified clear barriers during group discussions: visual and physical impairments, lack of technical skill, poor literacy skills, and cognitive problems faced by ABI survivors. Professionals identified potential problems associated with the use of BiH, such as difficulty switching between screens.

Opportunity

All stakeholders identified the need to have a smartphone as one of the most important enablers and any potential cost of the app as a significant barrier. Only 24% (9/37) said they would be willing to pay for the app, with a further 54% saying they would consider paying for the app depending on the price (Table 3). The groups identified a potential barrier to uptake being competition

Table 2 Summary of enablers and barriers identified by stakeholders mapped onto BCW behaviour components

	Enablers	ABI	Carers	Professionals		Barriers	ABI	Carers	Professionals
Capability	Physical ability to use smartphone	•	•	•	Capability	Visual and physical impairment	•	•	•
	Competent at using smartphone	•	•	•		Lack of technical skill	•		•
	Awareness of their problems		•	•		Poor literacy skills			•
	Able to use strategies	•		•		Cognitive problems e.g. switching between screens	•		•
Opportunity	Have a smartphone	•	•	•	Opportunity	Cost and competition from other apps	•	•	•
	Having the opportunity to personalise use	•	•	•		Losing smartphone and battery problems	•		
	Enables users to record symptoms as they happen	•		•		Technology not reliable e.g. loss of information if phone updated	•	•	
	Computerised record of use (e.g. to track goal attainment)			•		Incapability with existing systems i.e. will it sync with computer diary	•		•
	Offers opportunity to self-monitor and alter use	•		•		Work place restriction not allowing use	•		•
Motivation	Using a phone seen as 'normal' behaviour i.e. reduced stigma	•			Motivation	No interest in the use of technology or existing systems in place e.g. paper diary	•	•	•
	Potential to be personalised to individual needs	•	•	•		Do not see a use for it	•	•	•
	Motivated if they can see a use for it e.g. problem and solution system	•	•	•		Feeling the app is too complicated for them to use or learn to use			•
	Feeling confident to use the app	•				Loss of motivation and disengagement with rehabilitation process			•
	May allow the user to feel like they are taking control of their life again		•	•		Feeling as though they are being monitored	•		
	Do not want to use paper diary	•				Too time consuming to set up/edit	•	•	•
						Too many reminders may be annoying	•	•	•
						Lack of existing evidence/use in the ABI population	•	•	•

Summary of the barriers and enablers identified by ABI survivors, carers and professionals mapped onto the behaviour components of the BCW. The marked boxes indicate whether that stakeholder identified or discussed that barrier or enabler.

Table 3 Summary of questionnaire responses mapped onto BCW behaviour components

BCW component	Question/statement	Response options	Frequency	% total responses
Capability	Would you feel confident using the app? *Number scale of 1 (Definitely not) to 5 (Definitely) used.*	Definitely or almost	22/24	92%
		Maybe or somewhat	2/24	8%
	How appropriate is the app for a person with an ABI? *Number scale of 1 (Inappropriate) to 5 (Appropriate) used.*	Appropriate	6/25	24%
		Almost	11/25	44%
		Maybe	7/25	28%
		Less	1/25	4%
Motivation	When seeing the app for the first time, did it make you want to use of it? *Number scale of 1 (Definitely not) to 5 (Definitely) used.*	Definitely or almost	17/25	65%
		Maybe or less	6/25	23%
		Definitely not	2/25	8%
	What is/are the most appealing parts of the app?	Structured diary	30/41	73%
		Personalised problems and solutions	26/41	63%
		Traffic light system	22/41	54%
		Monitoring progress	15/41	37%
		Feedback online	13/41	32%
		Mentor/support	12/41	29%
	Can you see a use for the app?	Yes	39/41	95%
		No	2/41	5%
	What do you think the app could target or aid?	Memory problems	39/41	95%
		ADL	35/41	85%
		Independence	33/41	80%
		Managing routine	31/41	76%
		Problem solving	26/41	63%
		Self confidence	25/41	61%
		Anxiety/stress management	24/41	59%
		Behaviour monitoring	23/41	56%
		Anger/irritability	14/41	34%
		Goal setting	13/41	32%
		Depression	12/41	29%
Opportunity	Would you pay for the app?	Yes	9/37	24%
		Maybe	20/37	54%
		No	8/37	22%
	How long do you think you (or someone with ABI) would use the app for?	0–6 months	6/32	15%
		6–12 months	6/32	15%
		12+ months	20/32	49%
		Don't know	9/32	22%
	How appropriate is the training (i.e., ease of learning) to use the app? *Number scale of 1 (Inappropriate) to 5 (Appropriate) used.*	Appropriate	3/15	20%
		Almost appropriate	8 /15	53%
		Maybe	3 /15	20%
		Less	1 /15	7%
	How appropriate is the app when navigating different screens? *Number scale of 1 (Inappropriate) to 5 (Appropriate) used.*	Appropriate	4/20	20%
		Almost	12/20	60%
		Maybe	4/20	20%

from apps that have similar functions, but are free or have a one-off cost. Technological problems were identified as major barriers, specifically by individuals who were worried about loss of phones, the battery running down, compatibility with other systems and loss of data following phone updates. There was a concern about use in the work place, as for many people it is not appropriate to use a phone whilst working. With regards length of use, 49% (20/32) of stakeholders thought the app would be used by someone with ABI for more than 12 months and only 15% (6/32) felt it would be used as a short-term aid, between 0 and 6 months (Table 3). The initial questionnaire identified that 53% (8/15) of people felt that training required to use the app was largely suitable for the ABI population, but would need adapting to meet individual needs. Some stakeholders expressed a concern over the amount of time needed to set up, rather than learn to use BiH.

Motivation

Most people said they would be motivated if they could see a use for BiH (39/41, 95%); and after physically seeing the app, 65% (17/26) of people said they wanted to use it (Table 3). The questionnaire identified that most people (39/41, 95%) felt BiH would be useful for memory problems, to help with activities of daily living (35/41, 85%) and to support independence (33/41, 80%), such as taking responsibility of appointment planning. Although users in the focus group felt BiH would be useful for self-monitoring such as fatigue or anxiety levels, only 56% (23/41) said they thought it could help with behaviour monitoring. One interesting suggestion was to use the traffic light system to monitor positive behaviours, such as a feeling of wellbeing, rather than focusing on negative behaviours. All stakeholders identified the potential for personalisation to individual needs, one of the difficulties with existing technologies, as an important enabler to uptake. ABI survivors felt that using a mobile phone app as an assistive aid was viewed as 'normal' behaviour, i.e., reduced stigma, and would be a motivator for use (Table 2). The main barriers identified were the lack of interest in technology, not seeing a use for it and a lack of existing evidence of its use in ABI. ABI survivors were concerned about their privacy and a feeling of being monitored, and this was expressed as a potential barrier to uptake. Stakeholders felt that setting up the app may be time consuming and excessive reminders may be annoying.

Additional points were identified by stakeholders that did not map onto the components of the BCW. Most of these related to technical aspects of the app, something that is not well reflected by the BCW model. Stakeholders highlighted the inconvenience of having to access a computer to edit the diary and functions of the app, which could be a potential barrier to uptake. If individuals have difficulty remembering events, it is important that they can add or update events easily 'on the go'. If the system cannot be edited via the app, stakeholders felt BiH offered little additional use than a diary or the 'reminder' function on a standard smartphone. All stakeholders identified the need for voice recognition and the ability to verbally add things to the diary, along with having visual entries (e.g. adding pictures, diagrams and videos to diary entries, such as therapy exercises, making dinner, etc.). Professionals and carers suggested having an app specifically for mentor use, to monitor user activity without needing computer access. Professionals voiced concern over the use of the red button, the potential for it to be overused and who would be responsible for responding to it.

Discussion

Engagement methods

The aim of this study was to capture stakeholder views about the use of the smartphone app (BiH) in the ABI population. Both the BCW and existing technology questionnaires were used as the theoretical basis for the engagement activities. Views of ABI survivors, carers and professional were elicited through a combination of focus groups, presentations, and questionnaires. Our mixed method engagement approach provided us with useful feedback from stakeholders and enabled us to identify the importance of different opinions. The quantitative data obtained from questionnaires supported the qualitative feedback from discussions, the latter providing another dimension that would not be picked up with questionnaire responses alone. We thought the format of group engagement was helpful, as it gave stakeholders the opportunity to explore the app in more detail. Group situations promoted discussion about BiH, and stakeholders were keen to share their views about the app. The questionnaire provided useful quantifiable data, but was not completed by all.

Overall, we were able to engage well with various stakeholders, allowing us to obtain a broad range of feedback. We consulted with a stroke research group following completion of activities, who agreed that we had identified the correct stakeholders and our engagement format was appropriate. The stroke research group felt the questionnaire was suitable for the ABI population, but should be provided during focus groups or similar discussions. This would ensure stakeholders had the opportunity to explore the technology in greater depth before completing the questionnaire. Feedback from the research group reflected our findings regarding the success of focus groups, in comparison to conference presentations, where the environment did not lend itself to discussion and questionnaire completion.

Using the behaviour change wheel model

Behaviour change techniques (BCTs), defined as 'active components of an intervention designed to change behaviour' [45, 46], are specific, complex components of an intervention that are designed to change behaviour, that are observable and replicable [45]. As we focused on understanding behaviours and intervention functions, rather than techniques associated with changing behaviour, we found that certain stakeholder comments did not easily map onto the BCW, e.g., the potential uses of BiH. Behaviour change interventions operate within a social context, with effectiveness being the primary criteria to consider when implementing an intervention [45]. Assessing the potential use of BiH was difficult to map onto the BCW, along with the evaluation of specific technological aspects, e.g., was it visually appealing? Therefore, the use of existing technology-specific questionnaires was necessary, alongside the BCW components and APEASE criteria.

The behaviours required to use the app were more easily mapped onto the BCW, than the potential uses. We analysed our findings by mapping enablers and barriers on to the different BCW components (Table 2). Due to the type of intervention, we were less rigid with the definitions given in the BCW, thus making it easier to categorise feedback from stakeholders. This approach was used in a similar study evaluating the use of the model [47]. We recognised that not all components of the BCW are necessary when evaluating smart technology like BiH. The BCW with the addition of enablers and barriers, appears to be a useful format that could be replicated to evaluate similar engagement activities or interventions.

APEASE criteria

The APEASE criteria (see above) are important when evaluating interventions that aim to change behaviours, like BiH. All criteria were addressed during discussions, however stakeholders focused more on the 'practicability' and 'acceptability' aspects during focus groups, as this seemed to be most important. Practicability refers to how practical the technology would be in a real-life context and whether it is designed appropriately for the target population [34, 38, 45]. Individuals readily identified barriers and enablers that link with the practicality of use, which also mapped onto the capability and opportunity components of the BCW. Acceptability was addressed by all stakeholders via questionnaires and discussions. The acceptability of BiH differed between groups and the suggested improvements varied when speaking to ABI survivors and professionals. We were keen to ascertain whether BiH would be accepted by all stakeholders and what impact this would have on implementation. Other criteria were addressed, but some points seemed unimportant to ABI survivors and carers, such as the cost-effectiveness and unintended negative consequences of using the app. These stakeholders were interested in the potential cost of BiH for themselves or family members, but when questioned about the cost implications in the healthcare system, their feedback was minimal. As professionals did not attend focus groups, these criteria were somewhat overlooked in other engagement activities, where time and group size was a limiting factor. Therefore, we feel the BCW model needs to be fully considered prior to engaging with stakeholders and certain criteria should be prioritised depending on the group. The BCW may be used to inform qualitative interviews in further studies, which could serve as feasibility work to inform future implementation.

As previously mentioned, feedback highlighted the potential priorities for each stakeholder group. People with ABI mainly focused on the personal enablers and barriers associated with BiH uptake. They were interested in how useful and appropriate it would be for themselves, as well at the broader ABI population. This resonates with various studies, commonly stating a barrier to use is perceived usefulness and simplicity [22, 34, 48]. Professionals focused more on the clinical problems associated with using BiH (e.g. too complicated, misuse of the red button), but also the therapeutic benefits for their patients or clients. Carers were divided about their views on BiH, with some feeling it may reduce anxiety when allowing the person with ABI to have more independence, but others were concerned that it would add more pressure to their role. All stakeholders prioritised certain aspects as expected, but there was a consensus between groups regarding personalisation of the app, ability to use a smartphone, motivation to change from existing strategies. The latter has been addressed by various studies, highlighting the importance of personally relevant reminders to encourage use [6, 19, 22]. A systematic review by Ross et al., 2016 [39] presents various factors that influence the implementation of e-health technologies, like BiH. It identifies cost, complexity, adaptability, stakeholder engagement, training and education to all those involved as key factors in implementation. Our study has identified these barriers and enablers through stakeholder engagement at an early stage. We feel the data obtained appear to be a good representation of individuals that would potentially use or recommend the app.

Limitations

The study, however, had certain limitations as the iterative approach made it difficult to plan our engagement methods before starting the study. In retrospect, we should have used the BCW to design the questionnaire alongside the existing technology questionnaires, as this would have linked better with focus group discussions. Some BCW domains were not fully explored by questionnaires and discussions e.g. policy categories and intervention functions, as we chose to focus more on the behaviour components. Questionnaires did not capture all intervention and policy areas, as it would have taken too long to complete and may be a difficult concept for some people to grasp. This meant that we did not ask stakeholders about the potential to save money within rehabilitation services, or identify potential contraindications associated with BiH use. Professionals did however highlight potential problems associated with the app. Another limitation is that stakeholders had minimal time to use and experience BiH, therefore longer term use in a case study context would provide more useful and in depth feedback.

Future work

There is some indication that theory-based behavioural change interventions that have been led by theoretical domains framework (TDF) are more effective, than using behaviour change models alone (i.e. BCW) [49, 50]. The BCW used alongside TDF may provide better understanding of the nature of the intervention, and identify domains that could influence behaviour change [45, 50]. If we were to further this study, we could conduct single person interviews and use the TDF domain definitions to design interview questions. This approach could also be used in individual case studies.

Conclusion

Overall people were keen the use the Brain in Hand technology, but wanted it to be personalised, easy to use and inexpensive (and potentially free). They had concerns about practical issues such as losing the phone, who had access to the data, and losing the information if the phone updated. People who currently fear or avoid using technology did not see any benefits. The majority of stakeholders said they could see the benefit of this technology for themselves or others. The BCW is a useful tool for engagement, especially when designing questionnaires and discussion topic guides. The model may help researchers consider a wider perspective than just intervention functions and associated behaviours, especially when identifying barriers and enablers to use and recommendation. However, the BCW needs additional components that are specific to AT interventions. When designing a questionnaire for this type of stakeholder engagement, researchers need to consider additional technology aspects, such as visuals, design and language. Describing our engagement process should be of interest to others who are trying to evaluate interventions designed to change behaviour.

Abbreviations

ABI: Acquired brain injury; AT: Assistive technology; BCT: Behaviour change technique; BCW: Behaviour change wheel; BiH: Brain in Hand; COM-B: Capability, opportunity and motivation components of behaviour change model; HCP: Healthcare professional; MARS: Mobile Apps Rating Scale; mHealth: Mobile health; NHS: National Health Service UK; PDA: Personal digital assistant; SUS: System Usability Scale; TDF: Theoretical domains framework

Acknowledgements

The views expressed are those of the authors and not necessarily those of the MRC. We would like to acknowledge the contribution of all therapists, ABI survivors, carers and other volunteers that participated in the engagement activities.

Funding

Jade Kettlewell is a PhD student funded by a Hermes Fellowship, the University of Nottingham and Brain in Hand Ltd. This study presents research funded by a Medical Research Council (MRC) Proximity to Discovery award, reference number MC_PC_14121 awarded to authors KR and RdN. The funding bodies did not have any involvement in study design, data collection, analysis, interpretation of data or writing of the manuscript.

Authors' contributions

The study was designed and conducted by JK and JP, supported by KR and RdN. JK and JP contributed to the main writing up of the study findings, with additional input from authors KR and RdN. All authors critically reviewed the final version for publication. All authors read and approved the final manuscript.

Competing interests

The authors declare that they have no competing interests.

Author details

[1]Division of Rehabilitation and Ageing, School of Medicine, University of Nottingham, D1409, Medical School, Queens Medical Centre, Nottingham NG7 2UH, UK. [2]Division of Rehabilitation and Ageing, School of Medicine, University of Nottingham, B114, Medical School, Queens Medical Centre, Nottingham NG7 2UH, UK. [3]Rehabilitation Research (Long Term Conditions), Division of Rehabilitation and Ageing, School of Medicine, University of Nottingham, B102, Medical School, Queens Medical Centre, Nottingham NG7 2UH, UK. [4]Clinical Psychology & Neuropsychology, Division of Psychiatry & Applied Psychology, C22, Institute of Mental Health, Jubilee Campus, University of Nottingham, Nottingham NG7 2TU, UK.

References

1. Scottish Intercollegiate Guidelines Network, S. Brain injury rehabilitation in adults. Edinburgh: SIGN; 2013.
2. Tennant A, Headway. Acquired brain injury: the numbers behind the hidden disability; 2015. p. 9–11. http://www.headway.co.uk/
3. Parsonage, M., Traumatic brain injury and offending: an economic analysis. 2016, Centre for Mental Health. p 4 & 20 https://www.centreformentalhealth.org.uk/traumatic-brain-injury. Accessed Dec 2016.
4. Charters E, Gillett L, Simpson GK. Efficacy of electronic portable assistive devices for people with acquired brain injury: a systematic review. Neuropsychol Rehabil. 2015;25(1):82–121.
5. Jamieson M, JJ Evans, Assistive technology for executive functions, in Assistive technology for cognition: A handbook for clinicians and developers. London: Psychology Press; 2015. p. 81–92.
6. Ferguson S, Friedland D, Woodberry E. Smartphone technology: gentle reminders of everyday tasks for those with prospective memory difficulties post-brain injury. Brain Inj. 2015;29(5):583–91.

7. McDonald A, et al. Google calendar: a new memory aid to compensate for prospective memory deficits following acquired brain injury. Neuropsychol Rehabil. 2011;21(6):784–807.
8. De Joode EA, et al. Effectiveness of an electronic cognitive aid in patients with acquired brain injury: a multicentre randomised parallel-group study. Neuropsychol Rehabil. 2013;23(1):133–56.
9. Wilson BA, et al. Reducing everyday memory and planning problems by means of a paging system: a randomised control crossover study. J Neurol Neurosurg Psychiatry. 2001;70(4):477–82.
10. Jamieson M, et al. The efficacy of cognitive prosthetic technology for people with memory impairments: a systematic review and meta-analysis. Neuropsychol Rehabil. 2014;24(3–4):419–44.
11. Wilson BA, et al. Evaluation of NeuroPage: a new memory aid. J Neurol Neurosurg Psychiatry. 1997;63(1):113–5.
12. de Joode E, et al. Efficacy and usability of assistive technology for patients with cognitive deficits: a systematic review. Clin Rehabil. 2010;24(8):701–14.
13. Dewar, B.-K., et al., Assistive technology for memory, in Assistive Technology for Cognition: A handbook for clinicians and developers. London: Psychology Press; 2015. p. 31–41.
14. Boman IL, et al. Using electronic aids to daily living after acquired brain injury: a study of the learning process and the usability. Disabil Rehabil Assist Technol. 2007;2(1):23–33.
15. Baldwin VN, Powell T. Google calendar: a single case experimental design study of a man with severe memory problems. Neuropsychol Rehabil. 2015; 25(4):617–36.
16. O'Neill, B. and A. Gillespie, Assistive technology for cognition, in Assistive Technology for Cognition: A handbook for clinicians and developers. London: Psychology Press; 2015. p. 1–11.
17. Dowds MM, et al. Electronic reminding technology following traumatic brain injury: effects on timely task completion. J Head Trauma Rehabil. 2011; 26(5):339–47.
18. Gagnon MP, et al. m-Health adoption by healthcare professionals: a systematic review. J Am Med Inform Assoc. 2016;23(1):212–20.
19. Cruz G, et al. Text messages reduce memory failures in adults with brain injury: a single-case experimental design. Br J Occup Ther. 2016;79(10):598–606.
20. Tornas S, et al. Rehabilitation of executive functions in patients with chronic acquired brain injury with goal management training, external cuing, and emotional regulation: a randomized controlled trial. J Int Neuropsychol Soc. 2016;22(4):436–52.
21. Suffoletto B, et al. Mobile phone text messaging to assess symptoms after mild traumatic brain injury and provide self-care support: a pilot study. J Head Trauma Rehabil. 2013;28(4):302–12.
22. Jamieson M, et al. ForgetMeNot: active reminder entry support for adults with acquired brain injury, ACM CHI conference on human factors in computing systems; 2017. p. 6012–23.
23. Raiman L, Antbring R, Mahmood A. WhatsApp messenger as a tool to supplement medical education for medical students on clinical attachment. BMC Med Educ. 2017;17(1):7.
24. Ofcom. The UK is now a smarthphone society 2015 [cited 2017 June]; Available from: http://media.ofcom.org.uk/news/2015/cmr-uk-2015/.
25. Gillespie A, Best C, O'Neill B. Cognitive function and assistive technology for cognition: a systematic review. J Int Neuropsychol Soc. 2012;18(1):1–19.
26. Mahar C, Fraser K. Strategies to facilitate successful community reintegration following acquired brain injury (ABI). Int J Disabil Manag. 2011;6(01):68–78.
27. Dombovy ML, Olek AC. Recovery and rehabilitation following traumatic brain injury. Brain Inj. 1997;11(5):305–18.
28. Rimel RW, et al. Moderate head injury: completing the clinical Spectrum of brain trauma. Neurosurgery. 1982;11(3):344–51.
29. BritishPsychological Society, Clinical neuropsychology and rehabilitation services for adults with acquired brain injury, B.P.S.D.o. Neuuropsychology, Editor. UK: British Psychological Society; 2005.
30. Boman I, et al. Support in everyday activities with a home-based electronic memory aid for persons with memory impairments. Disabil Rehabil Assist Technol. 2010;5(5):339–50. 12p
31. Fish J, et al. Rehabilitation of executive dysfunction following brain injury: "content-free" cueing improves everyday prospective memory performance. Neuropsychologia. 2007;45(6):1318–30.
32. Jamieson M, et al. Issues influencing the uptake of smartphone reminder apps for people with acquired brain injury. In: Proceedings of the 17th International ACM SIGACCESS Conference on Computers & Accessibility; 2015. ACM.
33. de Joode EA, et al. Use of assistive technology in cognitive rehabilitation: exploratory studies of the opinions and expectations of healthcare professionals and potential users. Brain Inj. 2012;26(10):1257–66.
34. Wong D, et al. Smartphones as assistive technology following traumatic brain injury: a preliminary study of what helps and what hinders. Disabil Rehabil. 2017;39(23):2387-94.
35. VODG, Using assistive technology to support personalisation in social care. UK: The Voluntary Organisations Disability Group (VODG); 2013. p. 4–7, 22–23.
36. VODG, Technology is changing the way we live. Can it also transform the way we deliver adult social care? UK: The Voluntary Organisations Disability Group (VODG); 2016.
37. Michie S, van Stralen MM, West R. The behaviour change wheel: a new method for characterising and designing behaviour change interventions. Implement Sci. 2011;6(1):42.
38. West R, Michie S. A guide to development and evaluation of digital behaviour change interventions in healthcare. London: Silverback Publishing; 2016.
39. Ross J, et al. Factors that influence the implementation of e-health: a systematic review of systematic reviews (an update). Implement Sci. 2016; 11(1):146.
40. Hartzler A, et al. Stakeholder engagement: a key component of integrating genomic information into electronic health records. Genet Med. 2013; 15(10):792–801.
41. Liddell, A., S. Adshead, and E. Burgess Technology in the NHS: transforming the patient's experience of care.. 2008.
42. Johnson RB, Onwuegbuzie AJ, Turner LA. Toward a definition of mixed methods research. J Mixed Methods Res. 2007;1(2):112–33.
43. Stoyanov SR, Hides L, Kavanagh DJ, Zelenko O, Tjondronegoro D, Mani M. Mobile App Rating Scale: A New Tool for Assessing the Quality of Health Mobile Apps. JMIR mHealth and uHealth. 2015;3(1):e27.
44. Borsci S, Federici S, Lauriola M. On the dimensionality of the system usability scale: a test of alternative measurement models. Cogn Process. 2009;10(3):193–7.
45. Michie S, Atkins L, West R. The behaviour change wheel: a guide to designing interventions, vol. 23. London: Silverback Publishing; 2014. p. 145–50.
46. Wood CE, et al. Applying the behaviour change technique (BCT) taxonomy v1: a study of coder training. Transl Behav Med. 2015;5(2):134–48.
47. Connell LA, et al. Development of a behaviour change intervention to increase upper limb exercise in stroke rehabilitation. Implement Sci. 2015;10(1):1.
48. Evald L. Prospective memory rehabilitation using smartphones in patients with TBI: what do participants report? Neuropsychol Rehabil. 2015;25(2): 283–97.
49. Lawton R, et al. Using the Theoretical Domains Framework (TDF) to understand adherence to multiple evidence-based indicators in primary care: a qualitative study. Implement Sci. 2016;11:113.
50. Cane J, O'Connor D, Michie S. Validation of the theoretical domains framework for use in behaviour change and implementation research. Implement Sci. 2012;7(1):1.

5

Use of feedback to improve mental number line representations in primary care clinics

Rachel F. Eyler[1*], Sara Cordes[2], Benjamin R. Szymanski[3] and Liana Fraenkel[4,5]

Abstract

Background: As patients become more engaged in decisions regarding their medical care, they must weigh the potential benefits and harms of different treatments. Patients who are low in numeracy may be at a disadvantage when making these decisions, as low numeracy is correlated with less precise representations of numerical magnitude. The current study looks at the feasibility of improving number representations. The aim of this study was to evaluate whether providing a small amount of feedback to adult subjects could improve performance on a number line placement task and to determine characteristics of those individuals who respond best to this feedback.

Methods: Subjects from two outpatient clinic waiting rooms participated in a three phase number line task. Participants were asked to place numbers on a computerized number line ranging from 0 to 1000 in pre-test, feedback, and post-test phases. Generalized estimating equations were used to model log-transformed scores and to test whether 1) performance improved after feedback, and 2) the degree of improvement was associated with age, education level or subjective numeracy.

Results: There was an overall improvement in task performance following the feedback. The average percent absolute error was 7.32% (SD: 6.00) for the pre-test and 5.63% (SD: 3.71) for the post-test. There was a significant interaction between college education and post-test improvement. Only subjects without some college education improved with feedback.

Conclusions: Adults who do not have higher levels of education improve significantly on a number line task when given feedback.

Keywords: Numeracy, Mental number line, Calibration

Background

Patients are increasingly asked to take an active role in decision-making at all levels of their medical care. Examples of such decisions include choosing between competing health insurance plans, deciding whether to pursue cancer screening, or choosing between competing treatment options.

Extant data suggest that numerical aptitude influences patients' decision making. Patients with low numeracy, which can be measured either objectively (i.e., having a patient answer math problems) or subjectively (i.e., asking the patient how comfortable they feel with numbers), are at a disadvantage when making health-related decisions, as they have greater difficulty interpreting magnitudes of risk compared to those who are more numerate [1, 2]. For example, in a survey of women aged 40–50, participants overestimated the risk that they would develop and die of breast cancer within the next 10 years, with women who were lowest in objective numeracy making the largest overestimations [1]. Subjects with lower objective numeracy also tend to overestimate risks associated with medications [3]. In one survey where subjects were asked to consider a hypothetical cholesterol medication, when risk was presented numerically, 18% of the less numerate

* Correspondence: rachel.eyler@uconn.edu
[1]Department of Pharmacy Practice, University of Connecticut School of Pharmacy, 69 North Eagleville Road, Storrs, CT 06269, USA

subjects (as measured by an abbreviated objective numeracy scale [4]) overestimated the risk of taking the medication, compared to only 6% in the more numerate group [3]. Research has also demonstrated that subjects with low objective numeracy might overestimate benefits of testing and procedures, as seen in one study examining women's perceptions of the benefits related to mammography [2].

Much research has focused on presenting side effects in ways that may be more understandable to those who are low in numeracy. Indeed, visual aids such as icon arrays and bar graphs have been shown to increase understanding in patients who are low in numeracy [5–8]. However, recent data suggest that some visual aids may not be helpful to those who are also low in graphical literacy [9]. An alternative (or complementary) method may be to improve patients' understanding of numerical magnitudes by allowing them to calibrate their mental number line.

Over- or under-estimation of risk may be linked to distortion of a subject's intuitive representation of a mental number line [10]. This "mental number line" is traditionally observed via a number line placement task, in which individuals are asked to indicate where a given number would fall on a line with numeric endpoints (e.g., where 150 falls on a line with endpoints of 0 and 1000) [11]. Accuracy on this task has been found to correlate with mathematical achievement in children, numeracy, and more recently has been used to explore the law of diminishing marginal utility in economic decision-making [10, 12, 13].

Studies have shown that children demonstrate notable improvement in number line tasks with a small amount of feedback. For example, second graders who received feedback on the correct placement of 1–3 items had improved accuracy in 70% of number line problems, compared to just 36% for those who did not receive feedback [14]. Given this background, we sought to establish the feasibility of improving adult subjects' numerical representations. The aim of this study was to evaluate whether providing feedback to adult subjects improves performance on a number line placement task, and whether age, education level or subjective numeracy moderates the magnitude of improvement. Because of time constraints we used the subjective numeracy scale, which has been validated against objective numeracy measures and found to predict risk recall and consistent utility assessments [15].

Given the known influence of numeracy on this task, we hypothesized that adults with higher subjective numeracy would have smaller pre-intervention errors compared to adults with lower subjective numeracy. We also hypothesized that adults with higher subjective numeracy would already perform at or near their individual peak performances, and so performance on the number line task would reveal less improvement after the feedback trials compared to adults with lower subjective numeracy.

Although subjects who are highly educated are not necessarily high in numeracy [16], amount of education is related to an individuals' perception of magnitude [17]. Therefore we hypothesized that subjects who were more highly educated would also demonstrate smaller pre-intervention errors. Similar to subjects who are high in numeracy, we further hypothesized that adults with higher education levels would perform at or near their individual peak performance pre-intervention and so would demonstrate less improvement after the feedback compared to less educated adults.

Older adults may experience more difficulties processing information (especially numerical information) compared to their younger counterparts [18–20]. These differences are clinically important, as older adults tend to have more health-care related decisions to make. In one study, moderate to older-aged adults' willingness to take a medication was less influenced by numerical representations of the adverse effects than younger adults [3]. Given the potential for increased numerical processing difficulties, we hypothesized that older adults would perform worse on the pre-test task (i.e., make larger errors) and feedback would be less likely to improve performance in older, compared to younger, adults.

Methods

This study was submitted to the Yale Institutional Review Board, and was determined to be exempt. Subjects from two outpatient primary care clinic waiting rooms (both affiliated with a large academic medical center) participated in the tasks, and provided verbal consent before beginning. The research assistant approached patients consecutively. Subjects were not offered compensation for participation, and were considered eligible if they were at least 18 years of age and spoke English. Participants completed an 8-question subjective numeracy scale [21] before the tasks began. Computerized number line tasks were developed based on several studies performed with children and adults using the number line as an assessment of numerical understanding [11]. This work revealed that younger children initially place numbers along the line with logarithmic spacing, such that smaller numbers are placed further apart than larger numbers, while older children and adults (i.e., those who are more numerate) eventually place the numbers in a linear fashion. While there is debate regarding what this logarithmic-to-linear pattern may signify [11, 22, 23], it is agreed that the greatest difference in performance between individuals who are more or less numerate is observed for placements of smaller numbers, in the lower half of the range of values.

As such, studies in which participants have been given feedback on their performance on the number line have determined that children show the greatest improvements in number line performance when given feedback on their placement of values in the lower half of the line, in particular, for values around 150 when placing values on a 0–1000 line [24].

The computerized number line tasks were used to assess each subject's mental number line, and involved a "pre-test" phase, "feedback" phase, and "post-test" phase. In the pre-test phase, participants were asked to place eight numbers (5, 63, 119, 174, 287, 432, 641, 830, presented in random order) on a computerized number line ranging from 0 to 1000 (Fig. 1). In the feedback phase, participants were told that they were going to complete a similar task, but this time they would be able to see how "close or far" they were from the correct answer. Subjects placed an additional five numbers (169, 703, 147, 18, 156) on the number line, and the correct position was shown after each choice was made in order to provide participants with accurate feedback (Fig. 2). Finally, in the post-test phase participants were again asked to place the original eight numbers from the pre-test without feedback. The same numbers were presented to all subjects for consistency across participants, especially because there is evidence that error varies as a function of the particular values presented. At the end of the feedback phase, demographic information including age, gender, race, and level of education (less than high school, high school or equivalent, some college, college degree, or post graduate education) was collected.

Pre-test and post-test scores, reported as percent absolute error (PAE), were calculated as the average of the absolute differences between where the participant placed the number and the actual number, divided by the range of the number line (e.g., if the participant placed the number "150" on the line at the location

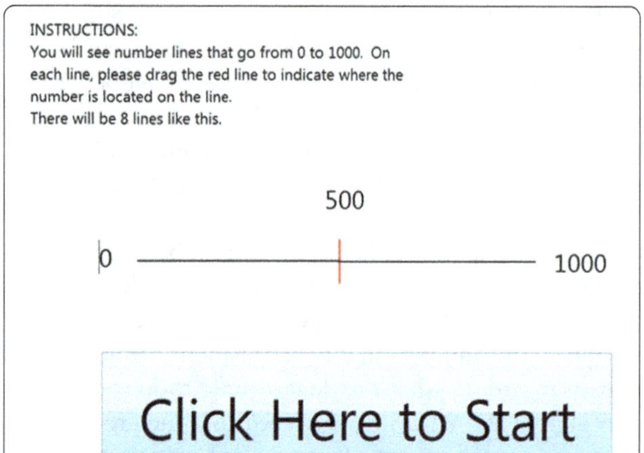

Fig. 1 Instruction screen for the pre-test phase

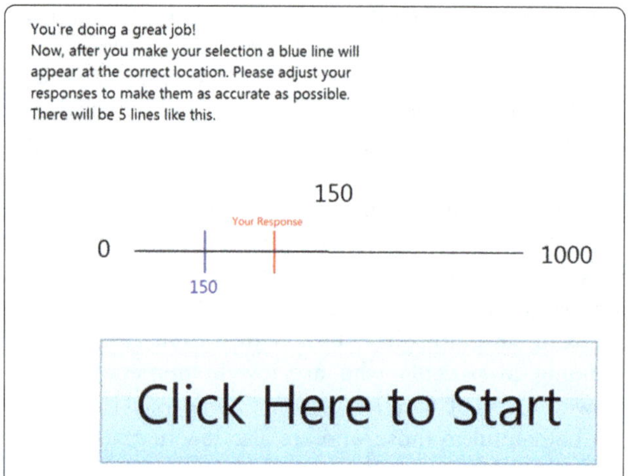

Fig. 2 Instruction screen for feedback phase

corresponding to a value of 250, the PAE would be computed as = |250–150| / 1000 = 0.1 or 10%). Thus, lower scores represent lower error and better performance on the number line task.

Repeated measures multivariate regression was used to model PAE. The model included age, education, subjective numeracy, and whether the participant had received feedback yet. As only 9 subjects had less than a high school education, the decision was made to group individuals into those who had completed high school or less versus those who completed at least some college. Generalized estimating equations (GEE) were used to account for within-subject correlation of pretest and posttest scores. Interaction terms between feedback and age, education, and numeracy allowed the effect of feedback to vary depending on the other variables. This model allowed us to evaluate which variables were associated with overall performance (i.e., variables that had equal effect on pretest and posttest scores) and which variables were differentially associated with improvement following feedback. Log-transformation of the outcome (PAE) was performed to account for non-constant error variance. The starting model was:

$$\begin{aligned}\log(PAE) = {} & \beta_0 + \beta_1 Age + \beta_2 Age \times Feedback \\ & + \beta_3 College + \beta_4 College \times Feedback \\ & + \beta_5 Numeracy + \beta_6 Numeracy \\ & \times Feedback + \beta_7 College \times Numeracy \\ & + \beta_8 College \times Numeracy \times Feedback \\ & + \beta_9 College \times Age + \beta_{10} College \times Age \\ & \times Feedback + \beta_{11} Feedback\end{aligned}$$

The variables in the regression model were as follows: Age was age in years, which was continuous and centered. Feedback was coded as 0 for pre-tests and 1 for post-tests. College Education was coded as 0 for people who did not complete high school and for people who only completed high school. It was coded as 1 for people who attended some college, graduated college, or had a postgraduate degree. Numeracy was the score on the subjective numeracy scale, which was continuous and centered. The dependent variable, lnPAE, was the natural log of the percent absolute error for the number line task. Using backward elimination, non-significant ($p > 0.10$) terms were removed from the model. The final model was:

$$\log(PAE) = \beta_0 + \beta_3 College + \beta_4 College \times Feedback + \beta_5 Numeracy + \beta_{11} Feedback$$

All analyses were performed in SAS version 9.4 (SAS Institute, Inc., Cary, NC).

Results

One hundred and one subjects participated. Of these, 59 (58.4%) were female, and 46 (45.5%) had at least some college education. The mean (SD) age was 55.1 (16.8) years and the mean (SD) subjective numeracy was 4.1 (1.1) out of a possible 6. We did not find a significant association between age and education (Fisher's exact $p = 0.552$) (Fig. 3). Thirty-seven (36.6%) participants were White, 56 (55.5%) were Black, and 8 (7.9%) were Hispanic.

There was an overall improvement (decrease in PAE) in number line task performance following the feedback training. The average PAE was 7.32% (SD: 6.00%) for the pre-test and 5.63% (SD: 3.71%) for the post-test (paired $t = 3.90$, DF = 100, $p < 0.001$).

In the multivariate log-transformed GEE model (see Table 1), some college education, and higher subjective numeracy were associated with lower PAEs on both pre- and post-test tasks. Age was not associated with number line performance, and was dropped from the final model. There was an overall decrease in PAE following feedback (β = − 0.27, 95%CI: -0.41 to − 0.14). We found no interaction between subjective numeracy and feedback, suggesting that the intervention had the same effect on individuals with high and low subjective numeracy. There was, however, a significant interaction between college education and feedback (β = 0.25, 95%CI: 0.06 to 0.44). Participants with college education had lower pre-test PAEs and did not significantly improve after feedback, while those without a college education tended to have higher pre-test PAEs and improved significantly following the feedback phase (see Fig. 4).

In the reduced model (Table 1), the intercept of 1.94 represents the expected value of lnPAE when all other variables are 0: that is, for a non-college educated (college = 0), averagely numerate (centered numeracy = 0) person taking the pre-test (feedback = 0). The signs of the parameter estimates for college education, numeracy, and feedback are all negative, which indicates that these are all associated with smaller lnPAE. The sign for the interaction between college education and feedback is positive, which means that the benefit of feedback is diminished in people with a college education.

Considered another way, the predicted pre-test lnPAE for a person with average subjective numeracy without a college education is 1.94. The predicted post-test lnPAE for a person with average subjective numeracy without a college education is 1.94–0.27 (the main effect of feedback) = 1.67. The predicted pre-test lnPAE for a person with average subjective numeracy with a college education is 1.94–0.44 (the main effect of college) = 1.50. Finally, the predicted post-test lnPAE for a person with

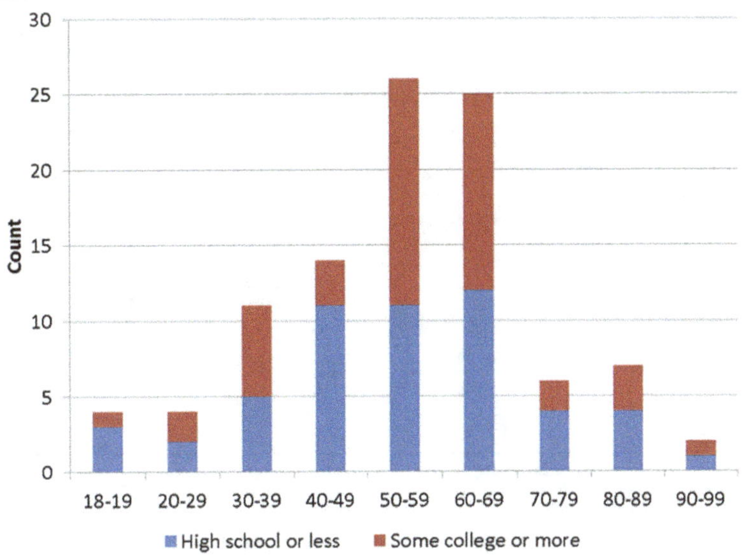

Fig. 3 Distribution of age and education

Table 1 Full and reduced multivariate models of variables associated with PAE

	Full Model			Reduced Model		
Parameter	Estimate	95% Confidence Interval	*p*-value	Estimate	95% Confidence Interval	*p*-value
Intercept	1.99	(1.73, 2.25)	< 0.001	1.94	(1.73, 2.16)	< 0.001
Age	0.01	(−0.01, 0.02)	0.344			
Age x Feedback	−0.01	(−0.02, 0.00)	0.102			
College Education	−0.47	(−0.77, − 0.16)	0.002	−0.44	(− 0.72, − 0.16)	0.002
College Education x Feedback	0.31	(0.09, 0.53)	0.006	0.25	(0.06, 0.44)	0.009
Numeracy	−0.01	(−0.04, 0.02)	0.560	−0.02	(− 0.03, − 0.01)	0.004
Numeracy x Feedback	−0.00	(− 0.02, 0.02)	0.715			
College Education x Numeracy	−0.02	(−0.05, 0.02)	0.386			
College Education x Numeracy x Feedback	−0.01	(−0.03, 0.02)	0.679			
College Education x Age	−0.01	(−0.02, 0.01)	0.299			
College education x Age x Feedback	0.01	(−0.00, 0.02)	0.115			
Feedback	−0.30	(−0.46, − 0.14)	< 0.001	−0.27	(− 0.41, − 0.14)	< 0.001

Note: continuous variables were centered

average subjective numeracy with a college education is 1.94–0.27 (the main effect of feedback) – 0.44 (the main effect of college) + 0.25 (the interaction between feedback and college) = 1.48.

In order to see whether the observed education effect was driven by individuals at the extremes (i.e., those who had not finished high school or those with post-graduate degrees), we plotted difference in PAEs (posttest – pretest) for each of the five education groups (Fig. 5). This did not appear to be the case, as those with a high school education appear to have improved slightly more than those who had not finished high school. All three groups with at least some college education had similar differences in PAE, which were all near zero. In an unadjusted paired t-test, subjects with a high school education or less ($n = 53$) lowered their PAE by 3.12 percentage points following feedback, from 9.67 to 6.55% ($t = 4.34$, df = 52, $p < 0.001$). Subjects who had completed some college or more ($n = 46$) had no significant improvement following feedback from 4.75 to 4.68%, a difference of – 0.07 percentage points ($t = 0.21$, df = 45, $p = 0.832$).

Finally, we assessed whether the effect of the feedback was stronger for smaller (< 300) numbers on the number line, as these were the values specifically targeted by the feedback. We calculated a PAE including only the 5

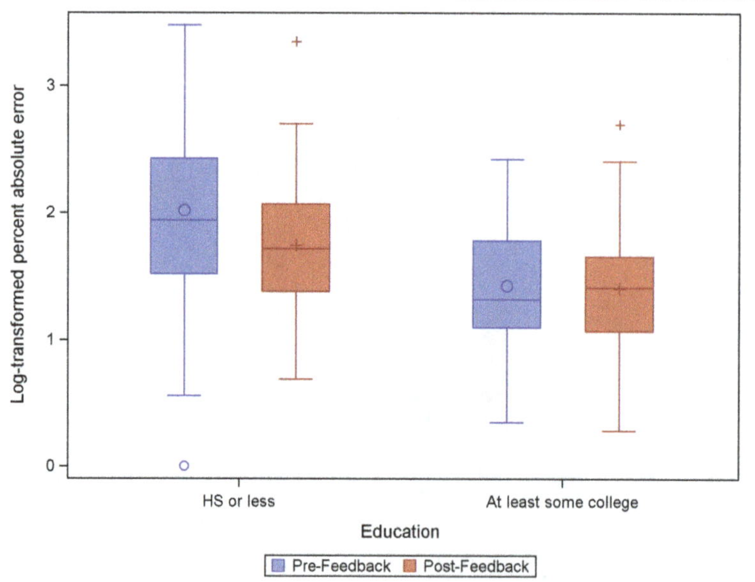

Fig. 4 Pre- and post-test Log-transformed percent absolute error by education status

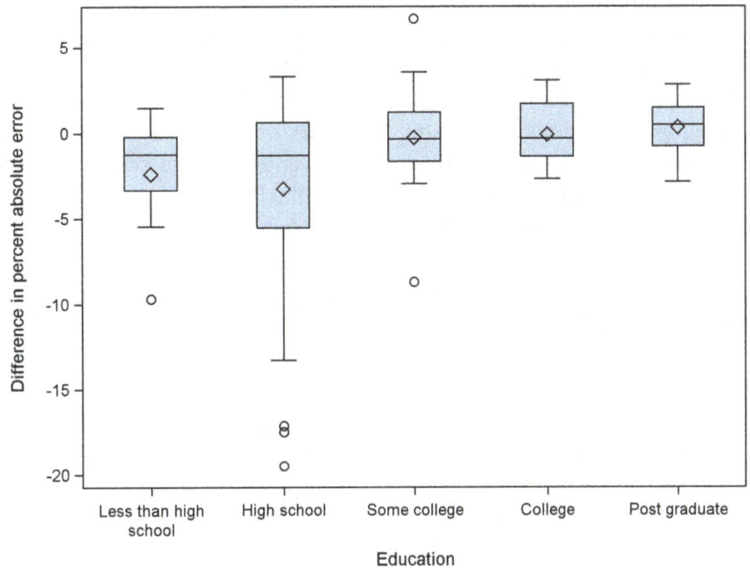

Fig. 5 Differences in percent absolute errors (posttest – pretest) by education.
*Note: Negative differences in percent absolute error indicate improved performance on the post-test

numbers that fell in the first third of the number line. For participants who did not complete high school the small-value PAE was 10.18% in the pre-test and 6.10% in the post-test for a decrease of 4.08 percentage points. For participants with at least some college education, the small-value PAE was 4.64% in the pre-test and 4.47 in the post-test for a decrease of 0.17 percentage points.

Discussion

In order for patients to make informed health-related decisions, they must be able to weigh risks and benefits. One aspect of understanding the magnitude of these risks and benefits is to understand the numerical values associated with the risks. Previous work has determined that the number line task assesses numerical magnitude understanding [14]. In this study we found that, as has been previously demonstrated in children, brief feedback significantly improves performance on a number-line task in adults without a college education.

We found significant main effects for college education and subjective numeracy on PAE, confirming our predictions that those with high numeracy and/or education would perform better on a number line task. Although these findings are not unexpected, they confirm that findings in the pediatric [17] and undergraduate population [12] can be expanded to a heterogeneous sample of adult patients in a primary care clinic who are the most likely to be making medical-related decisions. However, contrary to our prediction that older age would lead to lower number line performance, age had no effect on PAE. Younger and older participants performed equally well on the pre-test and had similar amounts of improvement following the feedback session. This may mean that cognitive inefficiencies that occur with aging have little impact on individual's understanding of numerical magnitudes and suggests that younger and older patients alike may benefit from a more detailed demonstration of numeric magnitude.

Interestingly, the only predictor of improvement was whether or not subjects had received at least some college education, presumably because subjects with a lower education level were able to improve with the feedback, while subjects with a higher education level were already performing near their individual peak performances before feedback was given. Importantly, education is a strong predictor of objective numeracy [25], which, in turn, is a strong predictor of one's ability to interpret medical risk information [1–3]. Our results suggest that the same individuals who are at risk for misinterpreting medical information could benefit from number line feedback training. This is motivation for further research into whether improving number line performance can also improve medical decision making itself.

Although the improvement of PAE found in our study is less than the 5–10 percentage points reported in children (who have much higher PAEs to start with) [24, 26], the improvement in PAE of 3.12 percentage points for adult subjects who did not attend college is encouraging. Additionally, subjects who did not attend college improved the most around their placement of small numbers (those < 300), with subjects improving by 4.1 percentage points when only the lowest 5 numbers were included. This finding aligns well with previous research suggesting that children and those who are low in numeracy are more likely to place numbers in a logarithmic fashion across the line (overestimating values at the beginning of the line) [11], and might explain why patients who are low in numeracy tend to overestimate risks (particularly risks with low likelihoods) associated with medications [3, 27]. In future studies we plan to assess whether this intervention may allow patients to more accurately assess the risk of side effects, so this is the area of the number line where it is most important to see the greatest impact (since these values correspond to the type of risks discussed in medical decisions).

Performance on a number line task may be a quick and easy way to identify patients who are in need of a more detailed discussion of the meanings of numbers. Findings in children do suggest that performance on a number line task is associated with measurable, real-world outcomes. Performance on the number line task has been strongly related to numeracy, math achievement, and economic decision-making [10, 12, 13]. We do not currently know if the improvements in the number line task seen with feedback can be translated into better medical decisions, but this will be an interesting area of further research. As many patients overestimate the risk of rare side effects, it is possible that giving the patients feedback regarding the actual location of the number may be beneficial. Feedback on the number line task - even with just 1–3 numbers - has not only been shown to quickly improve performance on the number line task, but also increased 7–9 year olds' ability to categorize numbers as "very small, small, medium, big, and very big." [24].

Future studies should evaluate whether completing a number line exercise prior to being presented with a clinical scenario could improve risk comprehension and decision making. Alternatively, patients could indicate their perceived risks of a medication on the number line, and subjects could receive real-time feedback on how accurately they charted these risks. Many subjects in this study did appear engaged during the study (even thinking of it as a challenge or game), so this method of discussing risk could present a more interactive approach to increasing risk understanding.

Limitations

Study limitations include the small study size and self-selection among the study population, as not everyone accepted our invitation to participate. The subjects' mental, cognitive, physical and emotional conditions in a busy waiting room could have affected their performance on this number line task, although it was reassuring that subjects were able to improve on the number line task despite these issues, as decision-making is also often made in these similar conditions.

Conclusions

Similar to findings in the pediatric population, adults without a college education can improve on a number line task when given a brief amount of feedback. Future research should evaluate the clinical utility of a feedback intervention to aid patients in their health-related decision making.

Abbreviations

GEE: Generalized Estimating Equations; PAE: Percent Absolute Error

Acknowledgements

The preliminary results of this study were presented at the 37th Annual Meeting of the Society for Medical Decision Making. St. Louis, MO (October 20, 2015).

Funding

This publication was supported by the National Institute of Arthritis and Musculoskeletal and Skin Diseases, part of the NIH, under Award Number AR060231-06 (Fraenkel). The content is solely the responsibility of the authors and does not necessarily represent the official views of the National Institutes of Health. The authors do not have any conflicts of interest related to the content of this manuscript.

Authors' contributions

RE, LF, and SC designed the study, RE led patient recruitment and data collection, BS led data analysis. All authors contributed to and approved the final manuscript.

Competing interests

The authors declare that they have no competing interests.

Author details

[1]Department of Pharmacy Practice, University of Connecticut School of Pharmacy, 69 North Eagleville Road, Storrs, CT 06269, USA. [2]Department of Psychology, Boston College, 300 McGuinn Hall, 140 Commonwealth Ave, Chestnut Hill, MA 02467, USA. [3]Department of Chronic Disease Epidemiology, Yale School of Public Health, 60 College Street, New Haven, CT 06510, USA. [4]Department of Medicine, Section of Rheumatology, Yale University School of Medicine, 300 Cedar Street, TAC #525, New Haven, CT 06520, USA. [5]VA Connecticut Healthcare System, West Haven, CT 06516, USA.

References

1. Black WC, Nease RF, Tosteson AN. Perceptions of breast cancer risk and screening effectiveness in women younger than 50 years of age. J Natl Cancer Inst. 1995;87:720–31.
2. Schwartz LM, Woloshin S, Black WC, Welch HG. The role of numeracy in understanding the benefit of screening mammography. Ann Intern Med. 1997;127:966–72.
3. Peters E, Hart PS, Tusler M, Fraenkel L. Numbers matter to informed patient choices a randomized design across age and numeracy levels. Med Decis Mak. 2014;34:430–42.

4. Weller JA, Dieckmann NF, Tusler M, Mertz C, Burns WJ, Peters E. Development and testing of an abbreviated numeracy scale: a Rasch analysis approach. J Behav Decis Mak. 2013;26:198–212.
5. Galesic M, Garcia-Retamero R, Gigerenzer G. Using icon arrays to communicate medical risks: overcoming low numeracy. Health Psychol. 2009;28:210–6. https://doi.org/10.1037/a0014474.
6. Fagerlin A, Ubel PA, Smith DM, Zikmund-Fisher BJ. Making numbers matter: present and future research in risk communication. Am J Health Behav. 2007;31:S47–56.
7. Lipkus IM, Hollands J. The visual communication of risk. J Natl Cancer Inst Monogr. 1999;25:149–63.
8. Peters E, Hibbard J, Slovic P, Dieckmann N. Numeracy skill and the communication, comprehension, and use of risk-benefit information. Health Aff (Millwood). 2007;26:741–8.
9. Garcia-Retamero R, Galesic M. Who proficts from visual aids: overcoming challenges in people's understanding of risks. Soc Sci Med. 2010;70:1019–25.
10. Schley DR, Peters E. Assessing "economic value" symbolic-number mappings predict risky and riskless valuations. Psychol Sci. 2014;25:753–61.
11. Siegler RS, Opfer JE. The development of numerical estimation evidence for multiple representations of numerical quantity. Psychol Sci. 2003;14:237–50.
12. Peters E, Slovic P, Västfjäll D, Mertz C. Intuitive numbers guide decisions. Judgm Decis Mak. 2008;3:619–35.
13. Siegler RS, Booth JL. Development of numerical estimation in young children. Child Dev. 2004;75:428–44.
14. Opfer JE, Siegler RS. Representational change and children's numerical estimation. Cogn Psychol. 2007;55:169–95.
15. Zikmund-Fisher BJ, Smith DM, Ubel PA, Fagerlin A. Validation of the subjective numeracy scale: effects of low numeracy on comprehension of risk communications and utility elicitations. Med Decis Mak. 2007;27:663–71.
16. Lipkus IM, Samsa G, Rimer BK. General performance on a numeracy scale among highly educated samples. Med Decis Mak. 2001;21:37–44.
17. Laski EV, Yu Q. Number line estimation and mental addition: examining the potential roles of language and education. J Exp Child Psychol. 2014;117:29–44.
18. Peters E, Hess TM, Västfjäll D, Auman C. Adult age differences in dual information processes: implications for the role of affective and deliberative processes in older adults' decision making. Perspect Psychol Sci. 2007;2:1–23. https://doi.org/10.1111/j.1745-6916.2007.00025.x.
19. Salthouse TA. The processing-speed theory of adult age differences in cognition. Psychol Rev. 1996;103:403–28.
20. Park DC, Lautenschlager G, Hedden T, Davidson NS, Smith AD, Smith PK. Models of visuospatial and verbal memory across the adult life span. Psychol Aging. 2002;17:299–320.
21. Fagerlin A, Zikmund-Fisher BJ, Ubel PA, Jankovic A, Derry HA, Smith DM. Measuring numeracy without a math test: development of the subjective numeracy scale. Med Decis Mak. 2007;27:672–80.
22. Barth HC, Paladino AM. The development of numerical estimation: evidence against a representational shift. Dev Sci. 2011;14:125–35.
23. Hurst M, Monahan KL, Heller E, Cordes S. 123s and ABCs: developmental shifts in logarithmic-to-linear responding reflect fluency with sequence values. Dev Sci. 2014;17:892–904.
24. Opfer JE, Thompson CA. The trouble with transfer: insights from microgenetic changes in the representation of numerical magnitude. Child Dev. 2008;79:788–804.
25. Galesic M, Garcia-Retamero R. Statistical numeracy for health: a cross-cultural comparison with probabilistic national samples. Arch Intern Med. 2010;170:462–8.
26. Thompson CA, Opfer JE. Costs and benefits of representational change: effects of context on age and sex differences in symbolic magnitude estimation. J Exp Child Psychol. 2008;101:20–51.
27. Fraenkel L, Cunningham M, Peters E. Subjective numeracy and preference to stay with the status quo. Med Decis Mak. 2015;35:6–11.

6

Heterogeneous network propagation for herb target identification

Kuo Yang[1], Guangming Liu[1], Ning Wang[1], Runshun Zhang[2], Jian Yu[1], Jianxin Chen[3*] and Xuezhong Zhou[1,4*]

From The 3rd China Health Information Processing Conference
Shenzhen, China. 24-25 November 2017

Abstract

Background: Identifying targets of herbs is a primary step for investigating pharmacological mechanisms of herbal drugs in Traditional Chinese medicine (TCM). Experimental targets identification of herbs is a difficult and time-consuming work. Computational method for identifying herb targets is an efficient approach. However, how to make full use of heterogeneous network data about herbs and targets to improve the performance of herb targets prediction is still a dilemma.

Methods: In our study, a random walk algorithm on the heterogeneous herb-target network (named heNetRW) has been proposed to identify protein targets of herbs. By building a heterogeneous herb-target network involving herbs, targets and their interactions and simulating random walk algorithm on the network, the candidate targets of the given herb can be predicted.

Results: The experimental results on large-scale dataset showed that heNetRW had higher performance of targets prediction than PRINCE (improved F1-score by 0.08 and Hit@1 by 21.34% in one validation setting, and improved F1-score by 0.54 and Hit@1 by 69.08% in the other validation setting). Furthermore, we evaluated novel candidate targets of two herbs (rhizoma coptidis and turmeric), which showed our approach could generate potential targets that are valuable for further experimental investigations.

Conclusions: Compared with PRINCE algorithm, heNetRW algorithm can fuse more known information (such as, known herb-target associations and pathway-based similarities of protein pairs) to improve prediction performance. Experimental results also indicated heNetRW had higher performance than PRINCE. The prediction results not only can be used to guide the selection of candidate targets of herbs, but also help to reveal the molecule mechanisms of herbal drugs.

Keywords: Heterogeneous herb-target network, Random walk, Herb target identification

Background

Target identification of herb medicine is the primary step toward investigating herbal molecular mechanism and improving clinical efficacy of treatment. Unlike allopathic Western Medicine, Traditional Chinese medicine (TCM) is characterized as holistic emphasizing on regulating the integrity of the human body [1]. The diverse herbal ingredients and multi-target molecular mechanism are critical characteristics of herb medicine [2, 3]. In recent years, herbal molecular mechanism studies mainly are focused on animal experiments, for example, Yu et al. [4] found that SP1 is potential target of turmeric by mice experiments. However, animal experiments not only cost a lot of times and manpower, but also are limited to the scale of minority herbs, which has caused enormous challenge for TCM researchers.

Network pharmacology emphasized the paradigm shift from "one target, one drug" to "network target, multicomponent therapeutics," highlighting a holistic thinking also shared by TCM [2, 5]. By integrating computational and experimental methods, network pharmacology provided a

* Correspondence: cjx@bucm.edu.cn; xzzhou@bjtu.edu.cn
[3]Beijing University of Chinese Medicine, Beijing 100029, China
[1]School of Computer and Information Technology and Beijing Key Lab of Traffic Data Analysis and Mining, Beijing Jiaotong University, Beijing 100044, China

new perspective of herb compatibility [6] and herbal molecular mechanism research [7]. On the one hand, plenty of medical associations data, i.e., drug-target associations (DrugBank [8] and Stitch [9]), phenotype-genotype associations (OMIM [10] and DO [11]), protein-protein interactions (String10 [12]) and human symptom-disease associations [13], provided abundant and valuable medical data, which can be applied to computational methods to predict herbal protein targets. On the other hand, plenty of prediction approaches based on network propagation have been widely applied to identify genetic associations, e.g., drugCIPHER-MS [14] for drug target identification, PRINCE [15], pgWalk [16] and Know-GENE [17] for disease gene identification and herb target prediction, which indicated that network propagation is an effective approach to figure out the problem of link prediction in complex network. In our previous work [3], we proposed a network-based herb target prediction algorithm integrating efficacy-based herb similarity, which implied efficacy-based herb similarity was better measure of herb correlation than herbal chemical-based similarity.

In TCM field, several curated databases involving the associations between herbal ingredients and targets, i.e. HIT [18], TCMID [19], have been established. Yet, the high credible dataset of herb-target associations is still incomplete. Therefore, developing effective approaches to identifying herbal protein targets has become a key step to decode molecular mechanism of herbs. Network pharmacology methods have been utilized to active ingredient-target networks of herbs that were responsible for the beneficial effects against hepatocellular carcinoma [20]. By integrating serum pharmacochemistry-based screening with high-resolution metabolomics analysis, Wang et al. [21] developed chinmedomics to identify the bioactive constituents of herbs and predicted action potential targets. Zhang et al. [22] proposed a computational strategy for network understanding of herb pharmacology via rapid identification of putative ingredient-target interactions in human structural proteome level. Liang et al. [23] proposed a holistic analysis method combines chemical and therapeutic properties with network pharmacology to decipher targets and ingredients of herbal formulae. Zhao et al. [24] introduced a system pharmacology model based on absorption filtering, network targeting and systems analyses to clarify the active compounds and therapeutic mechanisms of Bufei Jianpi formula.

Here, aiming at protein targets identification of herbs, a random walk algorithm [25] on heterogeneous herb-target network (heNetRW) was put forward (Fig. 1). By constructing a heterogeneous herb-target network and simulating random walk on the network, the candidate targets of the query herb can be predicted. In the experimental stage, two validation setting: NoTarget and HalfTarget situations were simulated to evaluate prediction performance of heNetRW. And the final results indicated that heNetRW has better performance than baseline algorithm PRINCE (improved F1-score by 0.08 and Hit@1 by 21.34% under NoTarget simulation, improved F1-score by 0.54 and Hit@1 by 69.08% under HalfTarget simulation). Furthermore, we evaluated novel candidate targets (not recorded in the benchmark) of

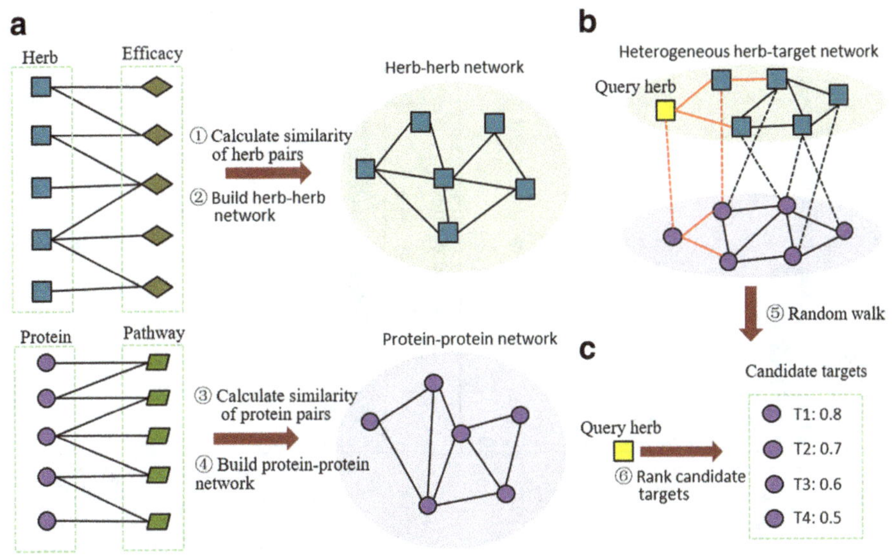

Fig. 1 The workflow of heNetRW. Based on herb-efficacy and protein-pathway associations, cosine similarities of herb pairs and protein pairs were calculated. Then the herb-herb network and protein-protein network (Fig. 1**a**), whose nodes represent herbs or proteins and edges represent shared efficacies or shared pathways, were built. Given a query herb, the random walk algorithm was simulated (red line) on the heterogeneous herb-target network (Fig. 1**b**). By ranking the candidate targets by correlation scores, candidate targets of a given herb can be identified (Fig. 1**c**)

rhizoma coptidis and turmeric by consulting recent published papers and conducting shortest path analysis, whose results manifested the correlativity between these candidate targets and query herbs.

Methods

Dataset

We integrated 1427 herbs were extracted from HIT [18] and Chinese pharmacopoeia (CHPA, 2015 edition) and 16,005 proteins from HIT and KEGG [26] databases. In the HIT database, there are associations between herbal ingredients and targets from medical literatures. By integrating herb-ingredient and ingredient-target associations, 23,453 associations between 1016 herbs and 1214 targets (see Additional file 1) were connected directly through 511 herbal ingredients. On average, each herb was associated with 23.08 targets, and each target was relevant to 19.32 targeted herbs (Fig. 2). The target number of 57.48% herbs was bigger than ten, which also verified multi-target mechanism of herbs. Otherwise, we collected 3487 herb-efficacy associations between 742 herbs and 360 efficacies from CHPA (see Additional file 2). 16,162 protein-pathway associations between 4794 proteins and 244 pathways (see Additional file 3) were also collected from KEGG database.

Similarity calculation of herb pairs and protein pairs

By building efficacy or target vectors and measuring the cosine value of these vectors, efficacy-based and target-based similarities of herb pairs can be calculated. For example, given m herbs and n related efficacies, every herb i can be represented by a vector of efficacy $V_i = (w_{i,1}, \ldots, w_{i,j}, \ldots, w_{i,n})$, where $w_{i,j} = 1$ if efficacy j belong to herb i, if not, $w_{i,j} = 0$. Then the efficacy-based similarity of herb x and y can be measured by the cosine value of their vectors (Eq. 1). Similarly, target-based herb similarities were also calculated.

$$Cos(V_x, V_y) = \frac{V_x \cdot V_y}{|V_x| \cdot |V_y|} \quad (1)$$

Similarly, by building vectors of pathways and herbs, and measuring the cosine value of these vectors, pathway-based and herb-based similarities of protein pairs also can be calculated.

Herb pairs with similar efficacies indicate similar targets

The basic assumption of heNetRW is that herb pairs with shared efficacies indicated shared targets, and protein pairs with shared pathways implied shared targeted herbs. Given an herb pair, we quantified the efficacy-based cosine similarity between the herb pair, and measured the target-based cosine similarity of the pair as the average pairwise similarity score. We partitioned the similarities of all herb pairs into 10 bins of equal size. The average target-based similarity of herb pairs in each bin can be calculated. Similarly, pathway-based and herb-based similarity of protein pairs were also measured.

To illustrate overlap results of herb pairs and protein pairs, we compared the overlap results with random shuffle [27]. We took herb pairs as an example. First of

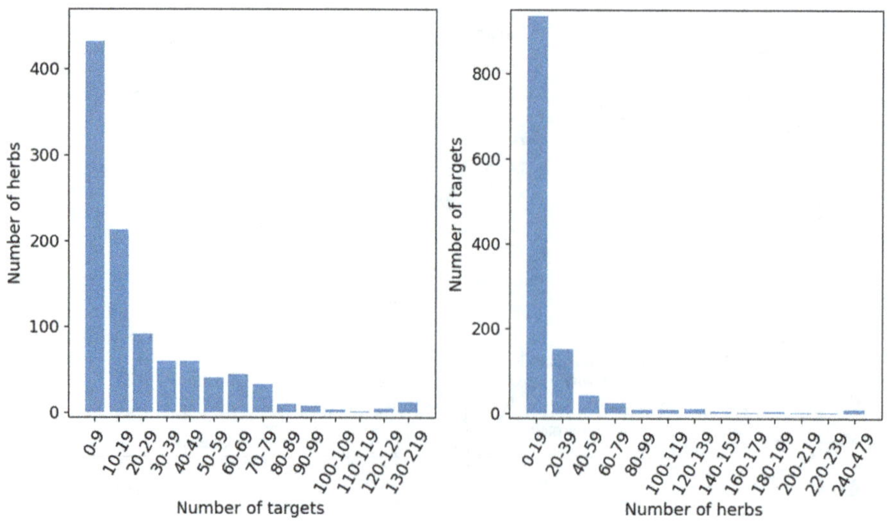

Fig. 2 The distribution of associations between herbs and targets. The target number distribution of herbs were shown in Fig. 2**a**. The horizontal axis represents number of targets, and the vertical axis represents the number of herbs with corresponding number of targets. Fig 2**b** showed the targeted herb number distribution of targets. The horizontal axis represents number of herbs, and the vertical axis represents the number of targets with corresponding number of targeted herbs

all, for herb pairs, remaining constant known efficacies of herbs, we shuffled randomly equal number of targets for each herb. Secondly, based on the random targets of herb pairs, the overlap results can be calculated. Finally, the above procedures were repeated for 100 times, and the average ratios of overlap results can be obtained.

Construction of herb-herb network and protein-protein network

Based on efficacy-based similarities of herb pairs, we constructed the herb-herb network, where nodes represent herbs and edges represent herb pairs with shared efficacies (that is, efficacy-based herb similarities are bigger than zero). The network we built may contain a large number of low confident edges between herbs pairs with small similarities. Therefore, only α neighbor herbs with the highest similarity scores for each herb were selected to build a more confident herb-herb network.

Similarly, by calculating pathway-based similarities of proteins, the protein-protein network also can be constructed. For a more confident protein-protein network, β neighbor proteins with the highest similarity scores for each protein were kept. The parameters α and β have been tuned to observe the influence of target prediction under different values of α and β.

Random walk on heterogeneous herb-target network to identify candidate targets

Given an herb-herb network, a protein-protein network and known herb-target associations, the heterogeneous herb-target network (HHGN) can be constructed, which included two type nodes: herb and protein nodes, and three type edges: herb-herb, protein-protein, and herb-target edges. Then the process that a random walker wandered on HHGN can be simulated to identify candidate targets of given herb.

For the HHGN, there are an herb layer, a protein layer, and interconnections between the two layers. The herb layer, which can be weighted by efficacy-based similarities of herbs, was composed of herbs and their relationships. The protein layer, which can be weighted by pathway-based protein similarity, was composed of proteins and their associations. Interconnections, which connected herb layer and protein layer, are composed of known associations between herbs and proteins. Hence, given a query herb, the random walker would start a journey on the HHGN with initial probability $p^{(0)}$. In next each step, the walker would select to start a new journey with the probability θ or select to move to neighbors of the current node with the probability $1-\theta$. For moving to neighbors, the walker would select to jump from the herb layer to the protein layer or vice versa with probability ϕ or select to wander in either the herb layer or the protein layer with the probability $1-\phi$. After a number of steps, the probability of each node on the HHGN would reach a steady state $p^{(t)}$, which can be used to measure the strength between the query herb and candidate targets.

Mathematically, HHGN is denoted by $I=(H,G,R)$, where $H=(h_{ij})_{m\times m}$ is the weight matrix of herb-herb network, $G=(g_{ij})_{n\times n}$ is the weight matrix of protein-protein network, $R=(a_{ij})_{m\times n}$ is the adjacency matrix of herb-protein network, and m and n is the numbers of herbs and proteins, respectively. The heNetRW is described as follows:

The heNetRW algorithm.

Input: $H, G, R, \theta, \varphi, \varepsilon$

1. Row normalize H to obtain $U=(u_{ij})_{m\times m}$, where $u_{ij}=h_{ij}/\sum_{j=1}^{m} h_{ij}$.
2. Row normalize G to obtain $V=(v_{ij})_{n\times n}$, where $v_{ij}=d_{ij}/\sum_{j=1}^{n} g_{ij}$.
3. Row normalize R to obtain $A=(r_{ij})_{m\times n}$, where $r_{ij}=a_{ij}/\sum_{j=1}^{n} a_{ij}$, $r_{ij}=0$ if $\sum_{j=1}^{n} a_{ij}=0$.
4. Row normalize R^T to obtain $B=(s_{ij})_{n\times m}$, where $s_{ij}=a_{ij}/\sum_{j=1}^{m} a_{ij}$, where $s_{ij}=0$ if $\sum_{j=1}^{m} a_{ij}=0$.
5. Set $T=\begin{pmatrix}(1-\varphi)U & \varphi A\\ \varphi B & (1-\varphi)V\end{pmatrix}$, row normalize T to get $W=(w_{ij})_{(m+n)\times(m+n)}$, where $w_{ij}=t_{ij}/\sum_{j=1}^{m+n} t_{ij}$
6. Initialize $p^{(0)}=((u^{(0)})^T,(v^{(0)})^T)^T$, $\omega=1000$
7. while $\omega>\varepsilon$:

    $p^{(t)}=(1-\pi)W^T p^{(t-1)}+\pi p^{(0)}$
    $\omega=L_1\ norm\ of\ \Delta p=p^{(t)}-p^{(t-1)}$
    t ++

Output : $p^{(t)}$

For the transition matrices A and B, r_{ij} and s_{ij} are the probability that the walker jumps from the i-th herb to the j-th protein and jumps from the i-th protein to the j-th herb, respectively. $u^{(0)}=(u^{(0)})_{m\times 1}$ and $v^{(0)}=(v^{(0)})_{n\times 1}$ are initial probabilities for the herb layer and the protein layer, respectively. $p^{(0)}$ represents the initial probability of every herb and protein. $p^{(t)}$ represents probability of nodes after t-th iteration of random walker, and Δp represents changed matrix of t-th and $(t-1)$-th iteration.

Finally, when the L_1 norm of matrix Δp is smaller than ε, the algorithm obtained steady-state probability $p^{(t)}$, and it contains the two part: herb scores $u^{(t)}$ and protein scores $v^{(t)}$, which can be regarded as predicted targets of the query herb. Sorting all the predicted proteins by the scores, the top n proteins of ranked list were selected as candidate proteins of the query herb.

Experimental setting and evaluation

We collected 1016 herbs with known targets, 120 of which only targeted one protein target and the remaining 896 herbs targeted more than one protein target. We filtered overlapped 261 herbs with known targets and known efficacies. In real world, there usually are two situations of target identification: (1) the query herb has no target; (2) the query herb has some targets. Therefore, we simulated the two situations: (1) predict all targets for the query herb whose all targets are removed (NoTarget); (2) predict left targets for the query herb whose half number of targets are randomly removed

(HalfTarget). Particularly, if the query herb only has one target, it only can be used to the first situation. If all known targets of the given herb were removed, and the given herb didn't have any herb neighbors in the heterogeneous herb-target network, the initial value $\boldsymbol{p}^{(0)}$ of the given herb will be zero, which would lead that the random walk algorithm would not spread nodes information to other nodes of the network. So when simulating NoTarget, 261 herbs with herbs and targets neighbors were selected as test herbs. And when simulating HalfTarget, we select 896 herbs with more than one known targets as test herbs. For the two situations: NoTarget and HalfTarget, heNetRW and PRINCE were evaluated by leave one out cross validation (LOOCV): remove all of known targets or half of known targets for the query herb and retain all of known targets for other herbs.

If the query herb had k known targets, the top k proteins of ranked proteins list will be selected as candidate targets of the query herb. For example, given the query herb rhizoma coptidis with 64 known targets, our algorithm would select the top 64 targets of ranked list as candidate targets. On the one hand, precision, recall and F1-score of every query herb were calculated by Eqs. 2 and 3, in which TP, FP and FN represent the numbers of true positives, false positives and true negatives, respectively. On the other hand, the top one hit (Hit@1) rate was also used to evaluate the algorithms. Hit@1 considers that the proportion of the query herbs, whose top one protein of ranked list is the known target of the query herb.

$$Precision = TP/(TP + FP); Recall = TP/(TP + FN) \quad (2)$$

$$F1 = \frac{2 \cdot Precision \cdot Recall}{Precision + Recall} \quad (3)$$

Shortest path analysis

To investigate the associations between candidate targets and known targets of given herbs, average shortest path length (ASPL) and shortest path length (SPL) distribution between them were conducted. First of all, the shortest path length $SPL(t, s)$ between candidate target t and known target s ($s \in$ the known targets set S) in the protein-protein interaction (PPI) network can be calculated. Then the ASPL can be calculated by the equation:

$$ASPL(t, S) = \frac{1}{|S|} \sum_{s \in S} SPL(t, s) \quad (4)$$

where $|S|$ represented the number of known targets. Otherwise, the distribution of all the SPLs was also calculated and compared with random shuffle. For the random experiment, candidate targets were selected randomly from the PPI network, and the SPL distribution between the candidate target and known targets was calculated. The above process was repeated for ten thousand times, finally, the average distribution of random candidate target and known targets can be obtained.

Results

Overview of heNetRW

The core idea of heNetRW is simulating random walk on a heterogeneous herb-target network to identify candidate targets of herbs. As illustrated in Fig. 1, firstly, based on herb-efficacy and protein-pathway associations, cosine similarities of herb pairs and protein pairs can be calculated. After that, the herb-herb network and protein-protein network were constructed. The weight of edges in the two networks depend on similarities of herb pairs or protein pairs. There are 741 nodes and 60,753 edges in herb-herb network (Table 1), whose average degree (the number of neighbors) is 163.98. The protein-protein network with 4794 nodes and 656,681 edges has a higher average node degree (= 273.95). Compared with herb-herb network (network density: 0.22), protein-protein network has the lower network density (=0.06). By integrating herb-herb network, protein-protein network and herb-target associations, the heterogeneous herb-target network (network density: 0.03), which is a very sparse network, can be constructed. Given a query herb, random walk algorithm on the heterogeneous network can be simulated to predict candidate targets. Sorting all predicted targets by correlation scores, the ranking list of candidate proteins can be obtained. LOOCV was used to evaluate the prediction performance. In addition, the PRINCE [3] algorithm, which is a state-of-the-art algorithm for herb target prediction, was adopted as the baseline algorithm in our experiments. With efficacy-based similarities of herb pairs, the PRINCE simulated network propagation on the PPI network to predict herb targets.

Herb pairs with similar efficacies indicate similar targets

The basic assumption of our method is that the herb pairs with shared efficacies implied shared targets, and

Table 1 The description of related networks

Network	Number of nodes	Number of edges	Average degree	Network density
Herb-herb network	741	60,753	163.98	0.22
Protein-protein network	4794	656,681	273.95	0.06
Heterogeneous herb-target network	6716	740,887	220.63	0.03

target pairs with shared pathways implied shared targeted herbs. To validate this assumption, we quantified efficacy-based and target-based similarities of herb pairs. And the overlap results were compared with results of random permutation using Fisher-Yates method [27]. Meanwhile, to validate whether protein pairs with similar pathways indicated similar targeted herbs, pathway-based and herb-based similarities of protein pairs also were adopted according to the same way. We selected 261 comon herbs with efficacies and targets as experimental herbs (Fig. 3a). The herb pairs with weak efficacy-based similarities (0.1–0.2) had weak target-based average similarity (0.18; Expected: 0.06±0.0013). Nevertheless, for the herb pairs with strong similarities (0.9–0.1), their target-based average similarity (0.60; Expected: 0.06±0.02) was also strong, which indicated herbs with more similar efficacies are more likely to have more similar targets. Similarly, for 789 proteins with pathways and targeted herbs (Fig. 3b), there were the similar results, which were proteins similarity bin from 0 to 0.1 (0.18; Expected: 0.07±0.0007) versus similarity bin from 0.9 to 1 (0.49; Expected: 0.08±0.01).

Target identification of herbs

In this study, we simulated two situations existed in the real world: NoTarget, the query herb with no known target (all of known targets as test targets); HalfTarget, the query herb with half of known targets (Half of known targets as train targets, the left targets as test targets). For the two settings: NoTarget and HalfTarget, we selected 261 herbs and 896 herbs as test herbs, respectively. Using LOOCV, the prediction performance of heNetRW was compared with PRINCE. Target prediction results (Table 2) implied that the performance of heNetRW was slightly better than PRINCE (improved F1-score by 0.08 and Hit@1 by 21.34%) under the NoTarget simulation. We also displayed F1-scores distribution of 261 test herbs with different number of test targets (known targets) (Fig. 4a). The distribution of F1-scores indicated that heNetRW (64.75% F1-scores bigger than 0.20) had better performance (p-value = 1.10e-8) than PRINCE (40% F1-scores bigger than 0.20). Under the HalfTarget simulation, heNetRW had much better performance than PRINCE (improved F1-score by 0.54 and Hit@1 by 69.08%). And the F1-scores distribution also implied heNetRW (70.87% F1-scores bigger than 0.40) has much better performance (p-value = 1.10e-249) than PRINCE (1.23% F1-scores bigger than 0.40). For the PRINCE, iteration algorithm would spread information of known nodes to other nodes in the PPI network. If the known nodes were isolated nodes in the PPI network, the information of the known nodes would not spread to other nodes, which would lead to poor prediction performance. But for the heNetRW algorithm, the information of known nodes still could spread to other nodes if there are neighbors (herb nodes or protein nodes) of these nodes in the heterogeneous herb-target network. The prediction results of PRINCE showed 67.30% F1-scores (12.17% for the heNetRW) was zero (Fig. 4b), which also implied heNetRW had a greater robustness than PRINCE. Otherwise, the prediction results also implied that under both the NoTarget and the HalfTarget, the query herbs with more test targets can lead to better

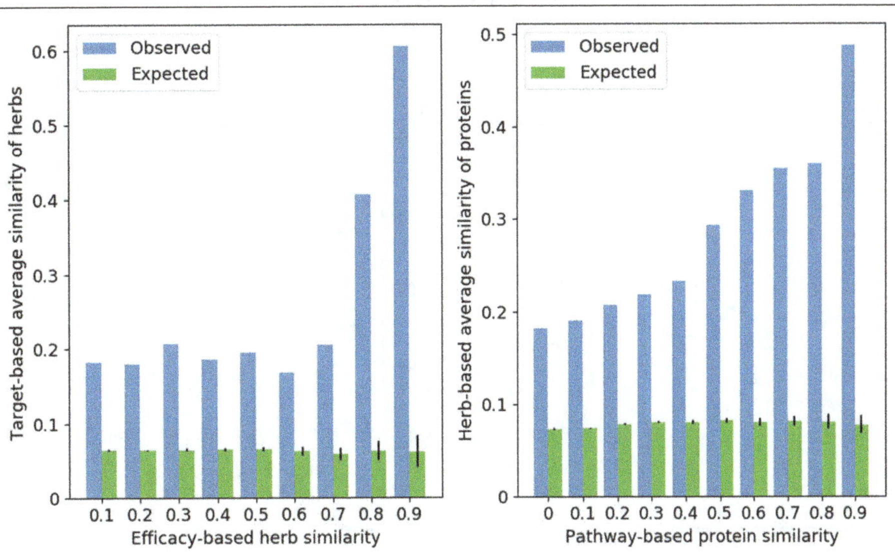

Fig. 3 Overlap analysis of herb pairs and protein pairs. Figure 3**a** Herb pairs with shared efficacies imply shared proteins. The horizontal axis represents efficacy-based similarity bins of herb pairs, and the vertical axis represents target-based average similarity of herb pairs under the corresponding efficacy-based herb similarity bins. The mazarine and green bar represent observed results and expected results of random permutation. Figure 3**b** Protein pairs with shared pathways imply shared targeted herbs. Similarly, the horizontal and vertical axis represent pathway-based similarity of protein pairs and herb-based average similarity of protein pairs under the corresponding bins

Table 2 The performance comparison of different prediction algorithms

Prediction simulation	Algorithm	Number of herbs	F1-score	Hit@1 (%)
NoTarget	PRINCE	260	0.16±0.17	29.23
	heNetRW	261	0.28±0.20	50.57
HalfTarget	PRINCE	896	0.05±0.10	6.70
	heNetRW	896	0.59±0.33	75.78

NoTarget and HalfTarget are two experimental simulations. PRINCE and heNetRW are prediction algorithms. Hit@1 represents the top one hit

performance of PRINCE. But for the heNetRW, more test targets of the query herb had a better performance under the NoTarget, and moderate quantity of test targets may have a better performance under the HalfTarget.

Parameters tuning of heNetRW

The prediction algorithm heNetRW had four parameters need to be tuned: the number α of selected neighbors for each herb in the herb-herb network, the number β of selected neighbors for each protein in the protein-protein network, the probability θ to start a new journey of random walk, and the probability ϕ to jump from the herb layer to the protein layer or vice versa. For NoTarget and HalfTarget simulations, the parameter α and β were tuned at the range from 20 to 100 (scale is 20), and the parameter θ and ϕ were tuned at the range from 0.1 to 0.9 (scale is 0.1) (Fig. 5). When one parameter was tuned, other three parameters remain unchanged. The prediction results indicated the algorithm is not sensitive to the parameters α, β, θ and ϕ under the NoTarget simulation (Fig. 5a and b). And under the HalfTarget simulation, the parameters α and β have little influence on improving prediction performance, small α and large β could make heNetRW have a better prediction performance (Fig. 5c). The parameters θ and ϕ have much influence on prediction performance of heNetRW (Fig. 5d). The larger parameter ϕ can lead to the better prediction performance. When the parameter θ is 0.4, heNetRW had better prediction performance.

Case study

We took prediction results of rhizoma coptidis and turmeric as an example (Table 3). For the NoTarget simulation, all of known targets of the given herb would be regarded as test targets. And half of known targets would be regarded as test targets for the HalfTarget simulation. Under the NoTarget, there were 35 known targets of rhizoma coptidis in the top 64 candidate targets (precision/recall/F1-score = 0.55) (Table 3). Also, we listed the top 20 candidate targets of rhizoma coptidis (Table 4). 16 of top 20 candidate target (precision = 0.80; recall = 0.22) were known targets (the bold targets in the Table 4) of rhizoma coptidis. To fully evaluate the performance of heNetRW, we consulted recent published papers to verify whether recent researches indicated the left 4 targets were associated to rhizoma coptidis. The researches of Han et al. [28] and Huang et al. [29] implied CYP3A4 (rank = 7) and ICAM1 (rank = 18) were related to rhizoma coptidis, respectively. For the turmeric with more test targets (152 known targets as test targets), 81 known targets appeared in the top 152 candidate targets (precision/recall/F1-score = 0.53). The entire top 20 predicted candidate targets (Table 4) were

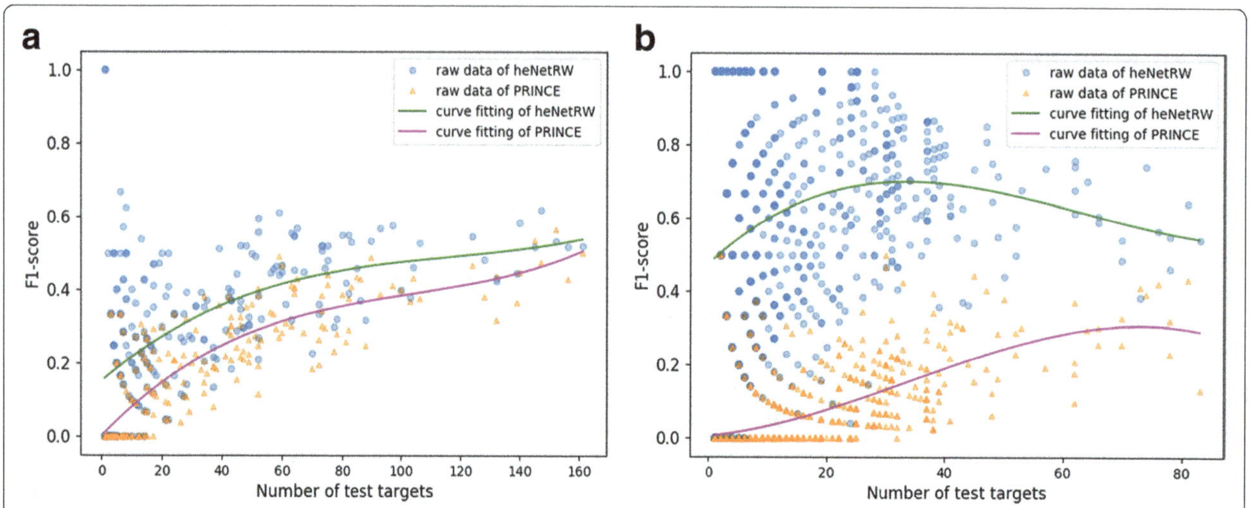

Fig. 4 F1-scores distribution of PRINCE and heNetRW. F1-scores distributions of heNetRW and PRINCE under the NoTarget and HalfTarget situations were showed, respectively (Fig. 4**a** and Fig. 4**b**). The horizontal axis represents number of test targets, and the vertical axis represents F1-scores of herbs with corresponding number of test targets. The circle point and triangle point represent the F1-scores of heNetRW and PRINCE. The green and pink line represent the curve fitting of heNetRW and PRINCE

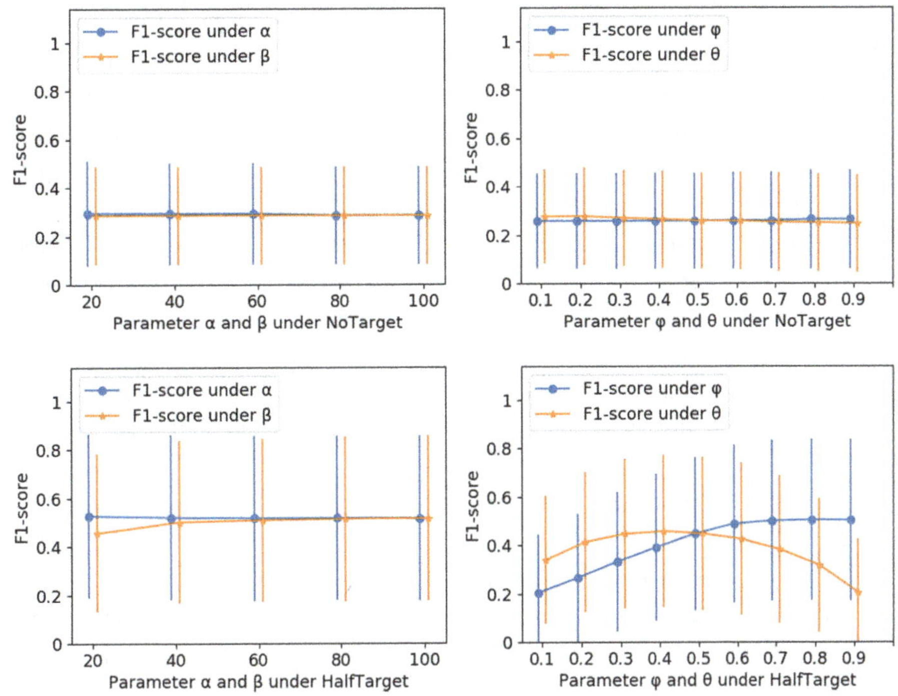

Fig. 5 Parameter tuning of heNetRW. Under NoTarget and HalfTarget simulations, the four heNetRW-related parameters α, β, θ and φ were tuned, and F1-scores (average and standard deviation) of prediction results were showed, respectively, as follows: Fig. 5**a** tuning parameters α and β under the NoTarget; Fig. 5**b** tuning parameters θ and φ under the HalfTarget; Fig. 5**c** tuning parameters α and β under the HalfTarget; Fig. 5**d** tuning parameters θ and φ under the HalfTarget

known targets of turmeric (precision = 1; recall = 0.13). As for the HalfTarget simulation, there were 24 and 43 known targets of rhizoma coptidis (precision/recall/F1-score = 0.75) and turmeric (precision/recall/F1-score = 0.57) in the top 32 and 76 candidate targets, respectively (Table 3). There were 17 known targets and 18 known targets of rhizoma coptidis (precision = 0.85; recall = 0.53) and turmeric (precision = 0.90; recall = 0.24) in the top 20 candidate targets, repectively (Table 5). Li et al. [30] revealed that coptisine reduced the expression of the MMP9 (rank = 16) at the mRNA level. By RT-qPCR and Western blot data, Wang et al. [31] showed that curcumol phosphorylated CDK2 (rank = 12) and CDK4 (rank = 14), which indicated that both of candidate

Table 3 The prediction performance of rhizoma coptidis and turmeric

Simulation	Herb	Number of Train targets	Number of test targets	Number of correct targets	Precision/recall/F1-score
NoTarget	Rhizoma coptidis	0	64	35	0.5469
	Turmeric	0	152	81	0.5329
HalfTarget	Rhizoma coptidis	32	32	24	0.75
	Turmeric	76	76	43	0.5658

PRINCE and heNetRW are algorithms of herb target prediction

targets are related to turmeric. For the left four candidate targets: SOD1 (NoTarget, rank = 8), HMOX1 (NoTarget, rank = 19), AKT1 (HalfTarget, rank = 12), and IL2 (HalfTarget, rank = 17), the average shortest path length (ASPL) and the distribution of shortest path length (SPL) analysis between these candidate targets and known targets of rhizoma coptidis (named KTofRC) were conducted (Fig. 6). Compared with random experiment (ASPL = 3.74±0.86), the ASPL between these candidate targets (SOD1: 2.60; HMOX1: 2.00; AKT1: 1.67; IL2: 1.92) and KTofRC indicated that these targets had strong interaction with KTofRC in the PPI network. The SPLs between these candidate targets and KTofRC were mainly distributed 1 and 2, e. g. for SOD1, HMOX1, AKT1 and IL2, 46.03%, 84.13%, 92.06% and 87.30% of SPLs with smaller than 3 (15.55% of SPLs for the random shuffle), which also implied that there were strong interaction between these targets and KTofRC.

Discussion

In genetic research, as a universal amplifier of genetic associations [32], network propagation methods, e.g. random walk [25], information diffusion [33] and electrical resistance [34], have been applied successfully to identify gene function [35], disease characterization [36], and drug targets [37]. In our study, a random walk algorithm on the heterogeneous herb-target network has been proposed to identify

Table 4 The top 20 candidate targets of rhizome coptidis and turmeric under the NoTarget

Rhizoma coptidis			Turmeric		
Rank	Candidate Target	Score	Rank	Candidate Target	Score
1	**CASP3**	0.4526	1	**CASP3**	0.2750
2	**RELA**	0.4109	2	**RELA**	0.2554
3	**PTGS2**	0.3834	3	**PTGS2**	0.2222
4	**TNF**	0.2988	4	**TNF**	0.1816
5	**NOS2**	0.2771	5	**BCL2**	0.1716
6	**BCL2**	0.2708	6	**NOS2**	0.1624
7	CYP3A4	0.2325	7	**BAX**	0.1403
8	SOD1	0.2132	8	**TP53**	0.1349
9	**BAX**	0.2096	9	**JUN**	0.1318
10	**CASP9**	0.1928	10	**CYP3A4**	0.1230
11	**IL6**	0.1846	11	**SOD1**	0.1182
12	**JUN**	0.1777	12	**FOS**	0.1165
13	**CDKN1A**	0.1701	13	**CASP9**	0.1158
14	**TP53**	0.1701	14	**VEGFA**	0.1141
15	**IL1B**	0.1658	15	**IL6**	0.1111
16	**VEGFA**	0.1612	16	**CDKN1A**	0.1106
17	**FOS**	0.1561	17	**NFKBIA**	0.0992
18	ICAM1	0.1558	18	**IL1B**	0.0926
19	HMOX1	0.1502	19	**MMP9**	0.0873
20	**MAPK1**	0.1358	20	**ICAM1**	0.0872

The bold candidate targets are known targets of given herbs

Table 5 The top 20 candidate targets of rhizome coptidis and turmeric under the HalfTarget

Rhizoma coptidis			Turmeric		
Rank	Candidate Target	Score	Rank	Candidate Target	Score
1	**PTGS2**	0.0311	1	**CASP3**	0.0657
2	**NOS2**	0.0285	2	**TNF**	0.0619
3	**BAX**	0.0259	3	**BCL2**	0.0518
4	**CASP9**	0.0252	4	**JUN**	0.0438
5	**CDKN1A**	0.0238	5	**VEGFA**	0.0424
6	**NFKBIA**	0.0220	6	**BAX**	0.0400
7	**FOS**	0.0212	7	**IL6**	0.0390
8	**CDK2**	0.0203	8	**MMP9**	0.0355
9	**VEGFA**	0.0202	9	**CASP9**	0.0334
10	**IL4**	0.0178	10	**AKT1**	0.0326
11	**BCL2L1**	0.0160	11	**CCND1**	0.0302
12	AKT1	0.0146	12	CDK2	0.0296
13	**HERC5**	0.0143	13	**MAPK1**	0.0282
14	**CDC2**	0.0135	14	CDK4	0.0269
15	**EIF6**	0.0132	15	**XDH**	0.0245
16	MMP9	0.0130	16	**SOD1**	0.0241
17	IL2	0.0126	17	**PRKCB**	0.0233
18	**MPO**	0.0121	18	**CYP3A4**	0.0213
19	**EGFR**	0.0120	19	**VCAM1**	0.0211
20	**HIF1A**	0.0118	20	**MYC**	0.0202

The bold candidate targets are known targets of given herbs

candidate targets for herbs. By building a heterogeneous herb-target network and simulating random walk on the network, the candidate targets of given herbs can be predicted. In the experiment stage, the NoTarget and HalfTarget situations were simulated to validate prediction performance of heNetRW. The final results indicated that heNetRW had better prediction performance than PRINCE.

There are two advantages of heNetRW algorithm. The algorithm PRINCE simulated random walk on the PPI network, and the initial nodes are known proteins of the herbs that are relevant to query herb. Nevertheless, for the heNetRW, random walk was simulated on the heterogeneous herb-target network, the initial nodes are targets that are relevant to known targets of the query herb and herbs that are relevant to the query herb. So with respect to PRINCE considering herb similarities and PPI associations, heNetRW considered more known information including known herb-target associations and pathway-based protein similarities. Experimental results also indicated more known information could make heNetRW have better prediction performance. Otherwise, by tuning parameters of heNetRW algorithm, we effectively controlled the trend of random walk to improve prediction performance. The prediction results can be used to guide the selection of candidate targets of herbs that have not been studied at present or find new protein targets of common herbs, which would help to reveal molecular mechanism of herbal drugs and improve treatment of complex diseases.

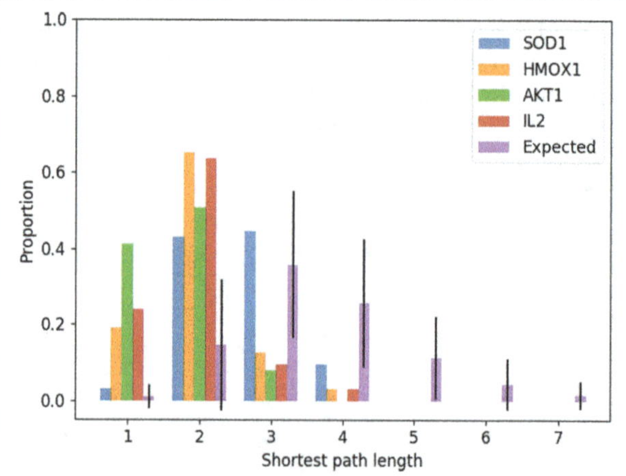

Fig. 6 Shortest path analysis of candidate targets of rhizoma coptidis. The horizontal axis represents shortest path length, and the vertical axis represents proportion of SPLs

In recent years, network embedding representation methods, e.g. deepwalk [38], LINE [39] and node2vec [40], have been widely applied to network classification [41] and link prediction [40]. By learning continue feature representations for nodes in networks, the node2vec algorithm can obtain a mapping of nodes to a low-dimensional space of features [40], which can be used to measure accurate similarity of nodes. In our study, the similarities of herb pairs and target pairs are based on efficacy-based and pathway-based cosine similarities, which only considered unilateral similarity of herb pairs or target pairs. In the future, by building heterogeneous herb-related (e.g. efficacies, indications and ingredients) network and target-related (e.g. pathways, GO terms and interactions) network, we will apply network embedding algorithm to obtain multi-dimensional similarity measure of herb pairs or target pairs. Otherwise, Under the NoTarget simulation, since initial nodes only contain herb nodes, not target nodes, the prediction performance of heNetRW was not well. To address the issue, known targets of herbs that are relevant to the query herb will be added to the set of initial nodes in the future.

Conclusions

Herb target identification is a critical step for revealing pharmacological mechanisms of herbal drugs and improving clinical treatment of diseases in TCM. In this study, we developed a heterogeneous network propagation method to identify herb targets. Based on two validation settings, our method was compared with the baseline method PRINCE. The experimental results indicated that our method had higher performance than PRINCE. We manually evaluated several candidate targets of two herbs, which is not in benchmark dataset, but have been confirmed by recent published papers. Therefore, the prediction results not only can be used to guide the selection of herbal candidate targets in wet lab, but also help to reveal molecule mechanisms of herbs.

Additional files

Additional file 1: – HIT_herb_target.xls. 23,453 herb-target associations between 1016 herbs and 1214 targets were collected and integrated from the HIT database. (XLS 1200 kb)

Additional file 2: – CHPA_herb_efficacy.xls. 3487 herb-efficacy associations between 742 herbs and 360 efficacies were collected from the Chinese pharmacopoeia (CHPA, 2015 edition). (XLS 200 kb)

Additional file 3: – KEGG_protein_pathway.xls. 16,162 protein-pathway associations between 4794 proteins and 244 pathways were collected from KEGG database. (XLS 896 kb)

Abbreviations

ASPL: average shortest path length; CHPA: Chinese pharmacopoeia; GO: gene ontology; HeNetRW: random walk method on heterogeneous herb-target network for herb target prediction; Hit@1: the top one hit; KTofRC: known targets of rhizome coptidis; LOOCV: leave one out cross validation; NoTarget and HalfTarget: validation settings for prediction algorithms; PPI: protein-protein interaction; SPL: shortest path length

Acknowledgements

Not applicable.

Funding

Publication of this article is supported by the Fundamental Research Funds for the Central Universities (K17JB00100, K17JB00230), the National Key Research and Development Program (2017YFC1703506), the National Science Foundation of China (61105055, 81230086), the Special Programs of Traditional Chinese Medicine (201407001, JDZX2015171), and the National Key Technology R&D Program (2013BAI02B01 and 2013BAI13B04).

Authors' contributions

Xuezhong Zhou and Jianxin Chen took charge of the entire research work. Kuo Yang conducted all of experiments, analyzed related data, and drafted the manuscript; Guangming Liu and Ning Wang were involved in collecting and analyzing data; Runshun Zhang and Jian Yu reviewed the methods and results and revised the manuscript. All authors read and approved the final manuscript.

Competing interests

The authors declare that they have no competing interests.

Author details

[1]School of Computer and Information Technology and Beijing Key Lab of Traffic Data Analysis and Mining, Beijing Jiaotong University, Beijing 100044, China. [2]Guanganmen Hospital, China Academy of Chinese Medical Sciences, Beijing 100053, China. [3]Beijing University of Chinese Medicine, Beijing 100029, China. [4]Data Center of Traditional Chinese Medicine, China Academy of Chinese Medical Sciences, Beijing 100700, China.

References

1. Li S. Network systems underlying traditional Chinese medicine syndrome and herb formula. Curr Bioinforma. 2009;4(3):188–96.
2. Li S, Fan TP, Jia W, Lu A, Zhang W. Network pharmacology in traditional Chinese medicine. Evid Based Complement Alternat Med. 2014;2014(1):138460.
3. Yang K, Zhou X, Zhang R, Liu B, Lei L, Zhang X, et al., Editors. Integrating herb effect similarity for network-based herb target prediction. International conference on biomedical engineering and informatics; 2016.
4. Yu J, Peng Y, Wu LC, Xie Z, Deng Y, Hughes T, et al. Curcumin down-regulates DNA methyltransferase 1 and plays an anti-leukemic role in acute myeloid leukemia. PLoS One. 2013;8(2):e55934.
5. Li S. Exploring traditional chinese medicine by a novel therapeutic concept of network target. Chinese Journal of Integrative Medicine. 2016;22(9):647–52.
6. Yang K, Zhang R, He L, et al. Multistage analysis method for detection of effective herb prescription from clinical data. Frontiers of Medicine. 2017;7:1–12.
7. Hopkins AL. Network pharmacology: the next paradigm in drug discovery. Nat Chem Biol. 2008;4(11):682.
8. Knox C, Law V, Jewison T, Liu P, Ly S, Frolkis A, et al. DrugBank 3.0: a comprehensive resource for 'omics' research on drugs. Nucleic Acids Res. 2011;39(Database issue):D1035.
9. Kuhn M, Von MC, Campillos M, Jensen LJ, Bork P. STITCH: interaction networks of chemicals and proteins. Nucleic Acids Res. 2008;36(Database issue):684–8.
10. Hamosh A, Scott AF, Amberger J, Bocchini C, Valle D, Mckusick VA. Online Mendelian inheritance in man (OMIM), a knowledgebase of human genes and genetic disorders. Nucleic Acids Res. 2005;33(1):514–7.
11. Kibbe WA, Arze C, Felix V, Mitraka E, Bolton E, Fu G, et al. Disease ontology 2015 update: an expanded and updated database of human diseases for linking biomedical knowledge through disease data. Nucleic Acids Res. 2015;43(Database issue):D1071.
12. Szklarczyk D, Franceschini A, Wyder S, Forslund K, Heller D, Huerta-Cepas J, et al. STRING v10: protein-protein interaction networks, integrated over the

tree of life. Nucleic Acids Res. 2015;43(Database issue):D447.
13. Zhou X, Menche J, Sharma A. Human symptoms-disease network. Nat Commun. 2014;5:4212.
14. Shiwen Zhao SL. Network-based relating pharmacological and genomic spaces for drug target identification. PLoS One. 2010;5(7):e11764.
15. Vanunu O, Magger O, Ruppin E, Shlomi T, Sharan R. Associating genes and protein complexes with disease via network propagation. PLoS Comput Biol. 2010;6(1):e1000641.
16. Rui J. Walking on multiple disease-gene networks to prioritize candidate genes. J Mol Cell Biol. 2015;7(3):214.
17. Le DH, Dang VT. Ontology-based disease similarity network for disease gene prediction. Vietnam. J Comput Sci. 2016;3(3):1–9.
18. Ye H, Ye L, Kang H, Zhang D, Tao L, Tang K, et al. HIT: linking herbal active ingredients to targets. Nucleic Acids Res. 2011;39(Database issue):D1055.
19. Xue R, Fang Z, Zhang M, Yi Z, Wen C, Shi T. TCMID: traditional Chinese medicine integrative database for herb molecular mechanism analysis. Nucleic Acids Res. 2013;41(Database issue):D1089.
20. Gao L, Wang X, Niu Y, Duan D, Yang X, Hao J, et al. Molecular targets of Chinese herbs: a clinical study of hepatoma based on network pharmacology. Sci Rep. 2016;6:24944.
21. Wang XJ, Zhang AH, Zhou XH. Liu Q, et al. An integrated chinmedomics strategy for discovery of effective constituents from traditional herbal medicine. Sci Rep. 2016;6:18997.
22. Zhang HP, Pan JB, Chi Z, Nan J, Hao W, Ji ZL. Network understanding of herb medicine via rapid identification of ingredient-target interactions. Sci Rep. 2014;4(1):3719.
23. X L, H L, S L. A novel network pharmacology approach to analyse traditional herbal formulae: the Liu-Wei-di-Huang pill as a case study. Mol BioSyst. 2014;10(5):1014.
24. Peng Z, Li J, Li Y, Tian Y, Wang Y, Zheng C. Systems pharmacology-based approach for dissecting the active ingredients and potential targets of the Chinese herbal Bufei Jianpi formula for the treatment of COPD. International Journal of Chronic Obstructive Pulmonary Disease. 2015;10(1):2633–56.
25. Tong H, Faloutsos C, Pan JY. Random walk with restart: fast solutions and applications. Knowl Inf Syst. 2008;14(3):327–46.
26. Kanehisa M, Goto S, Hattori M, Aokikinoshita KF, Itoh M, Kawashima S, et al. From genomics to chemical genomics: new developments in KEGG. Nucleic Acids Res. 2006;34(Database issue):354–7.
27. Snedecor GW. Statistical tables for biological, agricultural and medical research. By R. A. Fisher; F. Yates. Canadian Journal of Comparative Medicine & Veterinary Science. 1943;22(1):8.
28. Han YL, Yu HL, Li D, Meng XL, Zhou ZY, Yu Q, et al. In vitro inhibition of Huanglian [Rhizoma coptidis (L.)] and its six active alkaloids on six cytochrome P450 isoforms in human liver microsomes. Phytotherapy Research Ptr. 2011;25(11):1660–5.
29. Huang Z, Cai X, Li S, Zhou H, Chu M, Shan P, et al. Berberine-attenuated monocyte adhesion to endothelial cells induced by oxidized low-density lipoprotein via inhibition of adhesion molecule expression. Mol Med Rep. 2013;7(2):461–5.
30. Li J, Qiu DM, Chen SH, Cao SP, Xia XL. Suppression of human breast cancer cell metastasis by coptisine in vitro. Asian Pacific Journal of Cancer Prevention Apjcp. 2014;15(14):5747–51.
31. Wang J, Li XM, Bai Z, et al. Curcumol Induces Cell Cycle Arrest in Colon Cancer Cells via Reactive Oxygen Species and Akt/ GSK3β/cyclin D1 Pathway. J Ethnopharmacol. 2017;210:1.
32. Cowen L, Ideker T, Raphael BJ, et al. Network propagation: a universal amplifier of genetic associations. Nature Reviews Genetics. 2017;18(9):551.
33. Ben-Avraham D, Havlin S. Diffusion and reactions in fractals and disordered systems. Cambridge: University Press; 2000.
34. Doyle PG, Snell JL. Random Walks and Electric Networks. Mathematical Association of America. 1984;22(2):595–9.
35. Sharan R, Ulitsky I, Network-based SR. Prediction of protein function. Mol Syst Biol. 2007;3(1):88.
36. Cho DY, Kim YA, Przytycka TM. Chapter 5: network biology approach to complex diseases. PLoS Comput Biol. 2012;8(12):e1002820.
37. Csermely P, Korcsmáros T, Kiss HJ, London G, Nussinov R. Structure and dynamics of molecular networks: a novel paradigm of drug discovery: a comprehensive review. Pharmacol Ther. 2012;138(3):333–408.
38. PPerozzi B, Al-Rfou R, Skiena S. DeepWalk: online learning of social representations. Proceedings of the 20th ACM SIGKDD international conference on knowledge discovery and data mining. ACM. 2014:701–10.
39. Tang J, Qu M, Wang M, Zhang M, Yan J, and Mei Q. LINE: Large-scale information network embedding. Proceedings of the 24th International Conference on World Wide Web. ACM. 2015:1067–77.
40. Grover A, Leskovec J. node2vec: scalable feature learning for networks. Proceedings of the 22nd ACM SIGKDD international conference on knowledge discovery and data mining. ACM. 2016:855–64.
41. Li J, Zhu J, Zhang B. Discriminative deep random walk for network classification. Meeting of the Association for Computational Linguistics. 2016:1004–13.

7

Towards improving diagnosis of skin diseases by combining deep neural network and human knowledge

Xinyuan Zhang[1], Shiqi Wang[2], Jie Liu[2*] and Cui Tao[1*]

Abstract

Background: The emergence of the deep convolutional neural network (CNN) greatly improves the quality of computer-aided supporting systems. However, due to the challenges of generating reliable and timely results, clinical adoption of computer-aided diagnosis systems is still limited. Recent informatics research indicates that machine learning algorithms need to be combined with sufficient clinical expertise in order to achieve an optimal result.

Methods: In this research, we used deep learning algorithms to help diagnose four common cutaneous diseases based on dermoscopic images. In order to facilitate decision-making and improve the accuracy of our algorithm, we summarized classification/diagnosis scenarios based on domain expert knowledge and semantically represented them in a hierarchical structure.

Results: Our algorithm achieved an accuracy of 87.25 ± 2.24% in our test dataset with 1067 images. The semantic summarization of diagnosis scenarios can help further improve the algorithm to facilitate future computer-aided decision support.

Conclusions: In this paper, we applied deep neural network algorithm to classify dermoscopic images of four common skin diseases and archived promising results. Based on the results, we further summarized the diagnosis/classification scenarios, which reflect the importance of combining the efforts of both human expertise and computer algorithms in dermatologic diagnoses.

Keywords: Deep learning, Semantic data analytics, Image classification, Dermatology

Background

In biomedical informatics field, research has been done on using image-based artificial intelligence diagnosis system to help early detection of certain diseases, especially skin diseases [1, 2]. For pattern recognition and classification of clinical image, deep neural networks have been widely used. A recently published article in Nature provided an example for using a convolutional neural network (CNN) to disaggregate 2032 different kinds of skin diseases and tested its performance against 21 board-certified dermatologists [2]. The CNN performed on par with the experts, proving the feasibility of computer-aided diagnosis system. In the healthcare field, this system can potentially help healthcare providers make more effective diagnoses as a clinical decision support tool. There are multiple types of deep neural networks, including convolutional and recursive neural networks (CNN and RNN), etc. Some studies used deep neural networks to develop and modify image classification techniques [3–7]. Many previous studies showed promising results for both the reliability and accuracy of computer-aided decision support [8–10]. A subset of published articles examined the combination of human

* Correspondence: liujie04672@pumch.cn; cui.tao@uth.tmc.edu
[2]Department of Dermatology, Peking Union Medical College Hospital, Chinese Academy of Medical Sciences and Peking Union Medical College, Beijing, China
[1]School of Biomedical Informatics, The University of Texas Health Science Center at Houston, Huston, TX, USA

expertise and artificial intelligence [11, 12]. Nevertheless, we still need to better integrate human knowledge into artificial intelligence and to use artificial intelligence to extend human intelligence.

In our previous study, we classified four common cutaneous diseases based on dermoscopic images using deep learning algorithms [13]. This paper extended it by summarizing classification/diagnosis scenarios and semantically represented them in a hierarchical structure in hope to further facilitate decision-making and improve the accuracy of our algorithm. Four frequently seen skin diseases were selected for the study, melanocytic nevus, seborrheic keratosis (SK), basal cell carcinoma (BCC) and psoriasis. Melanocytic nevus is a very common benign cutaneous tumor. It can occur from infancy to old age, and the amount each person usually carries increases with age [14]. Seborrheic keratosis (SK), also known as basal cell papilloma, is due to the delayed maturation of benign epidermal cells. Melanocytic nevus and basal cell carcinoma both have deeper lesions, which must be accurately distinguished [15]. Basal cell carcinomas (BCC) is one of the most common human skin cancers, especially in the elderly. According to epidemiological studies, the incidence of BCC is increasing year by year, and the incidence in young people shows a gradual upward trend [16]. Psoriasis is a common and readily recurrent chronic inflammatory skin disease. Worldwide, the prevalence of psoriasis is 2–4%. It has a significant impact on the patient's health and even mental health [17]. Therefore, psoriasis is always one of the foci of dermatological research.

These four cutaneous diseases: basal cell carcinoma (BCC), melanocytic nevus, seborrheic keratosis (SK), and psoriasis, are epidermal malignant, melanocytic benign, epidermal benign, and non-neoplastic skin diseases respectively. It is noteworthy that the treatment of these four diseases is very different. If the diagnosis is incorrect or the diagnosis is delayed, it may lead to improper treatment, treatment delay, even no treatment [18]. Therefore, it is critical that the providers can make accurate diagnosis in time. If the artificial intelligence system can be used to automatically classify these four diseases, providers can benefit patients by diagnosing them more efficiently and accurately.

Methods

Dataset

The data used in this study originated from the dermatology department of Peking Union Medical College Hospital. The clinical database currently contains more than 28,000 dermoscopic images examined by MoleMax HD 1.0 dermoscopic devices. Our study was approved by the Ethics Committee of Institute of Peking Union Medical College Hospital, Chinese Academy of Medical Sciences. Informed consent was obtained from all participants.

Our experiment was developed based on a gold standard, where each image was rigorously reviewed by at least two experienced dermatologists before the diagnosis results were given. Figure 1 shows the annotation process. Figure 2 shows some examples of typical dermoscopic images. First, each dermoscopic image was reviewed by at least two experienced dermatologists. If consensus was reached, the resulting diagnosis was annotated. If not, a third dermatologist was consulted. If consensus was reached after discussion, the annotation reflected the agreed upon diagnosis. If not, the image was taken to the histopathological biopsy examination. In the end, each image was labeled with a disease name. As we have seen, this is a very time consuming and expensive process.

Training image selection

All together, our experiment dataset contains 1067 images from patients who visited the clinic between 2015 and 2017 with images of 418 melanocytic nevus, 291 seborrheic keratosis, 132 basal cell carcinoma, and 226 psoriasis dermoscopic, respectively. We used two datasets in the experiment. Dataset A consists all the images. Dataset B was a selected, evenly distributed dataset. 132 images were selected from each disease category, for a total of 528 images. Details are listed in Table 1.

Deep learning algorithm

We developed our algorithm based on GoogleNet Inception v3 code package which was pre-trained on over 1.28 million images [19]. We adjusted the final layer and used our datasets as input. The GoogleNet deep learning framework is a type of artificial neural network called CNN. It is inspired by a biological process called axonal transport or synaptic transmission, in which multiple neurons receiving signals partially overlap and cover the entire field [20]. CNNs have similar functions, where the calculated features are combined with each other. The simplified framework of the entire process is shown in Fig. 3. CNN is often used in real life for image or video recognition and natural language processing [21–23].

Each pixel in the input images was transformed into an element in matrices. For example, if an image has 864 pixels, multiplied by RGB layers, the number of elements in a matrix would be 2592. If there are 100 input images, the input matrix will have the dimension of 2592 * 100. This is also called the "Input Layer". Each image then went through the feature extraction process, during which the combination of convolutional and pooling layers was used. A feature map was obtained by applying a linear filter and a non-linear function to the input matrix. For example, the hidden layer A^k, where k is the kth feature map. The filters here consisted of its

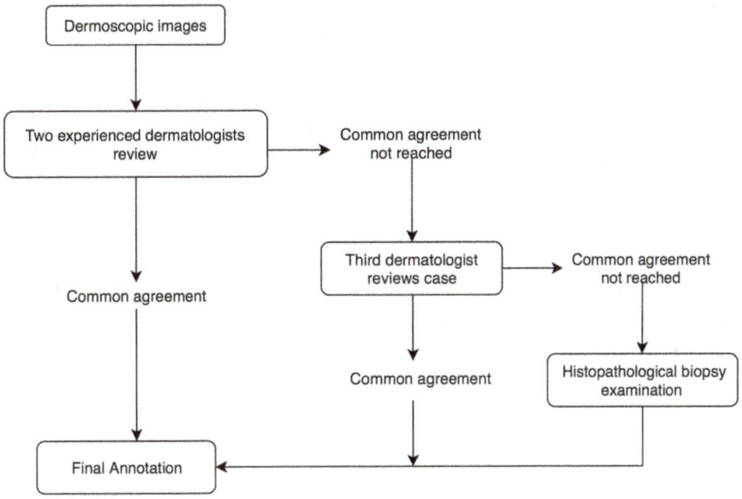

Fig. 1 Procedure for annotating the dermoscopic image

weight W^k and its bias b_k . The feature map A^k was calculated using Eq. 1 [24]. Then the calculated feature map from extraction was classified. Each hidden layer was composed of multiple feature maps. There are multiple hidden layers used in the model.

$$A_{ij}^{k} = \tanh\left(\left(W^k \cdot x\right)_{ij} + b_k\right) \quad (1)$$

The input layer is analogous to the receptive field of nerve cells. The hidden layer functions similarly to transmission down the axon, where the input signals are being processed. The terminal zone can be regarded as both the output layer and the receptive zone for the next cell, which is similar to the Inception 3 algorithm [19]. Data flows from left to the right. However, there is one difference between an artificial neural network and a biological one. Researchers developed backward error propagation to help tune the input activation functions, in which way the final layer of CNN was adjusted.

We ran the experiments using datasets A and B separately. Each data set was divided into training, validation and testing sets, in 8:1:1 ratio respectively. The prediction values were compared with the actual labels to update the final layer's weights W^k [19], as shown in Eq. 1. The validation set was separated from the training set to avoid over-fitting [25]. The calculated parameters from the training set were examined using the validation set to see whether they fit as well, and recalculated as needed. This process can help the model to memorize less of the irrelevant or unimportant details of the training images. A hold-out testing set was used to evaluate the accuracy of the whole process. Each image appears only once in each set.

The classification results by the algorithm can be used for diagnoses. Each test image was given a probability for each of the four disease categories, summing to 1. The highest probability was regarded as the classification category. Healthcare providers will also be able to receive more detailed information, in addition to just one

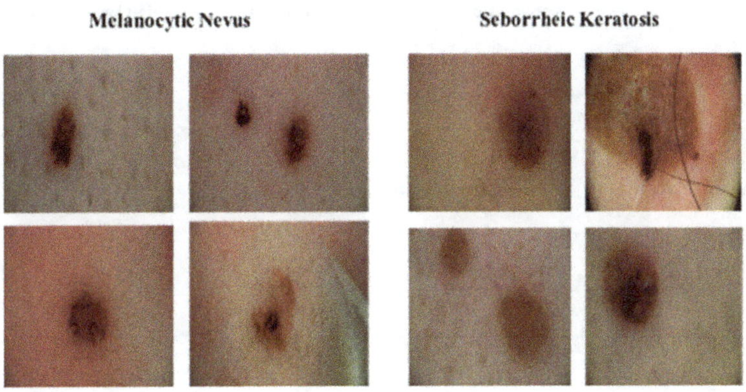

Fig. 2 Example of typical dermoscopic images

Table 1 Summary for datasets

Dataset A		Dataset B	
melanocytic nevus	418	melanocytic nevus	132
seborrheic keratosis (SK)	291	seborrheic keratosis (SK)	132
basal cell carcinoma (BCC)	132	basal cell carcinoma (BCC)	132
psoriasis	226	Psoriasis	132
Total number of images	1067	Total number of images	528

end result. These possibilities of the disease classifications can potentially be used to better perform semantic error analysis.

Evaluation and semantic error analysis

We also conducted an error analysis on misclassified images using dataset B. In order to get enough data for systematic analysis and remain the uniqueness of testing set, we used ten-fold cross validation to repeat the algorithms ten times. The summarized report of all the misclassified dermoscopic images for dataset B was then reviewed by domain experts (SW and JL). A thorough analysis was then conducted based on which a semantic classification of the misclassified images was generated.

Results

Results for deep learning algorithm

To avoid random errors, we repeated the experiment procedure ten times to obtain data for validation. All the experiments are evaluated on different testing sets. The average accuracy and standard deviation for ten results are shown in Table 2 for datasets A and B.

To further evaluate this method, we also calculated precision, recall, and F1 score for each disease (Tables 3 and 4). In order to prevent potential bias from uneven distribution of four diseases, we used a balanced distribution, which is data set B. The formulas were as follows.

$$Precision = \frac{true\ positive}{true\ positive + false\ positive} \tag{2}$$

$$\text{Recall} = \frac{true\ positive}{true\ positive + false\ negative} \tag{3}$$

$$F\text{-}measure = 2 \cdot \frac{precision \cdot recall}{precision + recall} \tag{4}$$

Categories for misclassified images

We then conducted an error analysis to summarize the reasons why certain images were misclassified by our algorithm. Two dermatologists and two informaticians reviewed these images and suggested possible causes for misclassifications. All the scenarios are summarized and represented using a hierarchical structure in Fig. 4. Figure 5 shows some examples of the misclassified cases.

As Fig. 4 shows, we have identified 4 major categories of possible error causes: "Characteristics of Disease", "Multiple Diseases", "Interference Factor" and "Accuracy of Algorithm".

Under the category "Characteristics of Disease", we further classified three subclasses: "Similar Characteristics", "Atypical Characteristics" and "Special Type". The category "Similar Characteristics" was defined to describe those errors caused by images that belong to different diseases but share similar features. These similar features could have affected the performance of the CNN classifier. The category "Atypical Characteristics" refers to those images that do not have typical features of the corresponding disease. For example, Fig. 5a is a regression lesion of

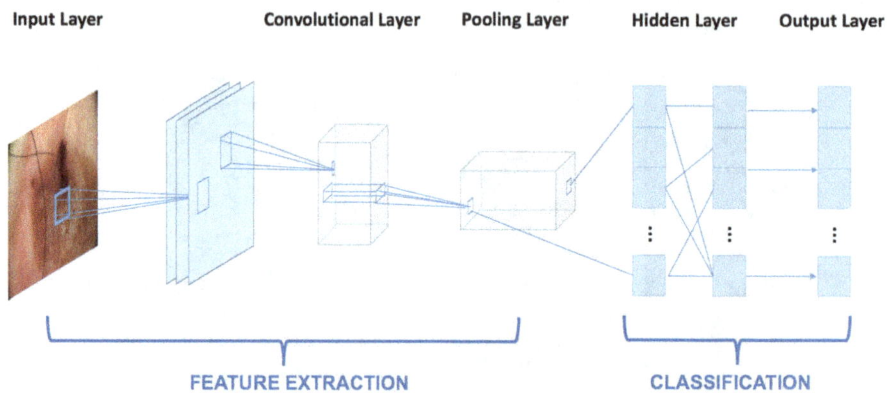

Fig. 3 A Simplified framework for deep neural networks

Table 2 Summary for accuracy and standard deviation

	Avg. Accuracy	Standard deviation
Dataset A	87.25%	2.24%
Dataset B	86.63%	5.78%

psoriasis vulgaris. The typical features of the disease such as dotted blood vessels were significantly reduced, leaving only inflammation. Therefore, the misclassification belongs to "Atypical Characteristic". The category "Special Type" defines the images that have abnormal features that usually do not appear in the corresponding disease. Figure 5b shows an example. This image was annotated as BCC but misclassified as melanocytic nevus. The image contains a large blue-gray oval nest and a leaf-like structure, but no branched blood vessels [17]. This case has many pigmented areas which covered most of the lesion. That may have been the cause of misdiagnosis.

The category "Multiple Diseases" refers to those misclassified images that contain lesions belonging to more than one disease. Image in Fig. 5c indicates both SK and BCC diseases and was classified by the algorithm to SK, but BCC lesions can also be seen in the image. The misclassification may be due to the fact that the pigmentation of SK is more obvious. In a subsequent study, we can preprocess the image to detect and separate multiple diseases.

"Hair/Line", "Air Bubbles/ Dermoscopic Gel" and "Brightness Unbalanced" are all the misclassified causes under the "Interference Factor" category. These factors would interfere with our algorithm when identifying the critical attributes during classification. The image in Fig. 5d is psoriasis, but misclassified to SK. The image does contain the dermoscopic findings of the corresponding disease, but there is an interference factor, hair. Human eyes can usually avoid the interference factor without losing the features of the lesion, but CNN considers hair as a key factor for classification.

Our algorithm itself can be improved. There are some images that couldn't be classified under any of the category above after reviewed by domain expert. Therefore, a category called "Accuracy of Algorithm" was added.

Table 3 Summary for Precision and Recall (Dataset B)

	BCC	melanocytic nevus	Psoriasis	SK
Precision	88.24%	89.06%	88.55%	79.07%
Recall	87.5%	88.37%	88.55%	80.31%
F-Measure	0.879	0.887	0.885	0.797

Table 4 Summary for classified Images (Dataset B)

Original annotation	Classified diseases			
	BCC	Melanocytic nevus	Psoriasis	SK
BCC	105	4	4	6
melanocytic nevus	4	114	1	9
Psoriasis	2	3	116	10
SK	9	8	10	102

Discussion

From Table 2, we can see that the average accuracy results are 87.25% for dataset A and 86.63% for dataset B. Since we only used a small portion of the images to train the algorithm, we believe our method is very promising. In addition, we can see that the results of dataset A and dataset B are not significantly different, so as a result, the deep learning algorithm can deal well with the unbalanced dataset. Moreover, the standard deviation of our results is about 2–5%, which can reflect the variation of accuracy. The relatively small number of images may be the reason.

The precision, recall, and f-measure values of SK are the lowest, while the other three diseases are all more than 87% on these measures (Table 3). As Table 4 shows, only 79.5% of the SK images were correctly classified. BCC with SK (15 images were misclassified) and melanocytic nevi with SK (17 images were misclassified) were often confused with each other. Previous studies also reported that they do have similar characteristics [26].

The categories of misclassification can facilitate future development of the system and help us to decide how to best incorporate human expertise. For some cases that our algorithm misclassified, it could be relatively easy for a human expert to make the right judgment. For example, for images with interference factors such as hair or air bubbles blocking the texture of skin lesions, human experts can often ignore the interfering factors and focus on the whole pattern, while a machine algorithm could accidently take those irrelevant factors as part of the features in training. There are techniques that can eliminate the hair factors automatically [27–29]. Nonetheless, the noise caused by the elimination process could generate more problems during automatic classification. Following the misclassification category, when an input picture was determined by the system under hair blocking category, we could attach it with semantic labels, such as the shape or edge of the lesions from the dermatologists to help with the classification.

Dermatologists will usually make a diagnosis based on more information than just the images themselves. For example, BCC occurs more commonly in elderly people [17], and high sun exposure can increase the risk of BCC in exposed body parts [30]. The occurrence of

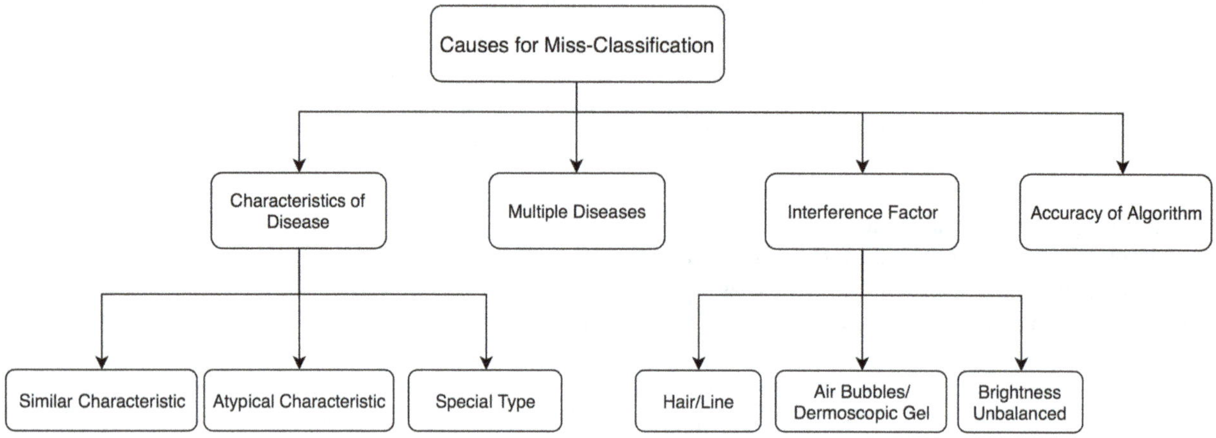

Fig. 4 Knowledge Representation Tree for decision making

psoriasis has two peaks, one at age 20 to 30 and the second at age 50 to 60. In addition, it was more commonly seen in non-Hispanic whites [18]. These kind of prior knowledge need to be embedded in the algorithms in the form of semantic labels with additional patients' data from EHR. These semantic features will incorporate more human knowledge to improve the accuracy of algorithm.

Our overarching goal is to develop a decision support system that can incorporate human knowledge into the process of artificial intelligence and then to use artificial intelligence to extend human capabilities. Our immediate next step is to improve our system by preprocessing the images and adding more semantic features. These improvements will be designed based on our defined semantic categories in Fig. 4. For example, we can modify the feature extraction computer algorithm to consider the atypical characteristics. If there were interference factor, we could attach the semantic labels as described before. Since we know the multiple diseases could be the reason for misclassification, preprocessing images to separate different lesions will be included in the model.

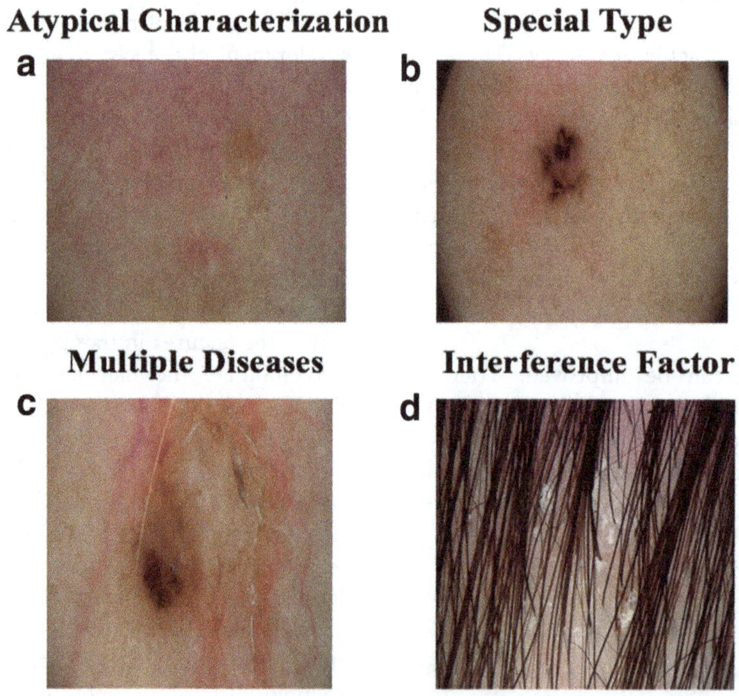

Fig. 5 Examples of misclassified images under categories of possible error causes: **a** "Atypical Characterizatioin", **b** "Special Type", **c** "Multiple Diseases" and **d** "Interference Factor"

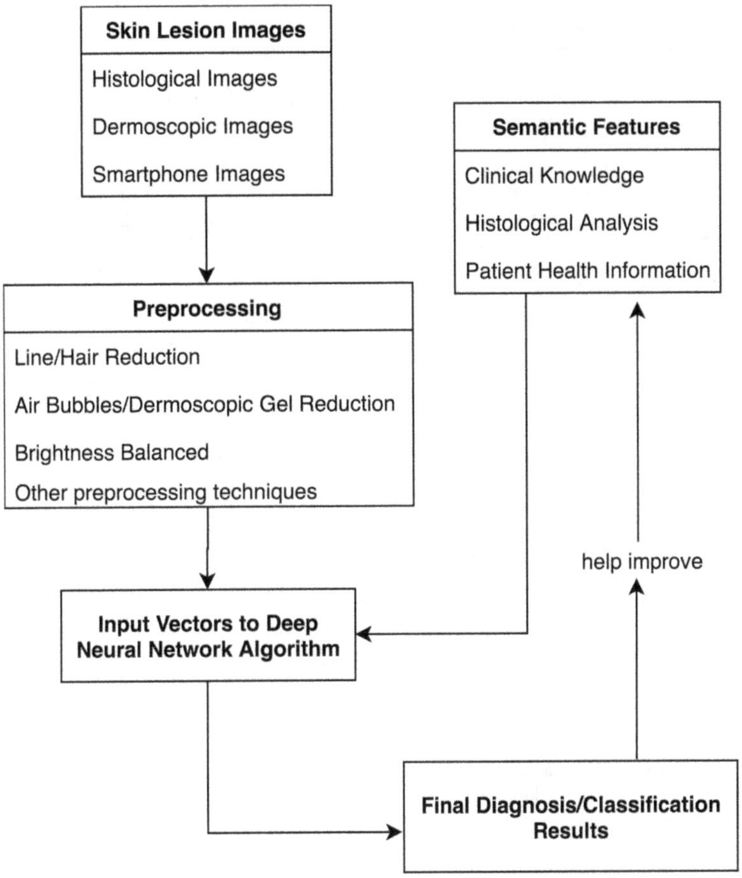

Fig. 6 Human intelligence joint with computer aided system

In addition, we will expand our dataset to test whether a larger dataset would result in better performance. We also plan to include more diseases and more types of images, such as histological images, smartphone images, etc. The ultimate goal is to deliver a decision support system to help clinicians make better diagnostic decisions and also create a patient-usable system which anyone can use with their mobile apps.

Conclusion

In this paper, we applied deep neural network algorithm to classify dermoscopic images of four common skin diseases. Dataset A (1067 images) has the accuracy of 87.25 ± 2.24% and dataset B (528 graphs distributed equally) has the accuracy of 86.63% ± 5.78%, which is promising.

A team of informaticians and dermatologists conducted a result analysis, especially for the misclassified images. Based on the result, we generated a hierarchical semantic structure (Fig. 6) to represent classification/diagnosis scenarios to further improve the algorithm to facilitate computer-aided decision support.

In a subsequent study, we would like to explore the method of integrating more human knowledge into our algorithm based on the result analysis. We will also make the system more extensive and scalable by handling larger datasets and more diseases and image types.

Abbreviations

BCC: Basal cell carcinoma; CNN: Convolutional Neural Network; SK: Seborrheic keratosis

Funding

The research was partially supported by the National Library of Medicine and National Institute of Allergy and Infectious Diseases of the National Institutes of Health under Award Number R01LM011829. Publication of this article was also supported by this grant.

Authors' contributions

Study concept: CT, JL, SW and XZ. Acquisition of data: SW and JL. Development of model: XZ. Analysis of data: XZ, SW and JL. Interpretation of results: all authors. Drafting the manuscript: XZ. Critical revision: all authors. All the authors read and approved the final version of the manuscript.

Competing interests

The authors declare that they have no competing interests.

References

1. Masood A, Ali Al-Jumaily A. Computer aided diagnostic support system for skin cancer: a review of techniques and algorithms. Int J Biomed Imaging. 2013;2013
2. Esteva A, Kuprel B, Novoa RA, Ko J, Swetter SM, Blau HM, Thrun S. Dermatologist-level classification of skin cancer with deep neural networks. Nature. 2017;542(7639):115–8.
3. Krizhevsky A, Sutskever I, Hinton GE. Imagenet classification with deep convolutional neural networks. Adv Neural Inf Process Syst. 2012;25:1097–105.
4. Ioffe S, Szegedy C. Batch normalization: accelerating deep network training by reducing internal covariate shift. Proc. 32nd. Int Conference on Machine Learning. 2015:448–56.
5. Szegedy C, et al. Going deeper with convolutions. Proc IEEE Conference on Computer Vision and Pattern Recognition. 2015:1–9.
6. Ramlakhan K, Shang Y. A mobile automated skin lesion classification system. 23rd IEEE International Conference on Tools with Artificial Intelligence (ICTAI). 2011:138–41.
7. He K, Zhang X, Ren S, Sun J. Deep residual learning for image recognition. In: Proceedings of the IEEE conference on computer vision and pattern recognition (pp. 770–778); 2016.
8. Rosado, B. et al. Accuracy of computer diagnosis of melanoma: a quantitative meta-analysis. Arch Dermatol 139, 361–367, discussion 366 (2003).
9. Burroni M, et al. Melanoma computer-aided diagnosis: reliability and feasibility study. Clin Cancer Res. 2004;10:1881–6.
10. Li B, Meng MQH. Computer-aided detection of bleeding regions for capsule endoscopy images. IEEE Trans Biomed Eng. 2009;56(4):1032–9.
11. Woods DD. Cognitive technologies: the design of joint human-machine cognitive systems. AI Mag. 1985;6(4):86.
12. Mnih V, Kavukcuoglu K, Silver D, Rusu AA, Veness J, Bellemare MG, et al. Human-level control through deep reinforcement learning. Nature. 2015;518(7540):529–33.
13. Zhang, X., Wang, S., Liu, L. & Tao, C. Computer-aided diagnosis of four common cutaneous diseases using deep learning algorithm. 2017 IEEE International Conference on Bioinformatics and Biomedicine (BIBM), Kansas City, MO, USA, pp. 1304–1306 (2017).
14. Hauschild A, Egberts F, Garbe C, Bauer J, Grabbe S, Hamm H, Schlaeger M. Melanocytic nevi. JDDG: Journal der Deutschen Dermatologischen Gesellschaft. 2011;9(9):723–34.
15. Braun RP, Ludwig S, Marghoob AA. Differential diagnosis of seborrheic keratosis: clinical and Dermoscopic features[J]. J Drugs Dermatol. 2017;16(9):835–42.
16. Scalvenzi M, Lembo S, Francia MG, Balato A. Dermoscopic patterns of superficial basal cell carcinoma. Int J Dermatol. 2008;47(10):1015–8.
17. Armstrong AW. Psoriasis. Jama Dermatology Patient Page. JAMA Dermatology September. 2017;153(9):2017.
18. Weenig RH, Davis MD, Dahl PR, Su WD. Skin ulcers misdiagnosed as pyoderma gangrenosum. N Engl J Med. 2002;347(18):1412–8.
19. Szegedy C, Vanhoucke V, Ioffe S, Shlens J, Wojna Z. Rethinking the inception architecture for computer vision. In: Proceedings of the IEEE conference on computer vision and pattern recognition (pp. 2818–2826); 2016.
20. Waxman SG. Chapter 2. Development and cellular constituents of the nervous system. Clinical neuroanatomy. 26th. New York: McGraw-Hill; 2010.
21. Krizhevsky A, Sutskever I, Hinton GE. Imagenet classification with deep convolutional neural networks. In: Advances in neural information processing systems (pp. 1097–1105); 2012.
22. LeCun Y, Bengio Y. Convolutional networks for images, speech, and time series. The handbook of brain theory and neural networks. 1995;3361(10):1995.
23. Egmont-Petersen M, de Ridder D, Handels H. Image processing with neural networks—a review. Pattern Recogn. 2002;35(10):2279–301.
24. DeepLearning 0.1 Documentation (2018) Convolutional Neural Netw (LeNet). Retrieved Sep 16, 2017, from http://deeplearning.net/tutorial/lenet.html.
25. Panchal G, Ganatra A, Kosta YP, Panchal D. Behaviour analysis of multilayer perceptronswith multiple hidden neurons and hidden layers. Int J Computer Theory and Engineering. 2011;3(2):332.
26. Minagawa A. Dermoscopy–pathology relationship in seborrheic keratosis. J Dermatol. 2017;44(5):518–24.
27. Abbas Q, Celebi ME, García IF. Hair removal methods: a comparative study for dermoscopy images. Biomedical Signal Processing and Control. 2011;6(4):395–404.
28. Jamil U, Khalid S, Akram MU. Digital image preprocessing and hair artifact removal by using Gabor wavelet. In: SoC design conference (ISOCC), 2016 international (pp. 215–216). IEEE; 2016.
29. George Y, Aldeen M, Garnavi R. Skin hair removal for 2D psoriasis images. In: Digital image computing: techniques and applications (DICTA), 2015 international conference on (pp. 1–8). IEEE; 2015.
30. Kricker A, Armstrong BK, English DR, Heenan PJ. Does intermittent sun exposure cause basal cell carcinoma? A case-control study in Western Australia. Int J Cancer. 1995;60(4):489–94.

8

Screening pregnant women for suicidal behavior in electronic medical records: diagnostic codes vs. clinical notes processed by natural language processing

Qiu-Yue Zhong[1*], Elizabeth W. Karlson[2], Bizu Gelaye[1], Sean Finan[3], Paul Avillach[1,3,4], Jordan W. Smoller[1,5], Tianxi Cai[6] and Michelle A. Williams[1]

Abstract

Background: We examined the comparative performance of structured, diagnostic codes vs. natural language processing (NLP) of unstructured text for screening suicidal behavior among pregnant women in electronic medical records (EMRs).

Methods: Women aged 10–64 years with at least one diagnostic code related to pregnancy or delivery (N = 275,843) from Partners HealthCare were included as our "datamart." Diagnostic codes related to suicidal behavior were applied to the datamart to screen women for suicidal behavior. Among women without any diagnostic codes related to suicidal behavior (n = 273,410), 5880 women were randomly sampled, of whom 1120 had at least one mention of terms related to suicidal behavior in clinical notes. NLP was then used to process clinical notes for the 1120 women. Chart reviews were performed for subsamples of women.

Results: Using diagnostic codes, 196 pregnant women were screened positive for suicidal behavior, among whom 149 (76%) had confirmed suicidal behavior by chart review. Using NLP among those without diagnostic codes, 486 pregnant women were screened positive for suicidal behavior, among whom 146 (30%) had confirmed suicidal behavior by chart review.

Conclusions: The use of NLP substantially improves the sensitivity of screening suicidal behavior in EMRs. However, the prevalence of confirmed suicidal behavior was lower among women who did not have diagnostic codes for suicidal behavior but screened positive by NLP. NLP should be used together with diagnostic codes for future EMR-based phenotyping studies for suicidal behavior.

Keywords: Natural language processing, Electronic medical records, Pregnancy, Suicidal behavior, Screening, Diagnostic codes, Clinical notes

Background

Suicide, a devastating event, is one of the leading cause of maternal deaths during pregnancy and the peripartum period [1, 2]. Early detection of pregnant women with nonfatal suicidal thoughts and behavior (hereafter referred to as suicidal behavior) presents an important opportunity for directing suicide prevention efforts to those at high risk for suicide and, therefore, can help to prevent maternal mortality [3–5]. However, low-cost, highly scalable methods to identify suicidal behavior are lacking. To date, studies have primarily relied on the International Classification of Diseases (ICD) billing codes using administrative or claims data to identify instances of suicidal behavior [5–9]. Suicidal behavior is often "under-coded" with only a small proportion of suicidal cases being detected by the ICD codes among all suicidal cases (i.e., low sensitivity) [10–13]. For example, a systematic review [9] reported that the sensitivity of one widely used ICD-9

* Correspondence: qyzhong@mail.harvard.edu
[1]Department of Epidemiology, Harvard T.H. Chan School of Public Health, Boston, MA 02115, USA

code category, suicide and self-inflicted injury (E950–E959), ranged from 13.8 to 65%. Using a large primary care database from the United Kingdom (UK), Thomas et al. [12] reported that the use of diagnostic codes to detect suicidal cases missed approximately three-quarters of the cases. The reported low sensitivity of billing codes for identifying suicidal behavior implies that a sizable portion of suicidal cases may be missed when case-finding relies on ICD codes alone. Therefore, expanded data collection methods for suicidal behavior are urgently needed to provide a foundation for prevention efforts [9, 14].

The increasing utilization of electronic medical records (EMRs) has provided unprecedented opportunities for identifying pregnant women with suicidal behavior. EMRs contain a ready repository of clinical and phenotypic information consisting of structured and unstructured data that can enable low-cost population-based studies [15, 16]. Structured data are entered by "clicking" on choices of lists, forms, or templates, including demographic data, laboratory test results, and diagnostic billing codes such as the aforementioned ICD codes [16–18]. Unstructured data—clinical data extracted from free-text such as physicians' notes and radiology reports—offers a valuable resource for defining clinical phenotypes [19–22]. The automated examination of a large volume of clinical notes requires the use of natural language processing (NLP) [23], a field of computational linguistics that allows computers to extract relevant information from unstructured human language [22]. NLP has been used successfully to identify patient cohorts for different phenotypes including treatment resistant depression, bipolar disorder, cerebral aneurysms, rheumatoid arthritis, Crohn's disease, ulcerative colitis, and diabetes [15, 23–32]. However, very few studies have used NLP to identify suicidal behavior in EMRs [10, 33, 34], and no study has reported any classification algorithm that is highly predictive of suicidal behavior.

Because of the low prevalence of suicidal behavior [4, 35], developing a phenotyping algorithm using the full EMR population would likely result in low positive predictive values (PPV) [36]. To address this, we first screened for patients with medical record information (structured or unstructured) suggestive of suicidal behavior and excluding those with no evidence of suicidal behavior [36]. The patients who screened positive for suicidal behavior would serve as a highly sensitive datamart and then can be used to develop highly predictive classification algorithms for suicidal behavior. Here, using EMRs from a large healthcare system (Partners HealthCare), we demonstrate that using diagnostic codes together with NLP can more effectively screen for pregnant women with a higher potential of suicidal behavior. We also compare the characteristics of patients identified by these two methods.

Methods

Data source and study population

We extracted data from the Partners HealthCare System Research Patient Data Registry (RPDR). The RPDR is a centralized clinical data warehouse for 4.6 million patients from two large academic medical centers (Massachusetts General Hospital [MGH] and Brigham and Women's Hospital [BWH]), as well as community and specialty hospitals in the Boston area. The RPDR includes structured and unstructured EMR information, including sociodemographic data, vital signs, laboratory and test results, problem list entries, prescribed medications, billing codes, and clinical notes for healthcare services provided within the system [37]. The Institutional Review Board of Partners HealthCare (Protocol Number: 2016P000775/BWH) and Harvard T.H. Chan School of Public Health (Protocol Number: IRB16–0899) approved all aspects of this study.

We initially identified women aged 10–64 years with at least one diagnostic code related to pregnancy or delivery (International Classification of Diseases-10 [ICD-10]: Z3A.*, O0.*- O9.*; ICD-9: 640.*- 679.*, V22.*, V23.*, V24.*, V27.*, V28.*; Diagnosis-Related Group [DRG]: 370–384) in the EMRs from January 1, 1996 to March 31, 2016, totaling 275,843 women (hereafter referred to as "datamart") included in the datamart (Fig. 1).

Suicidal behavior screened positive by diagnostic codes

We first screened for suicidal behavior based on diagnostic codes including the ICD codes and the Longitudinal Medical Record (LMR) codes. The LMR codes were assigned to problem list conditions in the ambulatory EMR system used across Partners HealthCare System. (Additional file 1: Table S1). In addition to the explicit diagnostic codes for suicidal ideation (e.g., ICD-9 V62.84) and suicide attempt (e.g., ICD-9 E95*), we also included additional sets of ICD code categories (poisoning by analgesics, antipyretics, and antirheumatics; poisoning by sedatives and hypnotics; and poisoning by psychotropic agents) with positive predictive value ≥0.8 for suicidal behavior, based on a previous study [4]. Among the 275,843 women with at least one diagnostic code related to pregnancy or delivery, 2433 women had at least one diagnostic code related to suicidal behavior, of which 196 had a diagnostic code that occurred during pregnancy, or within 42 days after abortion or delivery [38]. These 196 women, who screened positive for suicidal behavior based on diagnostic codes, hereafter will be referred to as the "diagnostic codes group" (Fig. 1).

Suicidal behavior screened positive by NLP-processed clinical notes

Among the 273,410 women without any diagnostic codes related to suicidal behavior, we randomly sampled

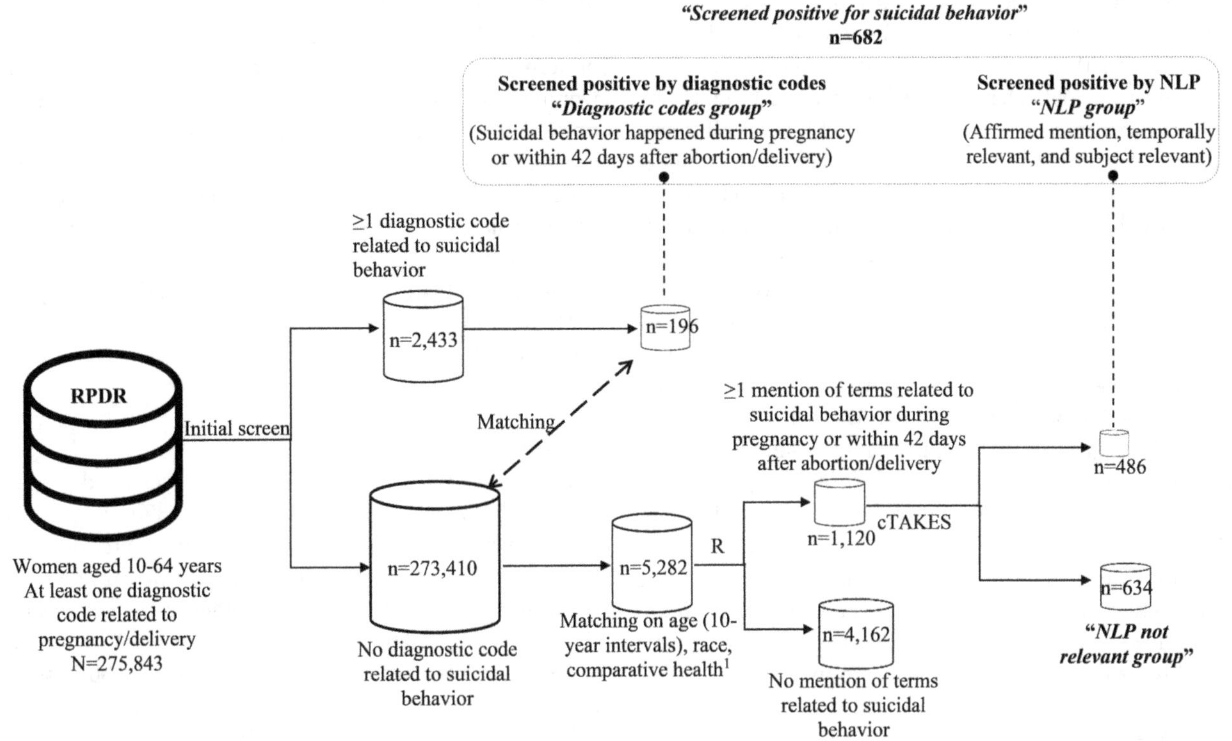

Fig. 1 Screening for suicidal behavior using diagnostic codes vs. NLP among pregnant women. Abbreviations: Natural Language Processing (NLP). [a] Comparative health: the total number of facts which included diagnostic codes for diseases, medications, and specific test results from hospital visits for each patient; it can be used as a proxy for healthcare utilization

a subset of women (N = 5880) who were matched for age (10-year intervals), race, and comparative health with the diagnostic codes group using a 1:30 matching ratio. The reason we chose the 1:30 ratio for subsequent NLP was twofold: (1) to provide a sample size that was large enough for a general view of distributions of CUIs, and (2) to minimize the NLP processing time. Comparative health, a proxy for healthcare utilization, was defined as the total number of observations in the medical records which included diagnostic codes for diseases, medications, and specific test results from hospital visits for each patient [39]. To comply with the IRB, Partners HealthCare employees (N = 598) were excluded, leaving 5282 women in the matched set. We then searched women's clinical notes and identified 1120 (21.2%) women with at least one mention of the terms related to suicidal behavior [12] (Additional file 1: Table S2) during pregnancy or within the 42 days after abortion or delivery [38].

We further processed the clinical notes of the 1120 women using the clinical Text Analysis and Knowledge Extraction System (cTAKES 3.2.3, http://ctakes.apache.org/) [40]. Based on the Unstructured Information Management Architecture (UIMA), cTAKES is a comprehensive clinical NLP tool that processes clinical notes and identifies terms. cTAKES maps the terms to a subset of the Unified Medical Language System (UMLS) Metathesaurus [41], the Systemized Nomenclature of Medicine-Clinical Terms (SNOMED-CT) [42], and assigns each term a UMLS concept unique identifier (CUI). cTAKES also extracts qualifying attributes (including negation, temporality, and subject status) associated with each CUI. As determined by cTAKES negation module [40], each CUI can be either affirmed (e.g., "patient reports feeling suicidal") or negated (e.g., "suicidal behavior: none"). Affirmed CUIs were considered as relevant for this analysis. cTAKES has a temporality module, *DocTimeRel* (Document Time Relation), to discover the temporal relation between a term and the document creation time [24]. The values for *DocTimeRel* include "before" (e.g., "patient attempted suicide when she was 14"), "after" (e.g., "She would not consider suicide an option if symptoms were to arise"), "overlap" (e.g., "patient states that she wants to kill herself"), and "before/overlap" (terms that started before document creation time and continue to the present [e.g., "patient endorses passive suicidal ideation since the birth of her baby"]). Terms tagged as "overlap" or "before/overlap" were considered as temporally relevant for this analysis. The *Subject* module indicates whether the patient or someone else (e.g., "mom attempted suicide") experiences the event. The values for the *Subject* module include "patient," "family member," "other," and "null." [43] The terms tagged as "patient" were considered as subject relevant for this analysis.

We created an expert-defined list of CUIs considered relevant to suicidal behavior (Additional file 1: Table S3). We included the distributions of attributes of the CUIs relevant to suicidal behavior in Additional file 1: Table S4.

To compensate for errors introduced by the NLP system, we calculated the proportion of affirmed, temporally relevant, and subject relevant CUIs related to suicidal behavior among all CUIs related to suicidal behavior for each woman and selected women with proportions that were greater than or equal to 0.25. This threshold was determined empirically with an aim to decrease false positives, while maintaining relatively low false negatives. From the NLP-processed clinical notes, we identified 486 pregnant women (hereafter referred to as the "NLP group") with CUIs related to suicidal behavior. Of note, the NLP group was screened positive by both term mentions related to suicidal behavior and cTAKES. The remainder (N = 634) who had at least one mention of the terms related to suicidal behavior during pregnancy or within the 42 days after abortion or delivery, but were not screened positive by the NLP are referred to as the "NLP not relevant group."

Reference group

We randomly sampled a subset of women aged 10–64 years with at least one diagnostic code related to pregnancy or delivery as the reference group. The reference group was matched with comparative health [39] for the diagnostic codes group using a 1:100 matching ratio. Since we did not need to process the clinical notes for reference group, we included a relatively larger sample size. After excluding Partners HealthCare employees, 17,183 women were included in the reference group.

Chart review to obtain estimates for prevalence of confirmed suicidal behavior

After the screening process, one of the authors (QYZ) manually reviewed the clinical notes for random samples of (1) 50 women from the diagnostic codes group (N = 196); (2) 100 women from the NLP group (N = 486); (3) 100 women from the NLP not relevant group (N = 634); and (4) 100 women who had neither diagnostic codes nor term mentions related to suicidal behavior (N = 4162). Based on the Columbia Classification Algorithm of Suicide Assessment (C-CASA), the reviewer assigned each woman a classification of either "with" or "without suicidal behavior" [44]. Women who had (1) completed suicide, (2) suicide attempt, (3) preparatory acts toward imminent suicidal behavior, or (4) suicidal ideation were considered as "with" suicidal behavior.

Statistical analysis

We compared the demographic and provider characteristics of pregnant women screened positive for suicidal behavior by the diagnostic codes versus NLP during encounters with suicidal behavior. We examined the distributions of demographic characteristics between pregnant women screened positive for suicidal behavior by the diagnostic codes versus NLP using the Chi-square test for categorical variables and Student's t-test for continuous variables. We reported the proportions of women who received diagnoses of psychiatric comorbidities at least once during or before the most recent encounter with suicidal behavior. Psychiatric comorbidities were defined using the ICD codes in Additional file 1: Table S5. All analyses were done using R [45].

Results

We identified 682 pregnant women who screened positive for suicidal behavior, of whom 196 (28.73%) were identified by diagnostic codes and 486 (71.26%) were identified by NLP. Based on manual chart review, the prevalence of confirmed suicidal behavior in women screened positive (PPV) by the diagnostic codes and by NLP in women without the diagnostic codes were 76.00 and 30.00%, respectively. The estimated number of confirmed suicidal behavior among the screen positive groups by the diagnostic codes and NLP would be 149 and 146, respectively. The prevalence of confirmed suicidal behavior was 1.00% among the NLP not relevant group. The prevalence of confirmed suicidal behavior was 0.00% among women who had neither diagnostic codes nor term mentions related to suicidal behavior. The approximate estimated prevalence of suicidal behavior in the reference group would be 2.76% (486 × 0.3/5282).

The demographic characteristics of women who screened positive for suicidal behavior by the diagnostic codes and NLP, respectively, are presented in Table 1. Compared with the NLP group, the diagnostic codes group was less likely to be Hispanic (33.33% vs. 28.57%), be married/common--law married/partnered (29.63% vs. 21.43%), report religious affiliation as Christian (45.47% vs. 38.27%), and have private insurance (44.65% vs. 32.14%); these women were more likely to be Black or African American (16.46% vs. 20.92%), be single (65.02% vs. 71.43%), and be insured by Medicaid (43.21% vs. 49.49%) and Medicare (6.17% vs. 9.18%).

Table 2 shows provider characteristics for participants' encounters (inpatient or outpatient visits) with suicidal behavior. For encounters with suicidal behavior, more than two-thirds of women in the diagnostic codes group (69.39%) visited the Emergency Department, whereas only 17.49% of women in the NLP group visited the Emergency Department. The proportions of women screened positive for suicidal behavior treated in an inpatient setting was higher among those in the diagnostic codes group (39.29%), as compared with those in the NLP group (19.55%).

Table 1 Demographic characteristics of pregnant women screened positive for suicidal behavior by diagnostic codes vs. NLP

Characteristics	Diagnostic codes (*N* = 196)		NLP[a](*N* = 486)		*P*-values[b]	Reference group[c](*N* = 17,183)	
	n	%	n	%		n	%
Age at the most recent pregnancy with suicidal behavior[d]	26.8 (6.9)		26.4 (6.2)		0.46	35.7 (8.3)[e]	
Age at the most recent pregnancy with suicidal behavior[d]					0.14		
< 16	4	2.04	2	0.41		38	0.22
[16, 18)	8	4.08	27	5.56		65	0.38
[18, 20)	16	8.16	53	10.91		205	1.19
[20, 35)	141	71.94	352	72.43		7594	44.19
≥ 35	27	13.78	52	10.70		9281	54.01
Language					0.51		
English	168	85.71	407	83.74		14,844	86.39
Spanish	21	10.71	66	13.58		1537	8.94
Other	7	3.57	13	2.67		802	4.67
Race/ethnicity					0.20		
Asian	7	3.57	8	1.65		1036	6.03
Black or African American	41	20.92	80	16.46		1837	10.69
Hispanic	56	28.57	162	33.33		2677	15.58
White	87	44.39	211	43.42		10,413	60.60
Other/Not recorded	5	2.55	25	5.14		1220	7.10
Religion					0.34		
Christian	75	38.27	221	45.47		5904	34.36
Catholic	63	32.14	162	33.33		6627	38.57
Islamic	5	2.55	8	1.65		451	2.62
Jewish	1	0.51	6	1.23		676	3.93
No preference/None	27	13.78	49	10.08		1275	7.42
Other/Unknown/Not recorded	25	12.76	40	8.23		2250	13.09
Marital status					0.15		
Married/Partner/Common law	42	21.43	144	29.63		10,816	62.95
Single	140	71.43	316	65.02		4675	27.21
Separated/Divorced/Widowed	9	4.59	15	3.09		1000	5.82
Other/Unknown	5	2.55	11	2.26		692	4.03
Vital status					0.04		
Deceased with date of death	2[f]	1.02	6[f]	1.23		168	0.98
Deceased with date of death unknown	4	2.04	1	0.21		35	0.20
Not reported as deceased	190	96.94	479	98.56		16,980	98.82
Veteran					0.12		
No	169	86.22	421	86.63		14,810	86.19
Yes	3	1.53	1	0.21		75	0.44
Unknown	24	12.24	64	13.17		2298	13.37
Insurance					0.03		
Medicaid	97	49.49	210	43.21		3097	18.02
Medicare	18	9.18	30	6.17		531	3.09

Table 1 Demographic characteristics of pregnant women screened positive for suicidal behavior by diagnostic codes vs. NLP *(Continued)*

Characteristics	Diagnostic codes (*N* = 196)		NLP[a](*N* = 486)		*P*-values[b]	Reference group[c](*N* = 17,183)	
Private Insurance	63	32.14	217	44.65		12,415	72.25
Self-pay	8	4.08	11	2.26		488	2.84
Other	10	5.10	18	3.70		652	3.79

Abbreviations: Natural language processing (*NLP*)
[a]Randomly sampled from women aged 10–64 years with at least one diagnostic code related to pregnancy or delivery, matching on age, race, comparative health with women screened positive for suicidal behavior by diagnostic codes using a 1:30 matching ratio
[b]For continuous variables, *P*-value was calculated using the Student's t test; for categorical variables, *P*-value was calculated using the Chi-square test.
[c]Randomly sampled from women aged 10–64 years with at least one diagnostic code related to pregnancy or delivery, matching on comparative health with women screened positive for suicidal behavior by diagnostic codes using a 1:100 matching ratio
[d]Mean (Standard deviation)
[e]Age at most recent date with diagnostic codes related to pregnancy or delivery
[f]None of the deaths occurred within 183 days after suicidal behavior

Psychiatric comorbidities were common among women with suicidal behavior (Table 3). Women screened positive for suicidal behavior by the diagnostic codes had higher psychiatric comorbidities including depression, schizophrenia, bipolar disorder, post-traumatic stress disorder (PTSD), and substance abuse. The distribution of care providers according to clinical specialties (Department of Psychiatry/Mental Health/Behavioral Health and Emergency Department) were similar across psychiatric comorbidities (Table 3).

Discussion

We demonstrated that the use of NLP along with term search substantially improved the sensitivity of screening suicidal behavior among pregnant women from a large EMR system. More than two-thirds of potential suicidal behavior and nearly half of confirmed suicidal behavior would have been missed if screening had relied solely on ICD codes. However, we observed that the PPV of NLP, the probability that a suicidal case identified by NLP was truly suicidal, was lower (30.00%) as compared to the diagnostic codes (76.00%). We found that women in the diagnostic codes group had more risk factors for suicidal behavior [46], including low socioeconomic status, being single, and psychiatric comorbidities as compared with those women in the NLP diagnostic group.

Table 2 Provider characteristics at encounters with suicidal behavior of pregnant women screened positive for suicidal behavior by diagnostic codes vs. NLP

Characteristics	Diagnostic codes (N = 196)		NLP (N = 486)		Reference group[a](N = 17,183)	
	n	%	n	%	n	%
Hospitals (ever)						
Massachusetts General Hospital	105	53.57	249	51.23	12,678	73.78
Brigham and Women's Hospital	95	48.47	250	51.44	12,800	74.49
Faulkner Hospital	0	0.00	1	0.21	4263	24.81
North Shore Medical Center	0	0.00	11	2.26	2659	15.47
Newton-Wellesley Hospital	0	0.00	4	0.82	5643	32.84
Spaulding Rehabilitation Hospital	0	0.00	2	0.41	1199	6.98
McLean Hospital	0	0.00	0	0.00	283	1.65
Clinics (ever)						
Emergency	136	69.39	85	17.49	9749	56.74
Psychiatry/Mental health/Behavioral health	7	3.57	221	45.47	2605	15.16
Obstetrics and Gynecology	12	6.12	18	3.70	11,386	66.26
Pediatrics	4	2.04	125	25.72	1253	7.29
Inpatient/outpatient (ever)						
Inpatient	77	39.29	95	19.55	14,116	82.15
Outpatient	157	80.10	407	83.74	17,055	99.26
Not recorded	0	0.00	46	9.47	9762	56.81

Abbreviations: Natural language processing (NLP)
[a]Provider characteristics during lifetime (ever)

Table 3 Psychiatric comorbidities of pregnant women screened positive for suicidal behavior by diagnostic codes vs. NLP

Psychiatric Comorbidities	Diagnostic codes (N = 196)		NLP (N = 486)		Reference group (N = 17,183)	
	n	%	n	%	n	%
Psychiatric Comorbidities						
Depression	171	87.24	353	72.63	5150	29.97
Schizophrenia	10	5.10	10	2.06	95	0.55
Bipolar	45	22.96	40	8.23	489	2.85
PTSD	58	29.59	76	15.64	590	3.43
Substance abuse	102	52.04	173	35.60	2332	13.57
Anxiety	100	51.02	259	53.29	5184	30.17
Psychiatric comorbidities at encounters to Department Psychiatry/Mental Health/Behavioral Health (ever)						
Depression	93	47.45	180	37.04	1536	8.94
Schizophrenia	7	3.57	4	0.82	43	0.25
Bipolar	18	9.18	26	5.35	234	1.36
PTSD	29	14.80	44	9.05	312	1.82
Substance abuse	43	21.94	36	7.41	177	1.03
Anxiety	30	15.31	113	23.25	1058	6.16
Psychiatric comorbidities at encounters to Emergency Department (Ever)						
Depression	128	65.31	80	16.46	608	3.54
Schizophrenia	6	3.06	2	0.41	22	0.13
Bipolar	25	12.76	8	1.65	76	0.44
PTSD	28	14.29	9	1.85	54	0.31
Substance abuse	74	37.76	57	11.73	652	3.79
Anxiety	51	26.02	42	8.64	660	3.84

Abbreviations: Natural language processing (*NLP*), post-traumatic stress disorder (*PTSD*)

Prior studies have attempted to identify patients with suicidal behavior in unstructured clinical notes. Using the UK Clinical Practice Research Datalink, Thomas et al. found that searching for terms related to suicide in general practice consultation records identified 10.7% of the suicidal cases that were missed by ICD diagnostic codes [12]. Anderson et al. [33] processed the History of Present Illness notes of 15,761 patients with at least one diagnostic code of depression in primary care clinical organizations. A rule-based NLP system was developed to search for positive mention or negation of suicidal behavior using a list of terms related to suicidal behavior. The proportion of patients with corresponding ICD diagnostic codes indicating suicidal ideation and suicide attempt in the notes were 3% and 19%, respectively. Haerian et al. [10] used an NLP tool, the Medical Language Extraction and Encoding System (MedLEE), to identify suicidal behavior in the EMRs for pediatric and adult inpatients. Of note, they used a list of CUIs with a specific focus on suicidal behavior by drug overdose, which was different from the CUI list we used in our study. In their study, 469 potential cases were identified by the ICD diagnostic codes, and 4087 were identified by the NLP algorithm after filtering out CUIs that were negated or associated with family history. The intersection of both ICD diagnostic codes and the NLP algorithm identified 260 potential cases. The positive predictive values for the ICD diagnostic codes and the NLP algorithm were similar (55% for ICD and 60% for NLP). Despite the different NLP tools used across EMR systems, these results consistently suggested that suicidal behavior was often documented in clinical notes without being assigned any diagnostic codes that were designed for billing purposes. Suicidal behavior is a complex phenotype coupled with many psychosocial problems, where clinical notes are often used to capture the complexity and diagnostic uncertainty [47, 48]. Incorporating information from unstructured clinical notes through NLP in our study, we were able to screen a significant number of patients with potential suicidal behavior that would otherwise not be found using structured data alone. However, the PPV of NLP used in the current study was lower than that of the diagnostic codes. Nonetheless, we identified a comparable number of suicidal cases (149 for diagnostic codes vs. 146 for NLP) when using only a subsample of women (5880 out of 273,410) without any diagnostic codes related to suicidal behavior for NLP. Despite the low PPV of NLP, considering the large number of pregnant women without diagnostic codes related to suicidal behavior (N = 273,410) and the fact that suicidal behavior was often documented in clinical notes, we maintain that NLP procedures may be used to identify more suicidal cases. Therefore, for future studies using EMR-based phenotyping for suicidal behavior, an optimal approach to increase screening sensitivity may best involve combining the application of NLP procedures with the diagnostic codes.

Only 30% of the women who screened positive for suicidal behavior by NLP were confirmed to be suicidal by chart review (PPV = 0.30). A large proportion of women who were not suicidal were screened positive for suicidal behavior by NLP. Similar to one previous study [10], the majority of the false positives came from the incorrect qualifying attributes based on our error analysis by manual review of the clinical notes from 100 women in the NLP group, in particular, negation associated with CUIs. Negation is a well-known challenge for processing unstructured clinical notes [49]. One study showed that approximately half of the conditions indexed in dictated reports were negated [50, 51]. For suicidal behavior, clinicians are likely to document both the presence and absence of suicidal behavior [10]. In the Partners HealthCare EMRs, we observed a major negation structure for suicidal behavior: terms related to suicidal behavior were followed by a colon and a negation word without any sentence punctuation (e.g., "suicidal behavior: none," "suicidal behavior: none reported," and "suicidal behavior: denied") (Additional file 1: Table S6). However, the standard cTAKES negation module NegEx [40, 52], a regular expression pattern matching algorithm that searches for predefined negation words around terms [53] was initially trained using the Intensive Care Unit discharge summaries [52], and is not able to recognize such negation structure [54]. Consequently, a considerable number of suicidal behavior terms that were negated were incorrectly identified as "affirmed." Further enhancement of the negation algorithm with training data pertaining specifically to suicidal behavior is required to decrease the false positives [49, 55]. Other common reasons leading to cTAKES miscoding women without suicidal behavior as suicidal (Additional file 1: Table S6) included (1) incorrect recognition of "before" as "overlap" by the *DocTimeRel* module (e.g., *DocTimeRel* module treated history of suicidal behavior as current suicidal behavior: "Suicide attempt/gesture: history of, hospitalized inpatient psych unit for suicide attempt in 1996"); (2) incorrect recognition of "family member" as "patient" by the *Subject* module (e.g., *Subject* module treated the suicidal behavior of patient's father as patient's: "Pt also identifies strongly with father, who was often aggressive toward others and threatened suicide"); (3) failure to identify section titles (e.g., "Suicidal Behavior Hx of Suicidal Behavior:") that do not describe the behavior of patients; and (4) failure to handle hypothetical conditions that temporally are neither recent nor historical (e.g., "If she has significant side effects from it such as lethargy/depression/irritability/suicidal thought, we will change it to LTG.").

We found that women in the diagnostic codes group had different characteristics as compared to women in the NLP group. On the one hand, these differences could be due to the lower prevalence of confirmed suicidal behavior in the NLP group. Therefore, developing highly predictive classification algorithms is needed for the NLP group. On the other hand, the differences between women screened positive for suicidal behavior by the diagnostic codes and NLP suggest that the two groups may differ with respect to the degree of suicide intent, methods used, and subsequent clinical management. Because a larger proportion of women screened positive by the diagnostic codes received inpatient care and were seen in the Emergency Department, they were likely to present as more severe cases of suicidal behavior with high suicide intent [56], requiring hospital admission and immediate care. In addition, the diagnostic codes for suicidal ideation (ICD-9: V62.82) were not used until October 2005 when the codes were introduced. Even after the codes became available, one study showed that suicidal ideation was less likely to be coded than suicide attempt [33]. These two factors (i.e., source of inpatient care and timing of availability of diagnostic codes) might have contributed to a disproportionate representation of more severe cases of suicidal behavior in the diagnostic codes group. In this scenario, women screened positive by the diagnostic codes may be a more relevant cohort for assessing patients at high risk for completed suicide [57], whereas women screened positive by NLP may be more relevant for investigating early identification of high-risk groups and suicide prevention interventions. Another possibility for the observed differences in characteristics, especially for psychiatric comorbidities, between the diagnostic codes group and the NLP group could be due to differential bias in coding: women with more risk factors were more likely to be coded for suicidal behavior.

There are several limitations of this study. First, the prevalence of confirmed suicidal behavior among women screened positive by NLP was only 30%. However, given the purpose of our study, which was to screen pregnant women with a higher potential of suicidal behavior and to develop a highly sensitive datamart for suicidal behavior, this low PPV might be tolerated. Nevertheless, using this highly sensitive datamart for suicidal behavior, future development of accurate classification algorithms using different machine learning techniques [58, 59] is clearly needed to identify true cases of suicidal behavior. Second, given the small sample size of women screened positive for suicidal behavior by the diagnostic codes, we did not further classify patients according to subtypes of suicidal behavior such as suicidal ideation and suicide attempt. Third, given that a woman was considered as screened positive for suicidal behavior only if she was screened positive by both term mention and NLP by cTAKES, it is possible that we might miss some women who did not pass the screening by term mentions related to suicidal behavior but would have been considered as screened positive by cTAKES. Fourth, we used 20 years of data from a single urban-regional EMR system that did not include patient visits outside this geographical area, time period, or network of hospitals. The generalizability of our results to patients in other healthcare systems may vary depending on the informatics infrastructure and local documentation practices [26]. Fifth, we focused on extracting facts expressed directly in the clinical notes (i.e., terms of suicidal behavior) using NLP. However, beyond extracting these basic facts, further research in studying other linguistic features, such as sentiment expressed in clinical notes (e.g., positive and negative emotions), and capturing the meaning of texts (e.g., word embedding [60–62]), may also be beneficial in identifying suicidal patients [63–67].

Conclusion

Our results illuminated the advantage of using NLP along with term search in EMRs to screen pregnant women for a complex, rare psychiatric phenotype. NLP substantially improved the sensitivity of screening for suicidal behavior in an obstetric population. We captured a group of pregnant women with potential suicidal behavior otherwise not reflected in the structured data. We also highlight the challenges of using NLP in screening pregnant women for suicidal behavior. Of note, NLP had lower PPV as compared with diagnostic codes. Improvement in the cTAKES modules, especially the negation module, may help to increase the PPV. For future studies using EMR-based phenotyping for suicidal behavior, an optimal approach may include combining NLP procedures with the diagnostic codes.

Our approach is the first to examine the large-scale use of NLP in suicidal behavior among pregnant women. The current study in our population of pregnant women was particularly challenging given the rarity of suicidal behavior, the stigma attached, the complexity of phenotypic assessment, and the historical misconception of the protective role of pregnancy in suicidal behavior [3, 68]. Because pregnancy is a time when women have frequent interactions with the healthcare system, EMR-based identification of pregnant women with suicidal behavior may be useful for future genetic, epidemiological, and clinical studies, presenting a valuable opportunity for healthcare providers to intervene promptly [5, 69].

Additional file

Additional file 1: Table S1. International Classification of Disease (ICD) codes and other diagnostic codes used to screen suicidal behavior. **Table S2.** Terms used to screen suicidal behavior in clinical notes. **Table S3.** Concept Unique Identifiers (CUIs) related to suicidal behavior. **Table S4.** Distributions of attributes of the Concept Unique Identifiers (CUIs) related to suicidal behavior among 1120 women. **Table S5.** International Classification of Disease (ICD) codes used to define psychiatric comorbidities. **Table S6.** Error analysis of false positive results from cTAKES to screen for suicidal behavior. (DOCX 36 kb)

Abbreviations

BWH: Brigham and women's hospital; C-CASA: Columbia classification algorithm of suicide assessment; cTAKES: clinical Text Analysis and Knowledge Extraction System; CUI: Concept unique identifier; DRG: Diagnosis-related group; EMRs: Electronic medical records; ICD: International classification of diseases; LMR: Longitudinal medical record; MedLEE: Medical language extraction and encoding system; MGH: Massachusetts general hospital; NLP: Natural language processing; PPV: Positive predictive values; RPDR: Research patient data registry; SNOMED-CT: Systemized nomenclature of medicine-clinical terms; UMLS: Unified medical language system

Acknowledgements

The authors are very grateful for the help of Leslie Howes at Harvard T.H. Chan School of Public Health, and the Harvard Catalyst Leadership Team during the planning and development of this research. The authors thank the Enterprise Research Infrastructure & Services at Partners HealthCare for the provision of computing resources. The authors also thank Laurie Bogosian and Stacey Duey of the Research Patient Data Repository at Partners HealthCare for the in-depth support. The authors thank Kathy Brenner for the help with editing this manuscript. This research was done as partial fulfillment of the requirements of a Doctor of Science degree by one of the authors (QYZ) in the Department of Epidemiology, Harvard T.H. Chan School of Public Health, Boston, MA, USA. One of the authors (QYZ) expresses appreciation to Dr. Michael Napolitano for his non-expert comments, and constant support and encouragement in completing this manuscript.

Funding

This research was supported by awards from the National Institutes of Health (the National Institute on Minority Health and Health Disparities: T37-MD001449; and the National Center for Research Resources (NCRR), the National Center for Advancing Translational Sciences (NCATS): 8UL1TR 000170–09). The NIH had no further role in study design; in the collection, analysis and interpretation of data; in the writing of the manuscript; and in the decision to submit the paper for publication.

Authors' contributions

QYZ (qyzhong@mail.harvard.edu), EWK (ekarlson@bwh.harvard.edu), BG (bgelaye@hsph.harvard.edu), PA (Paul_Avillach@hms.harvard.edu), JWS (jsmoller@hms.harvard.edu), TC (tcai@hsph.harvard.edu), and MAW (mawilliams@hsph.harvard.edu) conceived and designed the study. QYZ processed and analyzed the data with support from SF (Sean.Finan@childrens.harvard.edu). All authors interpreted the data. QYZ wrote the manuscript with input from all authors. All authors read and approved the final manuscript.

Competing interests

The authors declare that they have no competing interest.

Author details
[1]Department of Epidemiology, Harvard T.H. Chan School of Public Health, Boston, MA 02115, USA. [2]Department of Medicine, Division of Rheumatology, Immunology and Allergy, Brigham and Women's Hospital and Harvard Medical School, Boston, MA, USA. [3]Children's Hospital Informatics Program, Boston Children's Hospital, Boston, MA, USA. [4]Department of Biomedical Informatics, Harvard Medical School, Boston, MA, USA. [5]Psychiatric and Neurodevelopmental Genetics Unit, Massachusetts General Hospital, Boston, MA, USA. [6]Department of Biostatistics, Harvard T.H. Chan School of Public Health, Boston, MA, USA.

References

1. Oates M. Suicide: the leading cause of maternal death. Br J Psychiatry. 2003; 183:279–81.
2. Oates M. Perinatal psychiatric disorders: a leading cause of maternal morbidity and mortality. Br Med Bull. 2003;67:219–29.
3. Gelaye B, Kajeepeta S, Williams MA. Suicidal ideation in pregnancy: an epidemiologic review. Arch Womens Ment Health. 2016;19:741–51.
4. Barak-Corren Y, Castro VM, Javitt S, Hoffnagle AG, Dai Y, Perlis RH, et al. Predicting Suicidal Behavior From Longitudinal Electronic Health Records. Am J Psychiatry. 2017;174:154–62.
5. Zhong Q-Y, Gelaye B, Miller M, Fricchione GL, Cai T, Johnson PA, et al. Suicidal behavior-related hospitalizations among pregnant women in the USA, 2006-2012. Arch Womens Ment Health. Springer Vienna; 2016;19:463–472.
6. Gandhi SG, Gilbert WM, McElvy SS, El Kady D, Danielson B, Xing G, et al. Maternal and neonatal outcomes after attempted suicide. Obstet Gynecol. 2006;107:984–90.
7. Patrick AR, Miller M, Barber CW, Wang PS, Canning CF, Schneeweiss S. Identification of hospitalizations for intentional self-harm when E-codes are incompletely recorded. Pharmacoepidemiol Drug Saf. 2010;19:1263–75.
8. Simon GE, Savarino J. Suicide attempts among patients starting depression treatment with medications or psychotherapy. Am J Psychiatry. 2007;164:1029–34.
9. Walkup JT, Townsend L, Crystal S, Olfson M. A systematic review of validated methods for identifying suicide or suicidal ideation using administrative or claims data. Pharmacoepidemiol Drug Saf. 2012; 21(Suppl 1):174–82.
10. Haerian K, Salmasian H, Friedman C. Methods for identifying suicide or suicidal ideation in EHRs. AMIA Annu Symp Proc. 2012;2012:1244–53.
11. Colman I, Yiannakoulias N, Schopflocher D, Svenson LW, Rosychuk RJ, Rowe BH, et al. Population-based study of medically treated self-inflicted injuries. CJEM. 2004;6:313–20.
12. Thomas KH, Davies N, Metcalfe C, Windmeijer F, Martin RM, Gunnell D. Validation of suicide and self-harm records in the Clinical Practice Research Datalink. Br J Clin Pharmacol. 2013;76:145–57.
13. Lu CY, Stewart C, Ahmed AT, Ahmedani BK, Coleman K, Copeland LA, et al. How complete are E-codes in commercial plan claims databases? Pharmacoepidemiol Drug Saf. 2014;23:218–20.
14. US Public Health Service. The Surgeon General's Call to Action to Prevent Suicide. Washington, DC: US Public Health Service; 1999.
15. Castro VM, Minnier J, Murphy SN, Kohane I, Churchill SE, Gainer V, et al. Validation of electronic health record phenotyping of bipolar disorder cases and controls. Am J Psychiatry. 2015;172:363–72.
16. Jensen PB, Jensen LJ, Brunak S. Mining electronic health records: towards better research applications and clinical care. Nat Rev Genet. 2012;13:395–405.
17. Sinnott JA, Dai W, Liao KP, Shaw SY, Ananthakrishnan AN, Gainer VS, et al. Improving the power of genetic association tests with imperfect phenotype derived from electronic medical records. Hum Genet. 2014;133:1369–82.
18. de Lusignan S, van Weel C. The use of routinely collected computer data for research in primary care: opportunities and challenges. Fam Pract. 2006;23:253–63.
19. Bates DW, Evans RS, Murff H, Stetson PD, Pizziferri L, Hripcsak G. Detecting adverse events using information technology. J Am Med Inform Assoc. 2003;10:115–28.
20. Pakhomov SVS, Shah ND, Van Houten HK, Hanson PL, Smith SA. The role of the electronic medical record in the assessment of health related quality of life. AMIA Annu Symp Proc. 2011;2011:1080–8.
21. Fischer LR, Rush WA, Kluznik JC, O'Connor PJ, Hanson AM. Abstract C-C1-06: Identifying Depression Among Diabetes Patients Using Natural Language Processing of Office Notes. Clin Med Res. 2008;6:125–6.
22. Jha AK. The promise of electronic records: around the corner or down the road? JAMA. 2011;306:880–1.
23. Raymond Francis Sarmiento FD. Improving Patient Cohort Identification Using Natural Language Processing. In: MIT Critical Data, editor. Secondary Analysis of Electronic Health Records. Berlin, Germany: Springer International Publishing; 2016. p. 405–417.
24. Lin C, Karlson EW, Dligach D, Ramirez MP, Miller TA, Mo H, et al. Automatic identification of methotrexate-induced liver toxicity in patients with rheumatoid arthritis from the electronic medical record. J Am Med Inform Assoc. 2015;22:e151–61.
25. Castro VM, Dligach D, Finan S, Yu S, Can A, Abd-El-Barr M, et al. Large-scale identification of patients with cerebral aneurysms using natural language processing. Neurology. 2017;88:164–8.
26. Perlis RH, Iosifescu DV, Castro VM, Murphy SN, Gainer VS, Minnier J, et al. Using electronic medical records to enable large-scale studies in psychiatry: treatment resistant depression as a model. Psychol Med. Cambridge Univ Press; 2012;42:41–50.
27. Castro V, Shen Y, Yu S, Finan S, Pau CT, Gainer V, et al. Identification of subjects with polycystic ovary syndrome using electronic health records. Reprod Biol Endocrinol. 2015;13:116.
28. Castro VM, Apperson WK, Gainer VS, Ananthakrishnan AN, Goodson AP, Wang TD, et al. Evaluation of matched control algorithms in EHR-based phenotyping studies: a case study of inflammatory bowel disease comorbidities. J Biomed Inform. 2014;52:105–11.
29. Liao KP, Cai T, Gainer V, Goryachev S, Zeng-treitler Q, Raychaudhuri S, et al. Electronic medical records for discovery research in rheumatoid arthritis. Arthritis Care Res. 2010;62:1120–7.
30. Liao KP, Ananthakrishnan AN, Kumar V, Xia Z, Cagan A, Gainer VS, et al. Methods to Develop an Electronic Medical Record Phenotype Algorithm to Compare the Risk of Coronary Artery Disease across 3 Chronic Disease Cohorts. PLoS One. 2015;10:e0136651.
31. Ananthakrishnan AN, Cai T, Savova G, Cheng S-C, Chen P, Perez RG, et al. Improving case definition of Crohn's disease and ulcerative colitis in electronic medical records using natural language processing: a novel informatics approach. Inflamm Bowel Dis. 2013;19:1411–20.
32. Carroll RJ, Thompson WK, Eyler AE, Mandelin AM, Cai T, Zink RM, et al. Portability of an algorithm to identify rheumatoid arthritis in electronic health records. J Am Med Inform Assoc. 2012;19:e162–9.
33. Anderson HD, Pace WD, Brandt E, Nielsen RD, Allen RR, Libby AM, et al. Monitoring suicidal patients in primary care using electronic health records. J Am Board Fam Med. 2015;28:65–71.
34. Downs JM, Velupillai S, Gkotsis G, Holden R, Kikoler M, Dean H, et al. Detection of Suicidality in Adolescents with Autism Spectrum Disorders: Developing a Natural Language Processing Approach for Use in Electronic Health Records. Proc AMIA Symp [Internet]. 2017 [cited 2018 Mar 19]; Available from: https://kclpure.kcl.ac.uk/portal/en/publications/detection-of-suicidality-in-adolescents-with-autism-spectrum-disorders(2e703fc1-2f87-448e-abfc-14e36036c471)/export.html
35. Smoller JW. The use of electronic health records for psychiatric phenotyping and genomics. Am J Med Genet B Neuropsychiatr Genet [Internet]. 2017; Available from: https://doi.org/10.1002/ajmg.b.32548
36. Liao KP, Cai T, Savova GK, Murphy SN, Karlson EW, Ananthakrishnan AN, et al. Development of phenotype algorithms using electronic medical records and incorporating natural language processing. BMJ. 2015;350:h1885.
37. Wang SV, Rogers JR, Jin Y, Bates DW, Fischer MA. Use of electronic healthcare records to identify complex patients with atrial fibrillation for targeted intervention. J Am Med Inform Assoc. 2017;24:339–44.
38. World Health Organization. International Statistical Classification of Diseases and Related Health Problems. In: World Health Organization; 2004.
39. Murphy SN, Weber G, Mendis M, Gainer V, Chueh HC, Churchill S, et al. Serving the enterprise and beyond with informatics for integrating biology and the bedside (i2b2). J Am Med Inform Assoc. 2010;17:124–30.
40. Savova GK, Masanz JJ, Ogren PV, Zheng J, Sohn S, Kipper-Schuler KC, et al. Mayo clinical Text Analysis and Knowledge Extraction System (cTAKES): architecture, component evaluation and applications. J Am Med Inform Assoc. jamia.oxfordjournals.org. 2010;17:507–13.
41. Bodenreider O. The Unified Medical Language System (UMLS): integrating

biomedical terminology. Nucleic Acids Res. 2004;32:D267–70.
42. Donnelly KSNOMED-CT. The advanced terminology and coding system for eHealth. Stud Health Technol Inform. 2006;121:279–90.
43. Chikka VR, Mariyasagayam N, Niwa Y, Karlapalem K. Information Extraction from Clinical Documents: Towards Disease/Disorder Template Filling. Experimental IR Meets Multilinguality, Multimodality, and Interaction. Cham: Springer; 2015. p. 389–401.
44. Posner K, Oquendo MA, Gould M, Stanley B, Davies M. Columbia Classification Algorithm of Suicide Assessment (C-CASA): classification of suicidal events in the FDA's pediatric suicidal risk analysis of antidepressants. Am J Psychiatry. 2007;164:1035–43.
45. R Core Team. R: A language and environment for statistical computing. Vienna, Austria: R Foundation for Statistical Computing; 2014.
46. Turecki G, Brent DA. Suicide and suicidal behaviour. Lancet. 2016;387:1227–39.
47. Ford E, Carroll JA, Smith HE, Scott D, Cassell JA. Extracting information from the text of electronic medical records to improve case detection: a systematic review. J Am Med Inform Assoc. 2016;23:1007–15.
48. Ford E, Campion A, Chamles DA, Habash-Bailey H. "You don't immediately stick a label on them": a qualitative study of influences on general practitioners' recording of anxiety disorders. BMJ Open [Internet]. bmjopen.bmj.com; 2016; Available from: http://bmjopen.bmj.com/content/6/6/e010746.short
49. Wu S, Miller T, Masanz J, Coarr M, Halgrim S, Carrell D, et al. Negation's not solved: generalizability versus optimizability in clinical natural language processing. PLoS One. 2014;9:e112774.
50. Harkema H, Dowling JN, Thornblade T, Chapman WW. ConText: an algorithm for determining negation, experiencer, and temporal status from clinical reports. J Biomed Inform. 2009;42:839–51.
51. Chapman WW, Bridewell W, Hanbury P, Cooper GF, Buchanan BG. Evaluation of negation phrases in narrative clinical reports. Proc AMIA Symp. 2001:105–9.
52. Chapman WW, Bridewell W, Hanbury P, Cooper GF, Buchanan BG. A simple algorithm for identifying negated findings and diseases in discharge summaries. J Biomed Inform. 2001;34:301–10.
53. Sohn S, Wu S, Chute CG. Dependency Parser-based Negation Detection in Clinical Narratives. AMIA Jt Summits Transl Sci Proc. 2012;2012:1–8.
54. Garla V, Lo Re V III, Dorey-Stein Z, Kidwai F, Scotch M, Womack J, et al. The Yale cTAKES extensions for document classification: architecture and application. J Am Med Inform Assoc. 2011;18:614–20.
55. Gkotsis G, Velupillai S, Oellrich A, Dean H, Liakata M, Dutta R. Don't Let Notes Be Misunderstood: A Negation Detection Method for Assessing Risk of Suicide in Mental Health Records. In: Proceedings of the Third Workshop on Computational Lingusitics and Clinical Psychology. Association for Computational Linguistics; 2016. p. 95–105.
56. Crandall C, Fullerton-Gleason L, Aguero R, LaValley J. Subsequent suicide mortality among emergency department patients seen for suicidal behavior. Acad Emerg Med. 2006;13:435–42.
57. Chock MM, Bommersbach TJ, Geske JL, Bostwick JM. Patterns of Health Care Usage in the Year before Suicide: A Population-Based Case-Control Study. Mayo Clin Proc. 2015;90:1475–81.
58. Metzger M-H, Tvardik N, Gicquel Q, Bouvry C, Poulet E, Potinet-Pagliaroli V. Use of emergency department electronic medical records for automated epidemiological surveillance of suicide attempts: a French pilot study. Int J Methods Psychiatr Res [Internet]. Wiley Online. Library. 2017;26 Available from: https://doi.org/10.1002/mpr.1522
59. Walsh CG, Ribeiro JD, Franklin JC. Predicting Risk of Suicide Attempts Over Time Through Machine Learning. Clin Psychol Sci. SAGE Publications Inc. 2017;5:457–69.
60. Jagannatha AN, Yu H. Bidirectional RNN for Medical Event Detection in Electronic Health Records. Proc Conf. 2016;2016:473–82.
61. Mikolov T, Sutskever I, Chen K, Corrado GS, Dean J. Distributed Representations of Words and Phrases and their Compositionality. In: Burges CJC, Bottou L, Welling M, Ghahramani Z, Weinberger KQ, editors. Advances in Neural Information Processing Systems 26. Curran Associates, Inc; 2013. p. 3111–9.
62. Mikolov T, Chen K, Corrado G, Dean J. Efficient Estimation of Word Representations in Vector Space [Internet]. arXiv [cs.CL]. 2013. Available from: http://arxiv.org/abs/1301.3781
63. McCoy TH Jr, Castro VM, Roberson AM, Snapper LA, Perlis RH. Improving Prediction of Suicide and Accidental Death After Discharge From General Hospitals With Natural Language Processing. JAMA Psychiatry. 2016;73:1064–71.
64. Leonard Westgate C, Shiner B, Thompson P, Watts BV. Evaluation of Veterans' Suicide Risk With the Use of Linguistic Detection Methods. Psychiatr Serv. 2015;66:1051–6.
65. Roberts A. Language, Structure, and Reuse in the Electronic Health Record. AMA J Ethics. 2017;19:281–8.
66. Pestian J, Nasrallah H, Matykiewicz P, Bennett A, Leenaars A. Suicide Note Classification Using Natural Language Processing: A Content Analysis. Biomed Inform Insights. 2010;2010:19–28.
67. Pestian JP, Grupp-Phelan J, Bretonnel Cohen K, Meyers G, Richey LA, Matykiewicz P, et al. A Controlled Trial Using Natural Language Processing to Examine the Language of Suicidal Adolescents in the Emergency Department. Suicide Life Threat Behav. 2016;46:154–9.
68. Appleby L. Suicide during pregnancy and in the first postnatal year. BMJ. 1991;302:137–40.
69. Gold KJ, Singh V, Marcus SM, Palladino CL. Mental health, substance use and intimate partner problems among pregnant and postpartum suicide victims in the National Violent Death Reporting System. Gen Hosp Psychiatry. 2012;34:139–45.

9

Patient portal adoption and use by hospitalized cancer patients

Duaa Aljabri[1*], Adrian Dumitrascu[2], M. Caroline Burton[2], Launia White[3], Mahmud Khan[5], Sudha Xirasagar[5], Ronnie Horner[5] and James Naessens[4]

Abstract

Background: Portal use has been studied among outpatients, but its utility and impact on inpatients is unclear. This study describes portal adoption and use among hospitalized cancer patients and investigates associations with selected safety, utilization, and satisfaction measures.

Methods: A retrospective review of 4594 adult hospitalized cancer patients was conducted between 2012 and 2014 at Mayo Clinic in Jacksonville, Florida, comparing portal adopters, who registered for a portal account prior to hospitalization, with nonadopters. Adopters were classified by their portal activity during hospitalization as active or inactive inpatient users. Univariate and several logistic and linear regression models were used for analysis.

Results: Of total patients, 2352 (51.2%) were portal adopters, and of them, 632 (26.8%) were active inpatient users. Portal adoption was associated with patients who were young, female, married, with higher income, and had more frequent hospitalizations ($P < .05$). Active inpatient use was associated with patients who were young, married, nonlocals, with higher disease severity, and were hospitalized for medical treatment ($P < .05$). In univariate analyses, self-management knowledge scores were higher among adopters vs nonadopters (84.3 and 80.0, respectively; $P = .01$) and among active vs inactive inpatient users (87.0 and 83.3, respectively; $P = .04$). In regression models adjusted for age and disease severity, the association between portal behaviors and majority of measures were not significant ($P > .05$).

Conclusions: Over half of our cancer inpatients adopted a portal prior to hospitalization, with increased adoption associated with predisposing and enabling determinants (eg: age, sex, marital status, income), and increased inpatient use associated with need (eg: nonlocal residence and disease severity). Additional research and greater effort to expand the portal functionality is needed to impact inpatient outcomes.

Keywords: Adverse events, Cancer, Hospitalization, Portal, Satisfaction, Utilization

Background

Two decades ago, the National Academy of Medicine (formerly the Institute of Medicine) recommended implementation of electronic health records to improve quality of care in the United States [1]. Since then, health information technologies have been rapidly adopted, with a focus on providers rather than patients. In 1996, the Health Insurance Portability and Accountability Act legally allowed patients to access their own clinical records. However, record retrieval fees, illegible handwriting, and time delays hindered accessibility [2]. An additional challenge is the fragmented health system with many independently owned and operated health care service locations [3–5]. An integrated information system that aggregates and offers updated health information to patients through a single access point was needed. In 2009, the Health Information Technology for Economic and Clinical Health Act incentivized clinicians

* Correspondence: daljabri@email.sc.edu
[1]Department of Health Sciences Research, Mayo Clinic, Jacksonville, FL, USA

to provide patients with electronic access to clinical records through meaningful use rules, administered by the Centers for Medicare & Medicaid Services [6]. This incentive program remains the principal driver of patient portal development by funding nearly $30 billion in provider incentives to encourage appropriate use [7, 8]. Investigations where information access was offered via patient portals in the outpatient settings showed encouraging positive effects in patient satisfaction and self-management behaviors [4, 9–18]. However, providing patients access to information is important not only in home and outpatient settings, but also when patients are hospitalized [19].

When patients are able to see their own health information during the hospital stay, they become more informed, empowered to ask questions, and gain ownership of their health care [20, 21]. Despite daily bedside rounds, important patient informational needs may not be met due to the cost of reviewing tailored information with each patient individually [22]. Thus, the portal technology may provide opportunity for inpatients to meet informational needs, facilitate awareness, and improve understanding of their care during hospitalization and after discharge [2, 23]. Meeting informational needs could reduce uncertainties surrounding the care process, reduce information asymmetry between patients and providers, promote shared decision-making, and increase patient self-management and adherence to care [24, 25].

Unfortunately, assessments of patient portal use among hospitalized cancer patients are limited [8, 26–30]. For many patients, the hospital is a challenging and intimidating setting, compounded by unmet information needs and limited patient engagement [24, 31]. The rapid dynamic and pace of clinical care, changing medical teams, reliance on verbal communication, and absence of an established relationship with the care providers further challenge patients' effective participation in their own care [32, 33]. Additional affective and emotional challenges are faced by inpatients with cancer due to the nature of their disease, frequently uncertain outcomes of treatments, and the need to understand their multiple active conditions to make treatment decisions [34, 35]. In a study of breast cancer patients, those who desired an active role in treatment decision making also desired detailed information of their diagnosis, treatment procedures, and alternatives [36]. Similar information needs were vital to gynecologic and colorectal cancer patients who felt that information about the likelihood of cure, spread of disease, and treatment options were priorities for decision making [37]. Providing clinical information through patient portals may have the potential to transform the patient-physician relationship and help patients to become active in their disease management [38]. Recent documentation on hospital-based patient portals is encouraging [39–42]. Creber et al. published a protocol for developing a personalized inpatient portal at an urban academic medical center to improve cardiology inpatients engagement [2]. Greysen et al. conducted pilot interviews showing patients' enthusiasm for a tablet application that provides health information during their inpatient stay [43]. Vawdrey et al. assessed the patient-perceived efficacy of tablets to improve cardiothoracic surgery patients' engagement in care, showing a favorable response regarding usability of the application [19]. Several other studies assessed the feasibility of web-based applications to increase patient engagement in both pediatric and adult care [44–46]. Yet, the evaluation of patient portals among cancer inpatients is still limited, a knowledge gap addressed by this study. We hypothesized that patient adoption of a portal and active use during a hospital stay may be associated with greater patient safety, postdischarge care utilization and satisfaction, similar to outpatient settings. According to Karahanna et al., adoption and continued use represent different behaviors [47]. Adoption is the initial enrollment and signifies receptivity to the portal, while usage represents active engagement, continued use after adoption. Therefore we distinguish between these 2 behaviors and evaluate them separately. Our specific aims were to 1) identify the key patient factors predicting adoption and active inpatient use behaviors, and 2) examine the association between portal use behaviors and adverse events, post-discharge utilization (emergency visits and readmissions), and selected patient satisfaction measures (self-health management knowledge and satisfaction with the overall hospital experience).

Methods

Study setting and description of the portal

The site of the study was Mayo Clinic, Jacksonville, Florida (MCF), a large nonprofit, specialized tertiary care practice and medical research center with more than 1.3 million domestic and international patients seen each year. Physicians are salaried, not linked to care volume, thus reducing monetary incentives in patient treatment. MCF contracted with Cerner Solutions (Cerner Corp) to implement the patient portal and integrate it with the system-wide electronic health record in 2010. When patients schedule an appointment at MCF, they are invited to register for a portal account and are provided with information on why and how to register. With each appointment reminder, patients receive a reminder message to register for the portal. Portal invitations are also offered in all outpatient waiting areas and displayed on electronic screens around the clinic.

Once registered, patients' are able to access informational functions, such as viewing lab results, current medications, allergies, and diagnostic reports from clinic visits and hospitalizations, and administrative functions, such as paying bills, processing prescription refills, and

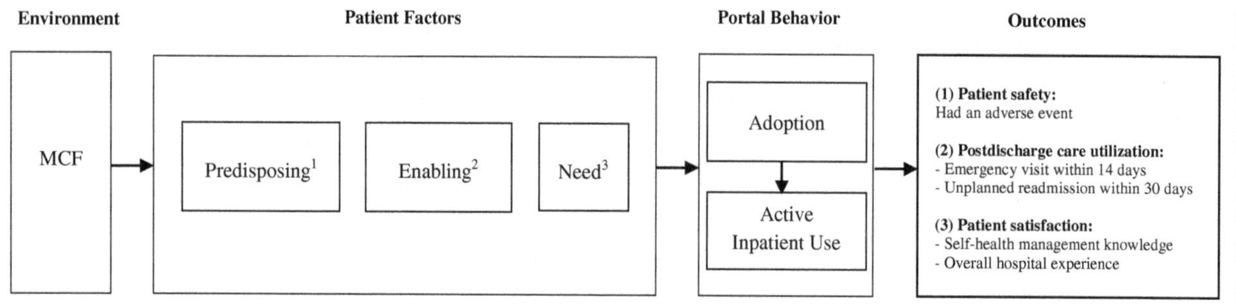

Fig. 1 Study Theoretical Model Derived from Andersen's Model of Healthcare Utilization. 1 Predisposing factors: age, sex, and race. 2 Enabling factors: marital status, employment status, health insurance type, and income. 3 Need factors: geographic area of residence, comorbidities, and frequency of hospitalizations. Additional need factors related to the admission: MSDRG type and APRDRG disease severity weight. APRDRG indicates All Patients Refined Diagnostic Related Group; MSDRG, Medicare Severity-Diagnosis Related Group

coordinating appointments. A Continuity of Care Document, a complete summary of patient current health status and history, is also available to view, download, or forward to physicians at other hospitals. Additional information on MCF patient portal is documented elsewhere [48]. Although the portal is designed for outpatients, some functions are applicable to inpatient health information needs during the hospital stay. Hospitalized patients potentially have time to access the portal when they are not occupied with diagnostic testing or other activities [49]. For example, the portal gives inpatients real-time access to laboratory results, admission notes, consultation reports, and surgical notes, to view on their own time and between bedside rounds. This functionality potentially facilitates patient communication and interaction with the health care team during their stay, and empowers the patient to be more attentive toward errors in documentation [20]. In addition, the medication function provides patients with information on the type and purpose of their medications, including in-hospital medication intake, which could enable patients to ask questions, review for accuracy, or report medication discrepancies [50, 51]. Before home discharge, a discharge summary and discharge instructions is uploaded to the portal, giving patients time to review closely and ensure their understanding of home self-management instructions. While the development of portal functionality for inpatients is in early stages, the offered content may still help patients become more activated and improve postdischarge care.

Study design and participants

This was a retrospective review of patients satisfying the following criteria: 1) adults 18 years of age or older, 2) cancer as a primary or secondary diagnosis at time of hospitalization identified through the *International Classification of Diseases, Ninth Revision* (ICD-9) codes, and 3) admitted to MCF between August 1, 2012, and July 31, 2014 ($N = 4594$). Per the unified theory of acceptance of use of technology, user acceptance and intention to use a technology is followed by actual use [52]. Therefore, we included the first hospitalization where a portal account had been established prior to admission to examine consequent inpatient use. If the patient had not established a portal account prior to any admission, then the first hospitalization in the study period was selected. Patients who had a portal account prior to admission were defined as *adopters*, and those without a portal account were *nonadopters*. Among adopters, inpatients who logged in their portal during the hospital stay were *active inpatient users* and those who never logged in were referred to as *inactive inpatient users*. The study was approved by the Mayo Clinic Institutional Review Board.

Study model

Our study was informed by Andersen's Model of Healthcare Utilization [53]. The model was initially developed in 1968 to understand health services use and later revised to include consumer satisfaction and dimensions of health status [54]. Shortly after the model was developed, health services use was portrayed as a health behavior influenced by multiple factors [55]. According to the World Health Organization, health behavior is defined as "any activity undertaken by an individual, regardless of actual or perceived health status, for the purpose of promoting, protecting or maintaining health, whether or not such behavior is objectively effective towards that end" [56]. Because the portal is a tool to maintain and promote health, we considered portal adoption and use as health behaviors that could be studied using Andersen's model. As shown in Fig. 1, we examined the influence of patients' characteristics in three major components: predisposing, enabling, and need factors, on portal adoption and use behaviors.

Measures

Environment and patient characteristics

In this study, we assumed that all study participants had a common environmental context, as all patients in

MCF received their care in the same structure. Predisposing determinants included age, sex, and race. Enabling determinants included marital status, employment status, health insurance type, and median income in the residential ZIP code less than Florida's state median income, a surrogate for socioeconomic status. Need factors included geographic area of residence, comorbidities, and frequency of hospitalizations in the study period. Additional need determinants related to the hospital admission included patient's disease severity weight as measured by the 3 M All Patients Refined Diagnosis Related Groups (APDRG) classification system, and whether the hospitalization was for medical or surgical treatment, based on the Medicare Severity-Diagnosis Related Group (MSDRG) codes [57].

Demographic data were extracted from the patient electronic health records. The ZIP code median income was obtained from the 2006–2010 American Community Survey and matched to the patient sample at the ZIP code level [58]. A count of comorbidities included in Charlson Comorbidity Index during the 12 months prior to hospitalization was documented [59].

Patient safety, utilization, and satisfaction

We examined selected patients' measures to investigate associations with portal use. For patient safety, we studied the occurrence or otherwise of provider-reported, in-hospital, adverse events, such as falls, accidental self-injuries, or other events related to the surgery, vascular, equipment or devices, medication, or skin events, obtained from quality management services. For postdischarge utilization, we examined the occurrence of emergency department visits within 14 days and unplanned readmissions within 30 days, both obtained from the hospital records. We measured patient satisfaction by obtaining data from the Hospital Consumer Assessment of Healthcare Providers and Systems (HCAHPS) survey. The survey is a validated instrument used since 2006 to assess patients' perspectives of hospital care, and distributed to a random sample of discharged patients between 2 days and 6 weeks after discharge [60]. While the survey included many important questions, we selected the relevant items with highest response. We measured *patient self-health management knowledge* with 2 questions: "When I left the hospital, I had a good understanding of the things I was responsible for in managing my health", and "When I left the hospital, I clearly understood the purpose for taking each of my medications", and measured *overall hospital satisfaction* with 1 question: "Using any number from 0 to 10, where 0 is the worst hospital possible and 10 is the best hospital possible, what number would you use to rate this hospital during your stay" [61]. Responses were transformed and averaged, resulting in a 0 to 100 linear-scaled score.

Data analysis

We described the characteristics of cancer patients according to their portal adoption and inpatient activity behaviors, and examined differences between groups using Pearson χ^2 and Wilcoxon nonparametric tests. Multivariate regression models were conducted to predict factors associated with portal adoption and active inpatient use, as well as to examine the association between selected outcomes and portal behaviors. All analyses were conducted in SAS Version 9.4 (SAS Institute Inc., Cary, North Carolina, USA), and significance was defined as $P < .05$.

Results

Participants, adopters, and active inpatient users

Of the 4594 study-eligible hospitalized patients with cancer, 2352 (51.2%) had a portal account prior to admission (ie, adopters), of whom 632 (26.8%) used the portal account during their hospital stay (ie, active inpatient users). Patient characteristics at admission were reported in Table 1. Significant differences in patient characteristics were present among portal adoption and inpatient use behaviors (Table 2). Adoption was influenced by a majority of predisposing and enabling factors, such as age, sex, race, marital status, employment status, income, and type of health insurance. While active inpatient use was similarly influenced by predisposing and enabling factors, such as age, race, and marital status, we found greater influence associated with need, such as having greater disease severity, being nonlocal, and admitted for medical rather than surgical treatment.

Bivariate associations of portal behaviors with adverse events, care utilization, and patient satisfaction

Bivariate associations of portal adoption with our selected measures (Table 3) showed that adopters had more emergency visits and readmissions than nonadopters, while reporting higher self-health management knowledge. Similarly, active inpatient users had more readmissions than inactive inpatient users, and marginally higher self-management scores. Logistic and linear regression analyses showed that after adjusting for age and disease severity, the association between portal behaviors and majority of our assessed measures were not significant (Table 4). Adverse events and overall hospital experience did not differ among groups in either univariate or multivariate regression analyses ($P > .05$).

Discussion

To date there remains a gap in the literature evaluating the use of inpatient portals among cancer patients. This study provides important information to clinicians, administrators, and researchers, on the key patient determinants associated with portal adoption and use. Prior

Table 1 Sample Baseline Characteristics by Portal Behavior[a]

Characteristics		Adopters ($n = 2{,}352$)	Nonadopters ($n = 2{,}242$)	*P* value	Active Inpatient Users ($n = 632$)	Inactive Inpatient Users ($n = 1{,}720$)	*P* value
Age group (years)	Mean (SD)	62.3 (14.0)	65.4 (14.8)	<.01[b]	60.2 (14.3)	63.0 (13.8)	<.01[b]
	≤44	259 (11.0)	191 (8.5)	<.01[c]	82 (13.0)	177 (10.3)	<.01[c]
	45-54	339 (14.4)	281 (12.5)		106 (16.8)	233 (13.5)	
	55-64	632 (26.9)	480 (21.4)		185 (29.3)	447 (26.0)	
	65-74	702 (29.8)	652 (29.1)		166 (26.3)	536 (31.2)	
	75-84	339 (14.4)	454 (20.2)		80 (12.7)	259 (15.1)	
	≥85	81 (3.4)	184 (8.2)		13 (2.1)	68 (4.0)	
Sex	Female	1,148 (48.8)	1,055 (47.0)	.25[c]	295 (46.7)	852 (49.5)	.22[c]
	Male	1,204 (51.2)	1,188 (53.0)		337 (53.3)	869 (50.5)	
Race	African American	121 (5.2)	273 (12.4)	<.01[c]	18 (2.9)	103 (6.1)	<.01[c]
	White	2,120 (91.3)	1847 (84.0)		575 (91.9)	1,545 (91.2)	
	Other	80 (3.4)	78 (3.5)		33 (5.3)	47 (2.8)	
Marital status	Married	1,786 (75.9)	1,454 (64.9)	<.01[c]	506 (80.1)	1,280 (74.4)	<.01[c]
	Single/divorced/widowed	566 (24.1)	788 (35.1)		126 (19.9)	440 (25.6)	
Employment status	Employed	739 (37.7)	547 (28.9)	<.01[c]	206 (38.1)	533 (37.5)	.79[c]
	Retired	836 (42.6)	935 (49.4)		208 (38.5)	628 (44.2)	
	Not employed/disabled	386 (19.7)	411 (21.7)		126 (23.3)	260 (18.3)	
Income	Below Florida median income	645 (28.3)	803 (37.2)	<.01[c]	167 (26.5)	478 (27.8)	.54[c]
	At or above Florida median income	1,707 (71.7)	1,439 (64.1)		465 (73.5)	1,242 (72.2)	
Health insurance	Commercial insurance/self pay	1,145 (48.7)	815 (36.4)	<.01[c]	339 (53.6)	806 (46.9)	<.01[c]
	Medicare/Medicaid/other government assistance	1,207 (51.3)	1,427 (63.6)		293 (46.4)	914 (53.1)	
Geographic area of residence	Nonlocal	521 (22.2)	493 (22.0)	.89[c]	166 (26.3)	335 (20.6)	<.01[c]
	Local	1,831 (77.8)	1,749 (78.0)		466 (73.7)	1,365 (79.4)	
Comorbidity [d]	None	1,115 (47.4)	1,052 (46.9)	.58[c]	289 (45.7)	826 (48.0)	.32[c]
	One or more	1,237 (52.6)	1,190 (53.1)		343 (54.3)	894 (52.0)	
Comorbidity type[e]	Congestive heart failure	145 (6.2)	171 (7.6)	.05[c]	51 (8.1)	94 (5.5)	.02[c]
	Peripheral vascular disease	322 (13.7)	338 (15.1)	.18[c]	83 (13.1)	239 (13.9)	.63[c]
	Cerebrovascular disease	165 (7.0)	224 (10.0)	<.01[c]	42 (6.6)	123 (7.2)	.67[c]
	Chronic pulmonary disease	262 (11.1)	256 (11.4)	.77[c]	61 (9.7)	201 (11.7)	.16[c]
	Mild liver disease	432 (18.4)	291 (13.0)	<.01[c]	129 (20.4)	303 (17.6)	.12[c]
	Diabetes mellitus	392 (16.7)	351 (15.7)	.35[c]	115 (18.2)	277 (16.1)	.23[c]
	Moderate/severe renal disease	196 (8.3)	179 (8.0)	.66[c]	53 (8.4)	143 (8.3)	.96[c]
	Moderate/severe liver disease	121 (5.1)	86 (3.8)	.03[c]	49 (7.8)	72 (4.2)	<.01[c]
Admission type based on MSDRG	Surgical	1,504 (63.9)	1,315 (58.7)	<.01[b]	348 (55.1)	1,156 (67.2)	<.01[b]
	Medical	848 (36.1)	927 (41.3)		284 (44.9)	564 (32.8)	
Frequency of hospitalizations, mean (SD)		1.8 (1.5)	1.4 (1.1)	<.01[b]	2.0 (1.7)	1.7 (1.4)	<.01[b]
APRDRG weight, mean, (median, SD)		2.5 (1.5, 2.9)	2.3 (1.5, 2.3)	.24[b]	3.1 (1.9, 3.6)	2.3 (1.4, 2.6)	<.01[b]

Abbreviations: APRDRG All Patients Refined Diagnosis Related Group, *MSDRG* Medicare Severity-Diagnosis Related Group

[a]Data are reported as No. (%) for count variables and mean (SD) for continuous variables

[b]Wilcoxon nonparmetric

[c]Pearson χ^2 test

[d]Comorbidity groups are not mutually exclusive as a patient may have more than 1 comorbidity diagnosis

[e]Comorbidity type was reported for diseases with > 5% of patients

Table 2 Logistic Regression Analysis Showing the Predictors of Portal Behaviors

Factors	Characteristics		Odds Ratio (95% CI)[a]	
			Adoption[b]	Active Inpatient Use[c]
Predisposing	Age	44-	**1.42 (1.03, 1.95)**	**1.89 (1.16, 3.06)**
		45-54	1.10 (0.82, 1.47)	**1.73 (1.10, 2.72)**
		55-64	1.22 (0.95, 1.57)	**1.48 (1.00, 2.19)**
		65-74 (reference)	1.00	1.00
		75-84	**0.71 (0.57, 0.87)**	1.08 (0.75, 1.56)
		85+	**0.36 (0.24, 0.54)**	0.77 (0.34, 1.75)
	Sex	Male (reference)	1.00	1.00
		Female	**1.26 (1.10, 1.45)**	0.97 (0.78, 1.21)
	Race	White (reference)	1.00	1.00
		African American	**0.34 (0.27, 0.45)**	**0.51 (0.29, 0.89)**
		Others	0.84 (0.58, 1.23)	1.39 (0.82, 2.37)
Enabling	Marital status	Divorced/single/widowed (reference)	1.00	1.00
		Married	**1.60 (1.37, 1.87)**	**1.49 (1.14, 1.94)**
	Employment	Employed (reference)	1.00	1.00
		Retired	1.04 (0.83, 1.30)	1.04 (0.75, 1.46)
		Not employed/disabled	**0.70 (0.57, 0.86)**	1.04 (0.77, 1.40)
	Health insurance	Commercial insurance (reference)	1.00	1.00
		Medicaid/Medicare	**0.76 (0.61, 0.95)**	1.07 (0.77, 1.50)
	Income	Below FL median income (reference)	1.00	1.00
		At or above FL median income	**1.39 (1.20, 1.60)**	1.10 (0.87, 1.39)
Need	Geographic area of residence	Local (reference)	1.00	1.00
		Nonlocal	1.13 (0.96, 1.33)	**1.34 (1.04, 1.71)**
	Comorbidities	None (reference)	1.00	1.00
		1+	1.05 (0.91, 1.21)	0.97 (0.77, 1.22)
	MSDRG type [d]	Surgical (reference)	-	1.00
		Medical	-	**2.17 (1.68, 2.78)**
	Frequency of hospitalizations		**1.43 (1.33, 1.55)**	1.08 (0.99, 1.19)
	APRDRG weight [d]		-	**1.13 (1.09, 1.17)**

Abbreviations: APRDRG All Patients Refined Diagnosis Related Group, *MSDRG* Medicare Severity-Diagnosis Related Group
[a]Bold values are statistically significant at $P<.05$. Odds ratios greater than 1 imply increased chance for behavior; less than 1 imply decreased chance for behavior
[b]Predictors for adoption: age, sex, race, marital status, employment status, income, health insurance type, and frequency of hospitalizations
[c]Predictors for active inpatient use: age, race, marital status, geographic area of residence, APRDRG weight, and MSDRG type
[d]Variables related to the hospital admission were not examined among adopters as the adoption behavior was established prior to admission

studies reported significant interest in patient portals among oncology populations [28, 29, 62]. Yet, to our knowledge, this is the first study to examine portal use in a large inpatient oncology cohort. In this sample, we found that portal adoption and use during hospitalization has reached modest levels and somewhat higher usage than published reports on inpatient portal use. Over half of our inpatient oncology population voluntarily adopted the portal before hospital admission and 27% actively used the portal during the stay. Dumitrascu et al. found that of 44.2% patients who had a portal account at the time of admission, only 20.8% accessed the portal during their stay [48]. Davis et al. found that of 34.4% registered portal patients, 23.4% used it while hospitalized [39]. Robinson et al. reported that 16% of surgical inpatients with a portal account used it while being in the hospital [63].

There were noteworthy differences in patient characteristics between adopters and nonadopters in a majority of predisposing and enabling factors. Portal adoption increased among patients who were female, married, and with higher income, and decreased among patients who were African American, unemployed, and had governmental health insurance. Interestingly, the likelihood of portal adoption was similar for patients aged 65 to 75 years as the middle-aged adults 45 to 55 years, contradicting popular beliefs that older patients were less

Table 3 Adverse Events, Postdischarge Care Utilization and Patient Satisfaction Among the portal Behavior Groups

Measures	Outcomes	Adopters ($n = 2352$)	Nonadopters ($n = 2242$)	P value	Active Inpatient Users ($n = 632$)	Inactive Inpatient Users ($n = 1720$)	P value
Patient safety	Had an adverse event, No. (%)	40 (1.7)	47 (2.1)	.36[a]	13 (2.1)	27 (1.6)	.42[a]
Postdischarge care utilization	Emergency visit within 14-days of discharge, No. (%)	272 (11.6)	214 (9.5)	.03[a]	75 (11.9)	197 (11.5)	.78[a]
	30-day unplanned r eadmission, No. (%)	299 (12.7)	222 (9.9)	<.01[a]	96 (15.2)	203 (11.8)	.03[a]
Patient satisfaction[c]	Understand responsibilities for self-health management, mean score (SD)	87.6 (19.6)	85.5 (20.1)	.02[b]	89.1 (18.4)	87.1 (20.0)	.22[b]
	Understand the purpose for taking each medication, mean score (SD)	90.0 (18.8)	87.8 (20.9)	.05[b]	91.8 (16.0)	89.4 (19.7)	.21[b]
	Aggregate self-health management knowledge score	84.3 (21.3)	80.0 (23.1)	<.01[b]	87.0 (19.2)	83.3 (21.9)	.05[b]
	Overall rating of the hospital stay, mean score (SD)	95.6 (9.1)	95.3 (10.3)	.75[b]	95.6 (10.5)	95.7 (8.6)	.56[b]

[a]Pearson χ^2 test
[b]Wilcoxon nonparametric
[c]Satisfaction survey was distributed to a random sample of discharges; thus, the sample size was as follows: adopters; $n = 788$, nonadopters; $n = 646$, active inpatient users; $n = 205$, and inactive inpatient users; $n = 577$

likely to engage in health technologies [64]. Portal adoption, however, considerably decreased among patients aged over 75 years. Similar to our findings, portal use among outpatient oncology patients was reported to be greater among younger, white patients, and those with upper aerodigestive malignancy diagnosis, greater disease severity, and case complexity [8]. Among nononcology populations, a similar digital divide was reported by age groups, race/ethnicity, income, and education [65–70]. Our findings showed higher portal adoption among those with more frequent hospitalizations, which was the only notable need determinant. Other studies have reported higher interest in the portal among those with more medical problems, greater severity of illness, or higher than average clinical need [10, 15, 71, 72].

Similarly, inpatient portal use increased with younger age and being married, but more influenced with need determinants. Active access was associated with residing outside the city of Jacksonville (nonlocals); suggesting that commuting patients found health information important to view during the stay. Additionally, access was greater among those with higher disease severity and those admitted for medical rather than surgical treatment. Medical admissions for cancer patients are usually associated with investigating the origin and cause of disease, or evaluating chemo or radiation treatments, compared to surgical admissions that involve typical procedural routines and surgical recovery that may fully occupy the patient's time in the hospital [73]. Because a cancer diagnosis is a stressful life event, patients'

Table 4 Association Between Patient Outcomes and Portal Behaviors: Results From Regression Models

	Independent Variables			
	Active Inpatient Users vs Nonadopters		Inactive inpatient Users vs Nonadopters	
Dependent Variables[a]	OR (95% CI)	P value	OR (95% CI)	P value
[adverse events = yes]	0.76 (0.40, 1.45)	.41	0.71 (0.44–1.16)	.17
[emergency visits = yes]	1.28 (0.97, 1.70)	.08	1.23 (1.00–1.51)	.08
[readmissions = yes]	1.60 (1.23, 2.08)	<.01	1.21 (0.99–1.48)	.06
Dependent Variables[a]	Beta Coefficient	P value	Beta Coefficient	P value
Self-health management knowledge	2.18	.07	1.15	.17
Overall hospital experience	0.16	.83	0.28	.60

[a]Five regression models were conducted adjusting for age and disease severity. Logistic regression was used for adverse events, emergency visits, and readmissions. Linear regression was used for self-health management knowledge and overall hospital experience scores

information-seeking behavior was thought to become more active, possibly as a coping strategy to overcome uncertainties [27, 29, 74].

Patient safety

Several studies have assumed that information technology systems have the potential to improve patient safety by identifying errors in medications and preventing adverse drug reactions. Yet, limited evidence exists regarding the effectiveness of a portal as a tool in reducing adverse events. One recent study by Kelly et al. found that 8% of parents with hospitalized children recognized errors in their child's medication list after using an inpatient portal application [46]. Further optimistic views about the ability of portals to reduce errors were derived from patient participation in care, where patients could notify clinicians of their medication allergies, unexpected toxicity symptoms, and lapses in care to prevent adverse events [50, 75–77]. Among surgical inpatients who were portal users, postoperative infection was their most frequent ICD-9 code, suggesting that experiencing a safety-event may activate patients to follow up their personal health information to avoid further complications [63]. In contrast to this evidence, our study did not find an association between portal adoption or use and adverse events. Likewise, a randomized controlled trial by Weingart et al. did not find sufficient evidence to support an association between adverse drug events and portal use [51]. Earlier research reported that patient history evaluation in cancer care is more focused, providing the patient an opportunity to recall medical and medication information to prevent errors. [78, 79] In addition, most adverse events at hospitals are underreported and the events in our data were limited to those reported by providers. A new initiative within the portal that is gaining popularity and has the potential to prevent errors is the OpenNotes national movement, which invites patients to read their clinicians' notes online and report back errors or safety concerns that, in turn, may avert mistakes from happening [80, 81]. Hence, it opens up a new possibility to engage patients as safety partners through their reported documentation errors.

Utilization

Studies that examined the effect of portal use on subsequent utilization of health services showed mixed results [10, 67, 82]. A study using propensity score matching found no difference between portal users and nonusers on clinical service utilization [83]. Among members of Kaiser Permanente, a retrospective study in the Northwest found that patient access to an online portal was associated with decreased rates of primary care office visits and phone calls [84], whereas the opposite was found by Palen et al. where portal users had higher rates of office visits, phone encounters, after-hour clinic visits, emergency department visits, and hospitalizations [85]. The assumption was that if patients could view personal health information, they will be more aware, able to manage their health, and need less emergency service or hospitalizations. This expectation was not validated in our study, suggesting that a portal technology may be a complementary technology and does not substitute for health services needs of oncology patients. Mayer et al. reported 77.2% of cancer patients' visits to the emergency department were due to pain, respiratory problems, and gastrointestinal issues, with 63.2% of those visits resulting in hospital admission [86]. Barbera et al. reported that 83.8% of cancer patients who died had visited the emergency department during their final 6 months of life with issues related to abdominal pain, dyspnea, pneumonia, fatigue, and pleural effusion [87]. Shapiro et al. found that those who had surgery during their index admission were 3 times more likely to be readmitted [88]. Weaver et al. examined cancer inpatients and found 48% of readmissions were within 1 to 2 days of discharge [89]. Donze et al. developed a predictive model and found that discharge from an oncology service was a significant predictor of unplanned readmission [90]. Similarly, a recent systematic review reported that comorbidities, older age, advanced disease, and index hospitalization length of hospital stay were significant predictors for readmission in oncology [91]. Thus, emergency department visits and readmissions may be influenced more by the nature of illness, treatment-related complications, and other such factors than avoidable reasons by portal use.

Patient satisfaction

Our findings suggest limited evidence of the relationship between patient satisfaction and portal use. Self-management knowledge scores appear to be considerably higher among both adopters and inpatient users in bivariate associations; however, in regression analyses, associations with satisfaction were somewhat attenuated and no longer statistically significant. Our interpretation of results needs to be cautiously taken as they were limited by the random selection of sample surveyed and the selection of self-management questions. In addition, we have no assessment of self-health management knowledge at baseline. Therefore, the association between portal use and self-health management knowledge may be confounded.

Prior research has shown inconsistent conclusions regarding associations between portal use and patient satisfaction; with wide variability in the offered portal features, the outcomes evaluated, and the populations studied [4, 10, 14, 31]. In addition, the potential of patient portals for patients with chronic conditions is documented, but relatively nascent for cancer [92].

Among chronically ill patients, the portal showed promise for improving diabetic patients' satisfaction with care, ability to self-manage, and adhering to treatments [93]. This has been accompanied by evidence of improved blood pressure control among people with newly diagnosed hypertension [94]. Patient portal access was also superior in general adherence and satisfaction with doctor-patient communication among patients with congestive heart failure [18, 95]. Yet, not all findings in the literature showed that patients with chronic conditions were amenable to improved outcomes with portal use [29, 96–98].

There are many potential recommendations to improve portal functions for inpatients. Hospitals often provide patients and families with standard information on disease and treatment options while being hospitalized, but that is not always enough [99]. An effective tool for awareness and self-management may include problem-solving support, regular education provision, treatment options with cost estimations that aid patient decision making, and consistent patients training on how to take responsibility for their own health [100].

It should be noted that emotional factors, such as anxiety or low self-efficacy, may dramatically influence self-management or symptom-coping behaviors [101, 102]. Of interest, some researchers suggest technology-based applications to provide recreational social supports to help patients cope with their illness. O'Leary et al. reported favorable patient perceptions toward games offered in the hospital-based portal [40]. The same was reported by Jameson et al., who indicated that electronic gaming can be a positive distraction away from pain [103]. Innovative social support approaches offering recreational avenues via the portal may attract more users, which in turn, may improve self-management, symptom-coping, and quality of life [104]. Thus, greater attention is needed to improve the portal content and functionality for inpatients to improve patient outcomes.

This study has a number of limitations. There is limited generalizability given that our oncology cohort was from a single center. Technology limitations restricted our analysis; we could not examine frequency of inpatient log-ins, or distinguish if a portal activity was carried out by the patient or a delegated family member. Further, it would be interesting to understand if there was a dose-response type curve associated with portal use but information on the extent of use was not available. Post-discharge utilization measures were limited to care utilization at MCF, with no data on utilization elsewhere. Conclusions regarding patient safety and satisfaction measures were limited by the range of variable values; adverse events were uncommon, and patient satisfaction was almost uniformly high among all patients. Finally, low response to the HCAHPS resulted in a small sub-sample size to analyze satisfaction, a major limitation, but no other measures were readily available. Despite these limitations, the study uncovered determinants of adoption and use behaviors among a large sample of hospitalized cancer patients. Additionally, it adds new information to the growing body of literature on inpatient engagement using acute care portals. Future research directions should investigate the extent of inpatient portal use, incorporate inpatient-centered education materials, and improve the portal with functions that add the most value for cancer inpatients.

Conclusions

We found that cancer patients had reached modest levels of portal adoption. While portal adoption increased with predisposing and enabling determinants (eg: age, sex, marital status, income), active inpatient use increased with need (eg: commute residence and high disease severity). While these findings should be cautiously interpreted, the study adds to the growing evidence that patient portals should be further addressed for inpatient care. Particularly, the study provides insights for the informatics research community and those interested in improving inpatient care and self-management support through technology.

Abbreviations

HCAHPS: Hospital Consumer Assessment of Healthcare Providers and Systems; ICD-9: International Classification of Diseases, Ninth Revision; MCF: Mayo Clinic Florida

Acknowledgments

The authors thank March Rucci and Lisa Nordan from the Center for the Science of Healthcare Delivery at Mayo Clinic in Florida for input and support to complete the study.

Funding

No funding was received from any external source.

Authors' contributions

DIA led the research and performed all analyses and interpretation of data. AGD and MCB participated in the conception and design of the study. LJW made substantial contributions to the data acquisition. DIA drafted the manuscript and MK, RH, SX, and JMN critically revised the manuscript for important intellectual content. JMN was the senior author, confirmed approach and provided editorial support on the internal drafts of the paper. All authors read and approved the final manuscript.

Competing interests

The authors declare that they have no competing interests.

Author details

[1]Department of Health Sciences Research, Mayo Clinic, Jacksonville, FL, USA. [2]Division of Hospital Internal Medicine, Mayo Clinic, Jacksonville, FL, USA. [3]Division of Biomedical Statistics and Informatics, Mayo Clinic, Jacksonville, FL, USA. [4]Department of Health Sciences Research, Mayo Clinic, Rochester, MN, USA. [5]Department of Health Services Policy and Management, University of South Carolina, Columbia, SC, USA.

References

1. Crossing the Quality Chasm. A new health system for the 21st century. In: Washington (DC): Institute of Medicine (US) committee on quality of health care in America; 2001.
2. Masterson Creber R, Prey J, Ryan B, Alarcon I, Qian M, Bakken S, et al. Engaging hospitalized patients in clinical care: study protocol for a pragmatic randomized controlled trial. Contemp Clin Trials. 2016;47:165–71.
3. Furukawa MF, King J, Patel V, Hsiao CJ, Adler-Milstein J, Jha AK. Despite substantial progress in EHR adoption, health information exchange and patient engagement remain low in office settings. Health Aff (Millwood). 2014;33:1672–9.
4. Kruse CS, Bolton K, Freriks G. The effect of patient portals on quality outcomes and its implications to meaningful use: a systematic review. J Med Internet Res. 2015;17:e44.
5. Rittenhouse DR, Ramsay PP, Casalino LP, McClellan S, Kandel ZK, Shortell SM. Increased health information technology adoption and use among small primary care physician practices over time: a National Cohort Study. Ann Fam Med. 2017;15:56–62.
6. CMS. Electronic health records incentive programs. 2017. http://www.cms.gov/Regulations-and-Guidance/Legislation/EHRIncentivePrograms/index.html. Accessed 23 Feb 2018.
7. Blumenthal D. Launching HITECH. N Engl J Med. 2010;362:382–5.
8. Gerber DE, Laccetti AL, Chen B, Yan J, Cai J, Gates S, et al. Predictors and intensity of online access to electronic medical records among patients with cancer. J Oncol Pract. 2014;10:e307–12.
9. Ammenwerth E, Schnell-Inderst P, Hoerbst A. The impact of electronic patient portals on patient care: a systematic review of controlled trials. J Med Internet Res. 2012;14:e162.
10. Goldzweig CL, Orshansky G, Paige NM, Towfigh AA, Haggstrom DA, Miake-Lye I, et al. Electronic patient portals: evidence on health outcomes, satisfaction, efficiency, and attitudes: a systematic review. Ann Intern Med. 2013;159:677–87.
11. Hibbard JH, Greene J, Overton V. Patients with lower activation associated with higher costs; delivery systems should know their patients' 'scores'. Health Aff (Millwood). 2013;32:216–22.
12. Greene J, Hibbard JH. Why does patient activation matter? An examination of the relationships between patient activation and health-related outcomes. J Gen Intern Med. 2012;27:520–6.
13. Hibbard JH, Mahoney ER, Stock R, Tusler M. Do increases in patient activation result in improved self-management behaviors? Health Serv Res. 2007;42:1443–63.
14. Neuner J, Fedders M, Caravella M, Bradford L, Schapira M. Meaningful use and the patient portal: patient enrollment, use, and satisfaction with patient portals at a later-adopting center. Am J Med Qual. 2015;30:105–13.
15. Ralston JD, Carrell D, Reid R, Anderson M, Moran M, Hereford J. Patient web services integrated with a shared medical record: patient use and satisfaction. J Am Med Inform Assoc. 2007;14:798–806.
16. Osborn CY, Mayberry LS, Wallston KA, Johnson KB, Elasy TA. Understanding patient portal use: implications for medication management. J Med Internet Res. 2013;15:e133.
17. Horvath M, Levy J, L'Engle P, Carlson B, Ahmad A, Ferranti J. Impact of health portal enrollment with email reminders on adherence to clinic appointments: a pilot study. J Med Internet Res. 2011;13:e41.
18. Ross SE, Moore LA, Earnest MA, Wittevrongel L, Lin CT. Providing a web-based online medical record with electronic communication capabilities to patients with congestive heart failure: randomized trial. J Med Internet Res. 2004;6:e12.
19. Vawdrey DK, Wilcox LG, Collins SA, Bakken S, Feiner S, Boyer A, et al. A tablet computer application for patients to participate in their hospital care. AMIA Annu Symp Proc. 2011;2011:1428–35.
20. Gentles SJ, Lokker C, McKibbon KA. Health information technology to facilitate communication involving health care providers, caregivers, and pediatric patients: a scoping review. J Med Internet Res. 2010;12:e22.
21. Walker DM, Sieck CJ, Menser T, Huerta TR, Scheck McAlearney A. Information technology to support patient engagement: where do we stand and where can we go? J Am Med Inform Assoc. 2017;24:1088–94.
22. Bickmore TW, Pfeifer LM, Jack BW. Taking the time to care: empowering low health literacy hospital patients with virtual nurse agents. Proceedings of the SIGCHI Conference on Human Factors in Computing Systems (CHI '09). 2009; doi: https://doi.org/10.1145/1518701.1518891.
23. Roberts S, Chaboyer W, Gonzalez R, Marshall A. Using technology to engage hospitalised patients in their care: a realist review. BMC Health Serv Res. 2017;17:388.
24. Kaziunas E, Hanauer DA, Ackerman MS, Choi SW. Identifying unmet informational needs in the inpatient setting to increase patient and caregiver engagement in the context of pediatric hematopoietic stem cell transplantation. J Am Med Inform Assoc. 2016;23:94–104.
25. Prey JE, Restaino S, Vawdrey DK. Providing hospital patients with access to their medical records. AMIA Annu Symp Proc. 2014;2014:1884–93.
26. Borosund E, Cvancarova M, Moore SM, Ekstedt M, Ruland CM. Comparing effects in regular practice of e-communication and web-based self-management support among breast cancer patients: preliminary results from a randomized controlled trial. J Med Internet Res. 2014;16:e295.
27. Cahill JE, Lin L, LoBiondo-Wood G, Armstrong TS, Acquaye AA, Vera-Bolanos E, et al. Personal health records, symptoms, uncertainty, and mood in brain tumor patients. Neurooncol Pract. 2014;1:64–70.
28. Pai HH, Lau F, Barnett J, Jones S. Meeting the health information needs of prostate cancer patients using personal health records. Curr Oncol. 2013;20:e561–9.
29. Wiljer D, Leonard KJ, Urowitz S, Apatu E, Massey C, Quartey NK, et al. The anxious wait: assessing the impact of patient accessible EHRs for breast cancer patients. BMC Med Inform Decis Mak. 2010;10:46.
30. Wiljer D, Bogomilsky S, Catton P, Murray C, Stewart J, Minden M. Getting results for hematology patients through access to the electronic health record. Can Oncol Nurs J. 2006;16:154–64.
31. Woollen J, Prey J, Wilcox L, Sackeim A, Restaino S, Raza ST, et al. Patient experiences using an inpatient personal health record. Appl Clin Inform. 2016;7:446–60.
32. O'Leary KJ, Kulkarni N, Landler MP, Jeon J, Hahn KJ, Englert KM, et al. Hospitalized patients' understanding of their plan of care. Mayo Clin Proc. 2010;85:47–52.
33. Olson DP, Windish DM. Communication discrepancies between physicians and hospitalized patients. Arch Intern Med. 2010;170:1302–7.
34. Beckjord EB, Arora NK, McLaughlin W, Oakley-Girvan I, Hamilton AS, Hesse BW. Health-related information needs in a large and diverse sample of adult cancer survivors: implications for cancer care. J Cancer Surviv. 2008;2:179–89.
35. Kowalski C, Lee SY, Ansmann L, Wesselmann S, Pfaff H. Meeting patients' health information needs in breast cancer center hospitals - a multilevel analysis. BMC Health Serv Res. 2014;14:601.
36. Hack TF, Degner LF, Dyck DG. Relationship between preferences for decisional control and illness information among women with breast cancer: a quantitative and qualitative analysis. Soc Sci Med. 1994;39:279–89.
37. Beaver K, Booth K. Information needs and decision-making preferences: comparing findings for gynaecological, breast and colorectal cancer. Eur J Oncol Nurs. 2007;11:409–16.
38. Tang PC, Ash JS, Bates DW, Overhage JM, Sands DZ. Personal health records: definitions, benefits, and strategies for overcoming barriers to adoption. J Am Med Inform Assoc. 2006;13:121–6.
39. Davis SE, Osborn CY, Kripalani S, Goggins KM, Jackson GP. Health literacy, education levels, and patient portal usage during hospitalizations. AMIA Annu Symp Proc. 2015;2015:1871–80.
40. O'Leary KJ, Sharma RK, Killarney A, O'Hara LS, Lohman ME, Culver E, et al. Patients' and healthcare providers' perceptions of a mobile portal application for hospitalized patients. BMC Med Inform Decis Mak. 2016;16:123.
41. Pell JM, Mancuso M, Limon S, Oman K, Lin CT. Patient access to electronic health records during hospitalization. JAMA Intern Med. 2015;175:856–8.
42. Dalal AK, Dykes PC, Collins S, Lehmann LS, Ohashi K, Rozenblum R, et al. A web-based, patient-centered toolkit to engage patients and caregivers in the acute care setting: a preliminary evaluation. J Am Med Inform Assoc. 2016;23:80–7.
43. Greysen SR, Khanna RR, Jacolbia R, Lee HM, Auerbach AD. Tablet computers for hospitalized patients: a pilot study to improve inpatient engagement. J Hosp Med. 2014;9:396–9.

44. Maher M, Hanauer DA, Kaziunas E, Ackerman MS, Derry H, Forringer R, et al. A novel health information technology communication system to increase caregiver activation in the context of hospital-based pediatric hematopoietic cell transplantation: a pilot study. JMIR Res Protoc. 2015;4:e119.
45. Runaas L, Hanauer D, Maher M, Bischoff E, Fauer A, Hoang T, et al. BMT roadmap: a user-centered design health information technology tool to promote patient-centered Care in Pediatric Hematopoietic Cell Transplantation. Biol Blood Marrow Transplant. 2017;23:813–9.
46. Kelly MM, Hoonakker PL, Dean SM. Using an inpatient portal to engage families in pediatric hospital care. J Am Med Inform Assoc. 2017;24:153–61.
47. Karahanna ESD, Chervany NL. Information technology adoption across time: a cross-sectional comparison of pre-adoption and post-adoption beliefs. MIS Q. 1999;23:183–213.
48. Dumitrascu AG, Burton MC, Dawson NL, Thomas CS, Nordan LM, Greig HE, et al. Patient portal use and hospital outcomes. J Am Med Inform Assoc. 2017;0:1–7.
49. Chu ES, Hakkarinen D, Evig C, Page S, Keniston A, Dickinson M, et al. Underutilized time for health education of hospitalized patients. J Hosp Med. 2008;3:238–46.
50. Wasson JH, MacKenzie TA, Hall M. Patients use an internet technology to report when things go wrong. Qual Saf Health Care. 2007;16:213–5.
51. Weingart SN, Carbo A, Tess A, Chiappetta L, Tutkus S, Morway L, et al. Using a patient internet portal to prevent adverse drug events: a randomized, controlled trial. J Patient Saf. 2013;9:169–75.
52. Venkatesh VMMGDG, Davis FD. User acceptance of information technology: toward a unified view. MIS Q. 2003;27:425–78.
53. Andersen R. A behavioral model of families' use of health services. Chicago: Center for Health Administration Studies, University of Chicago; 1968.
54. Andersen R, Newman JF. Societal and individual determinants of medical care utilization in the United States. Milbank Q. 2005;83 https://doi.org/10.1111/j.468-0009.2005.00428.x.
55. Andersen RM. Revisiting the behavioral model and access to medical care: does it matter? J Health Soc Behav. 1995;36:1–10.
56. Nutbeam D. Health promotion glossary. Health Promotion (Oxford, England). 1986;1:113–27.
57. 3M Health Information Systems. All patients refined diagnosis related groups (APR-DRGs). Version 20.0. Methodology Overview. 2003. https://www.hcup-us.ahrq.gov/db/nation/nis/APR-DRGsV20MethodologyOverviewandBibliography.pdf. Accessed 23 Feb 2018.
58. United States Census Bureau. American Community Survey (ACS). https://www.census.gov/programs-surveys/acs.
59. Charlson ME, Pompei P, Ales KL, MacKenzie CR. A new method of classifying prognostic comorbidity in longitudinal studies: development and validation. J Chronic Dis. 1987;40:373–83.
60. Agency for Healthcare Research and Quality. HCAHPS Survey. http://www.hcahpsonline.org/en/survey-instruments. Accessed 23 Feb 2018.
61. Agency for Healthcare Research and Quality. HCAHPS Fact Sheet CAHPS Hospital Survey. http://www.hcahpsonline.org/globalassets/hcahps/facts/hcahps_fact_sheet_november_2017a.pdf. Accessed 11 Feb 2017.
62. Yu PP. The evolution of oncology electronic health records. Cancer J. 2011; 17:197–202.
63. Robinson JR, Davis SE, Cronin RM, Jackson GP. Use of a patient portal during hospital admissions to surgical services. AMIA Annu Symp Proc. 2016;2016:1967–76.
64. Smith SG, Pandit A, Rush SR, Wolf MS, Simon C. The association between patient activation and accessing online health information: results from a national survey of US adults. Health Expect. 2015;18:3262–73.
65. Goel MS, Brown TL, Williams A, Cooper AJ, Hasnain-Wynia R, Baker DW. Patient reported barriers to enrolling in a patient portal. J Am Med Inform Assoc. 2011;18(Suppl 1):i8–12.
66. Smith SG, O'Conor R, Aitken W, Curtis LM, Wolf MS, Goel MS. Disparities in registration and use of an online patient portal among older adults: findings from the LitCog cohort. J Am Med Inform Assoc. 2015;22:888–95.
67. Irizarry T, DeVito Dabbs A, Curran CR. Patient portals and patient engagement: a state of the science review. J Med Internet Res. 2015;17:e148.
68. Ancker JS, Barron Y, Rockoff ML, Hauser D, Pichardo M, Szerencsy A, et al. Use of an electronic patient portal among disadvantaged populations. J Gen Intern Med. 2011;26:1117–23.
69. Gordon NP, Hornbrook MC. Differences in access to and preferences for using patient portals and other eHealth technologies based on race, ethnicity, and age: a database and survey study of seniors in a large health plan. J Med Internet Res. 2016;18:e50.
70. Yamin CK, Emani S, Williams DH, Lipsitz SR, Karson AS, Wald JS, et al. The digital divide in adoption and use of a personal health record. Arch Intern Med. 2011;171:568–74.
71. Phelps RG, Taylor J, Simpson K, Samuel J, Turner AN. Patients' continuing use of an online health record: a quantitative evaluation of 14,000 patient years of access data. J Med Internet Res. 2014;16:e241.
72. Miller H, Vandenbosch B, Ivanov D, Black P. Determinants of personal health record use: a large population study at Cleveland Clinic. J Healthc Inf Manag. 2007;21:44–8.
73. Numico G, Cristofano A, Mozzicafreddo A, Cursio OE, Franco P, Courthod G, et al. Hospital admission of cancer patients: avoidable practice or necessary care? PLoS One. 2015;10:e0120827.
74. Catt S, Chalmers A, Fallowfield L. Psychosocial and supportive-care needs in high-grade glioma. Lancet Oncol. 2008;9:884–91.
75. Weingart SN, Cleary A, Seger A, Eng TK, Saadeh M, Gross A, et al. Medication reconciliation in ambulatory oncology. Jt Comm J Qual Patient Saf. 2007;33:750–7.
76. Basch E, Artz D, Dulko D, Scher K, Sabbatini P, Hensley M, et al. Patient online self-reporting of toxicity symptoms during chemotherapy. J Clin Oncol. 2005;23:3552–61.
77. Hibbard JH, Peters E, Slovic P, Tusler M. Can patients be part of the solution? Views on their role in preventing medical errors. Med Care Res Rev. 2005;62:601–16.
78. Adler HM. The history of the present illness as treatment: who's listening, and why does it matter? J Am Board Fam Pract. 1997;10:28–35.
79. Rosenzweig MQ, Gardner D, Griffith B. The history and physical in Cancer care: a primer for the oncology advanced practitioner. J Adv Pract Oncol. 2014;5:262–8.
80. Esch T, Mejilla R, Anselmo M, Podtschaske B, Delbanco T, Walker J. Engaging patients through open notes: an evaluation using mixed methods. BMJ Open. 2016;6:e010034.
81. Delbanco T, Walker J, Bell SK, Darer JD, Elmore JG, Farag N, et al. Inviting patients to read their doctors' notes: a quasi-experimental study and a look ahead. Ann Intern Med. 2012;157:461–70.
82. Pillemer F, Price RA, Paone S, Martich GD, Albert S, Haidari L, et al. Direct release of test results to patients increases patient engagement and utilization of care. PLoS One. 2016;11:e0154743.
83. Meng D, Palen TE, Tsai J, McLeod M, Garrido T, Qian H. Association between secure patient-clinician email and clinical services utilisation in a US integrated health system: a retrospective cohort study. BMJ Open. 2015;5: e009557.
84. Zhou YY, Garrido T, Chin HL, Wiesenthal AM, Liang LL. Patient access to an electronic health record with secure messaging: impact on primary care utilization. Am J Manag Care. 2007;13:418–24.
85. Palen TE, Ross C, Powers JD, Xu S. Association of online patient access to clinicians and medical records with use of clinical services. JAMA. 2012;308: 2012–9.
86. Mayer DK, Travers D, Wyss A, Leak A, Waller A. Why do patients with cancer visit emergency departments? Results of a 2008 population study in North Carolina. J Clin Oncol. 2011;29:2683–8.
87. Barbera L, Taylor C, Dudgeon D. Why do patients with cancer visit the emergency department near the end of life? CMAJ. 2010;182:563–8.
88. Shapiro JS, Humeniuk MS, Siddiqui MA, Bonthu N, Schroeder DR, Kashiwagi DT. Risk factors for readmission in patients with Cancer Comanaged by hospitalists. Am J Med Qual. 2017;32:526–31.
89. Weaver C, Schiech L, Held-Warmkessel J, Kedziera P, Haney E, DiLullo G, et al. Risk for unplanned hospital readmission of patients with cancer: results of a retrospective medical record review. Oncol Nurs Forum. 2006;33:E44–52.
90. Donze J, Aujesky D, Williams D, Schnipper JL. Potentially avoidable 30-day hospital readmissions in medical patients: derivation and validation of a prediction model. JAMA Intern Med. 2013;173:632–8.
91. Bell JF, Whitney RL, Reed SC, Poghosyan H, Lash RS, Kim KK, et al. Systematic review of hospital readmissions among patients with Cancer in the United States. Oncol Nurs Forum. 2017;44:176–91.

92. Coughlin SS, Prochaska JJ, Williams LB, Besenyi GM, Heboyan V, Goggans DS, et al. Patient web portals, disease management, and primary prevention. Risk Manag Healthc Policy. 2017;10:33–40.
93. Ralston JD, Hirsch IB, Hoath J, Mullen M, Cheadle A, Goldberg HI. Web-based collaborative care for type 2 diabetes: a pilot randomized trial. Diabetes Care. 2009;32:234–9.
94. Manard W, Scherrer JF, Salas J, Schneider FD. Patient portal use and blood pressure control in newly diagnosed hypertension. J Am Board Fam Med. 2016;29:452–9.
95. Earnest MA, Ross SE, Wittevrongel L, Moore LA, Lin CT. Use of a patient-accessible electronic medical record in a practice for congestive heart failure: patient and physician experiences. J Am Med Inform Assoc. 2004;11:410–7.
96. Wagner PJ, Dias J, Howard S, Kintziger KW, Hudson MF, Seol YH, et al. Personal health records and hypertension control: a randomized trial. J Am Med Inform Assoc. 2012;19:626–34.
97. Grant RW, Wald JS, Schnipper JL, Gandhi TK, Poon EG, Orav EJ, et al. Practice-linked online personal health records for type 2 diabetes mellitus: a randomized controlled trial. Arch Intern Med. 2008;168:1776–82.
98. Price M, Bellwood P, Kitson N, Davies I, Weber J, Lau F. Conditions potentially sensitive to a personal health record (PHR) intervention, a systematic review. BMC Med Inform Decis Mak. 2015;15:32.
99. Holmstrom I, Roing M. The relation between patient-centeredness and patient empowerment: a discussion on concepts. Patient Educ Couns. 2010; 79:167–72.
100. Lovell MR, Luckett T, Boyle FM, Phillips J, Agar M, Davidson PM. Patient education, coaching, and self-Management for Cancer Pain. J Clin Oncol. 2014;32:1712–20.
101. Lev EL. Bandura's theory of self-efficacy: applications to oncology. Sch Inq Nurs Pract. 1997;11:21–37. discussion 9-43
102. Haugland T, Wahl AK, Hofoss D, DeVon HA. Association between general self-efficacy, social support, cancer-related stress and physical health-related quality of life: a path model study in patients with neuroendocrine tumors. Health Qual Life Outcomes. 2016;14:11.
103. Jameson E, Trevena J, Swain N. Electronic gaming as pain distraction. Pain Res Manag. 2011;16:27–32.
104. Foster C, Breckons M, Cotterell P, Barbosa D, Calman L, Corner J, et al. Cancer survivors' self-efficacy to self-manage in the year following primary treatment. J Cancer Surviv. 2015;9:11–9.

10

Algorithm-based decision support for symptom self-management among adults with Cancer: results of usability testing

Mary E. Cooley[1*], Janet L. Abrahm[2], Donna L. Berry[3], Michael S. Rabin[4], Ilana M. Braun[2], Joanna Paladino[2], Manan M. Nayak[1] and David F. Lobach[5,6]

Abstract

Background: It is essential that cancer patients understand anticipated symptoms, how to self-manage these symptoms, and when to call their clinicians. However, patients are often ill-prepared to manage symptoms at home. Clinical decision support (CDS) is a potentially innovative way to provide information to patients where and when they need it. The purpose of this project was to design and evaluate a simulated model of an algorithm-based CDS program for self-management of cancer symptoms.

Methods: This study consisted of three phases; development of computable algorithms for self-management of cancer symptoms using a modified ADAPTE process, evaluation of a simulated model of the CDS program, and identification of design objectives and lessons learned from the evaluation of patient-centered CDS. In phase 1, algorithms for pain, constipation and nausea/vomiting were developed by an expert panel. In phase 2, we conducted usability testing of a simulated **s**ymptom **a**ssessment and **m**anagement **i**ntervention for self-care (SAMI-Self-Care) CDS program involving focus groups, interviews and surveys with cancer patients, their caregivers and clinicians. The Acceptability E-scale measured acceptability of the program. In phase 3, we developed design objectives and identified barriers to uptake of patient-centered CDS based on the data gathered from stakeholders.

Results: In phase 1, algorithms were reviewed and approved through a consensus meeting and majority vote. In phase 2, 24 patients & caregivers and 13 clinicians participated in the formative evaluation. Iterative changes were made in a simulated SAMI-Self-Care CDS program. Acceptability scores were high among patients, caregivers and clinicians. In phase 3, we formulated CDS design objectives, which included: 1) ensure patient safety, 2) communicate clinical concepts effectively, 3) promote communication with clinicians, 4) support patient activation, and 5) facilitate navigation and use. We identified patient barriers and clinician concerns to using CDS for symptom self-management, which were consistent with the chronic care model, a theoretical framework used to enhance patient-clinician communication and patient self-management.

Conclusion: Patient safety and tool navigation were critical features of CDS for patient self-management. Insights gleaned from this study may be used to inform the development of CDS resources for symptom self-management in patients with other chronic conditions.

Keywords: Rule-based clinical decision support, Symptom management, Patient engagement, Patient self-management, Cancer

* Correspondence: mary_cooley@dfci.harvard.edu
[1]The Phyllis F. Cantor Center, Dana-Farber Cancer Institute, 450 Brookline Avenue, Boston, MA 02115, USA
Full list of author information is available at the end of the article

Background

Patient-centered healthcare is one of six aims to improve the United States healthcare system [1]. One facet of patient-centered care is engaging patients and encouraging self-management, especially in the context of chronic illness. Self-management programs that provide coaching and education, and are supported by timely information, facilitate patient engagement [2, 3].

Given the frequency of symptoms from cancer and its treatment, it is essential that patients (and their caregivers) understand how to self-manage symptoms and when to call their clinicians for advice. McCorkle and colleagues [3–5] noted that most patients with cancer try to self-manage their care and that developing system-level interventions to support self-management is essential for quality cancer care. Evidence-based strategies to assist patients with self-management include: education, telephone consultations, Internet tools for tracking disease-specific parameters, and coaching [3, 6–13]. Such interventions targeted information management, medications, psychological consequences of illness, lifestyle, social support, communication, accessing services, and setting goals [14–16]. Self-management interventions decreased the severity of pain [17], fatigue [18], and depression [19]. Web-based interventions, featuring self-monitoring, education and coaching of patients combined with summaries of patient-reported data delivered to clinicians, led to improvement in symptom distress and quality of life [12, 16, 20]. Evidence suggests that reporting symptoms to clinicians alone may not be sufficient. A project in which patients receiving chemotherapy reported on symptoms using an automated phone system failed to impact care. Even though symptoms of moderate to severe intensity were reported, clinicians did not provide patients with management guidance [10].

Considering the variability of clinician response to symptom reports, an optimal approach to enhance self-management includes providing patient-specific, real-time, actionable information. Supplying Clinical Decision Support *(CDS)* directly to patients may enhance their ability to self-manage symptoms. *CDS* "provides individuals with person-specific information, intelligently filtered or presented at appropriate times, to enhance health" [21]. Four studies have described rule-based CDS tools for cancer patients. [12, 20, 22, 23] In two studies, CDS was used to identify the presence of a symptom using an algorithm with a single decision node that generated general recommendations for symptom management [12, 22]. In studies by Berry and colleagues [24] and Weaver, [23] the focus was self-care support and identifying symptoms to report to clinicians. Berry and colleagues [12] found that Web-based coaching of patients to report symptom experiences verbally resulted in more frequent reports during clinic visits, but the investigators did not document how often a participant called the clinic to ask for help. Ruland et al. [20] developed a Web-based resource that assisted patients with assessing symptoms, finding information, communicating with clinic personnel and provided self-management advice. This tool was evaluated and showed a slight decrease in symptom distress for patients [20] but the CDS component was not evaluated independently for its effect. A follow-up study determined that communication with nurses was the most valued component [25].

The present study extends the literature by reporting on the design and formative evaluation of an algorithm-based simulated model of a patient-centered CDS program that facilitates cancer symptom self-management, provides advice on when patients should contact their clinicians, and includes coaching information about what to tell them. The goals of the project were to develop computable algorithms for pain, constipation and nausea/vomiting in phase 1, conduct iterative usability testing of the simulated CDS program called the **S**ymptom **A**ssessment and **M**anagement **I**ntervention for **Self-Care** (SAMI-Self-Care) with patients, their caregivers and clinicians in phase 2, and develop design objectives and identify barriers to uptake of patient-centered CDS based on the data gathered from stakeholders, which included members of an expert panel, patients, caregivers, and their clinicians in phase 3.

Methods

We employed a convergent, parallel, mixed methods design, [26] in which we collected qualitative and quantitative data in parallel, analyzed it separately, and then merged all data during interpretation, to evaluate the acceptability of a simulated algorithm-based CDS program for cancer symptom self-management. This study was conducted at Dana-Farber Cancer Institute (DFCI) and approved by the Institutional Review Board (IRB), Protocol number-12-300.

Phase 1: Algorithm-based CDS intervention development

In order to develop the patient-centered CDS algorithms, we used a modified ADAPTE process [27–29] consisting of five steps; 1) identify expert panels to develop and evaluate the computable algorithms, 2) develop groups to work on each symptom and synthesize the literature, 3) convene groups to translate evidence-based information into computable algorithms for each symptom, 4) conduct peer review on the content of the algorithms before convening a multidisciplinary consensus meeting, and 5) hold a multidisciplinary panel meeting to review, modify and approve the algorithms.

The study team identified areas of expertise that were critical for developing and evaluating an algorithm-based CDS tool for symptom self-management. Individuals with the desired expertise were identified through existing professional relationships or through recommendations of colleagues. The identified individuals were invited to join the panel by the principal investigator (MEC) and included: stakeholders with expertise in clinical care (oncologists, palliative care experts, psychiatrists, and oncology nurses), information systems (experts in CDS, patient data collection, health communication, and graphic design), care delivery process (experts in workflow, quality improvement, and health equity), as well as patients and caregivers.

Our expert panel drew from evidence-based resources and worked with CDS experts to develop computable algorithms that would enable self-management of pain, constipation, and nausea/vomiting. Overall, the expert panel met four times for 4 h each time to review the algorithms developed by the research team. The symptoms chosen were the most common reasons for urgent care among cancer patients and identified as important targets for symptom management by patients and their caregivers in a previous study that explored patient preferences for CDS to enhance clinical care [30]. Our process of developing algorithms was based on our previous work that adapted evidence-based guidelines for clinicians [31]. Similar to our previous work, multidisciplinary groups were formed for each symptom and serial meetings were held to develop the initial algorithms. Once the algorithms were completed, a group meeting with the members of the research team and the expert panel was held to review, modify and approve the algorithms. For each symptom, characteristics were identified to direct self-management. Characteristics of pain included descriptors of neuropathic or somatic pain, and a measure of intensity (moderate, severe). Features of nausea/vomiting included chemotherapy-induced, radiation-induced, chemoradiation-induced, acid reflux, vertigo, recent narcotic increase, anticipation of chemotherapy, and constipation. Characteristics of constipation included frequency and consistency of stool.

Phase 2: Usability testing

In order to refine the algorithm content and the simulated SAMI-Self-Care tool display and function iteratively, we used a collaborative-participatory approach. This approach engaged stakeholders in a shared co-designing process and helped ensure that the product will meet real-life needs and be adopted [32, 33]. The team formulated a scenario for a symptom management dilemma that would allow patient users to traverse the self-care management algorithms so that self-management recommendations could be generated. Cognitive testing was performed for each algorithm by reviewing the content displayed on an iPad with patients and their caregivers to ensure that these questions were clear, understandable, and relevant, and that the response options were appropriate prior to initiating the iterative usability testing. Cognitive testing of items is recommended as a standard approach to the development process as it allows one to ascertain whether participants understand items on a questionnaire and allows for iterative changes before finalizing questions [34].

This patient-vetted algorithm content was given to the Dana-Farber Harvard Comprehensive Cancer Center Health Communication Core. The Core developed a mockup of the SAMI-Self-Care using interactive PDF files to simulate the function of the CDS tool based on expert panel input and clinical informatics literature [35, 36]. The PDF files imitated the functionality of a Website and allowed participants to experience the "look and feel" of a potential operational CDS system on an iPad. This approach provided a practical and economical approach to usability testing, especially during formative stages of development when iterative refinement is necessary. The Health Communication Core also designed reports containing self-management recommendations to elicit feedback from participants regarding report content and appearance. A series of focus groups or interviews were conducted to elicit feedback about the CDS program. Using a multi-methods approach (i.e. focus groups and interviews) is appropriate when the intent is to gather information that is focused on specific goals and questions, which in this case was participant response about the usability of an algorithm-based CDS program [37]. We used a combination of methods to provide flexibility to participants to be able to participate in the usability sessions. We used the same facilitator to conduct the focus groups and interviews and used an interview guide to elicit information about the usability and acceptability of the SAMI-Self-Care CDS program.

Based on feedback from the expert panel, patients, caregivers, and clinicians, we iteratively created three successive versions of the SAMI-Self-Care program. Figures 1, 2, 3, 4 show the iterative development of the self-management report that was generated for participants based on responses to the questions and algorithm-based CDS. Feedback from the usability testing was used to inform the changes that were made to the CDS program and the self-management report (see results).

Participant recruitment

Patients were identified through medical records at DFCI under a waiver of consent authorization, and names were submitted to their clinicians for approval to contact patients, as required by the IRB. Eligible patients were age ≥ 18, English speaking, and had received cancer treatment within the past 6-months. All approved patients were sent an initial letter describing the study and inviting them to participate. Patients received two follow-up calls if they didn't respond to the letter. Patients identified caregivers to invite to participate in the study. Eligible caregivers

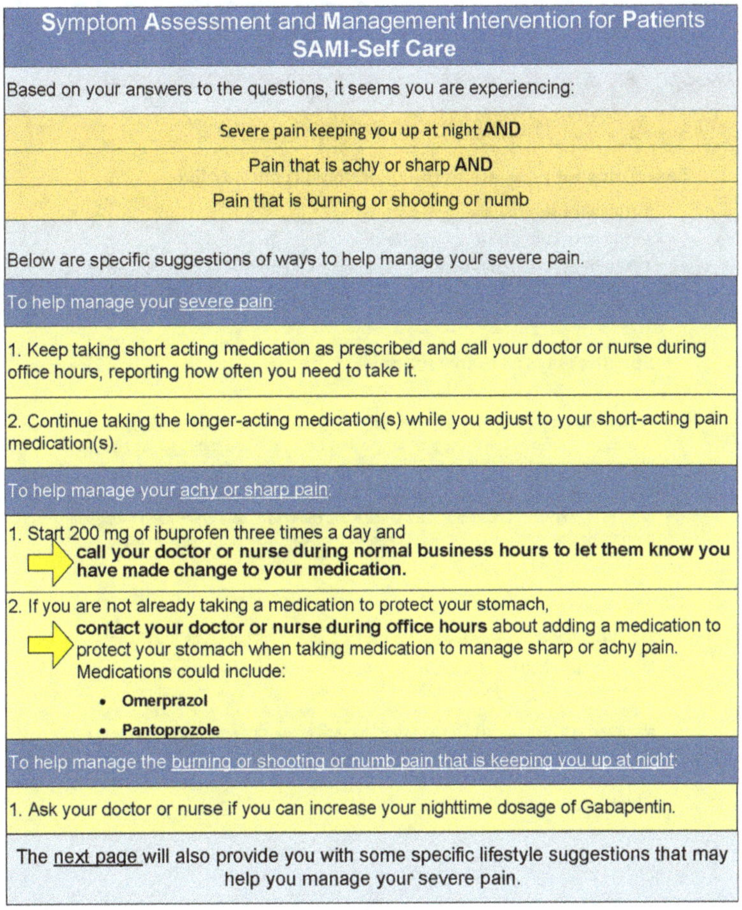

Fig. 1 Initial SAMI-Self Care report

were age ≥ 18 years and provided care to a patient who received cancer treatment within the past 6-months. Deliberate efforts were made to sample across a range of diagnoses, educational backgrounds, ages, genders, and races. All participants signed consent forms at the time of participation. Each participant received $50 for completing the study.

Clinicians in ambulatory oncology included physicians, nurse practitioners, physician assistants, and registered nurses. Clinicians were identified through clinic rosters. An invitation to participate in the study was emailed to eligible clinicians. Two follow-up emails were sent if no response was received. Clinicians were recruited for either focus groups or interviews depending on their schedules. Clinicians received an invitation letter describing the study but signed consent was waived by the IRB. Each clinician received $100 for completing the study.

Focus group and interview processes

Focus groups and interviews were held separately for clinicians and patients/caregivers. Focus groups included up to five participants; interviews included one or two participants and were held in a convenient conference room at DFCI. Meetings for clinicians lasted about 30 min whereas those for patients and caregivers lasted 45–60 min. One symptom was addressed per session. Using a script, the facilitator queried patients, caregivers and clinicians about the algorithm content of the SAMI-SC programs for constipation, pain, and nausea/vomiting, and asked about the "look and feel" of the materials for pain and nausea/vomiting. The topics for patients and caregivers focused on the: 1) visual appeal, 2) format and navigation, 3) understandability of written content and terminology, and 4) wording of self-management suggestions. The topics for the clinicians focused on 1) a review of the patient self-management algorithms, 2) review of the simulated SAMI-Self-Care CDS program, and 3) feedback about ways to improve the algorithms and/or simulated model. Patients/caregivers and clinicians reported demographic data using a standardized survey.

The number of sessions per symptom was determined by evidence of content saturation and absence of new common responses [38]. With patients/caregivers, we conducted six sessions for pain, seven sessions for nausea/

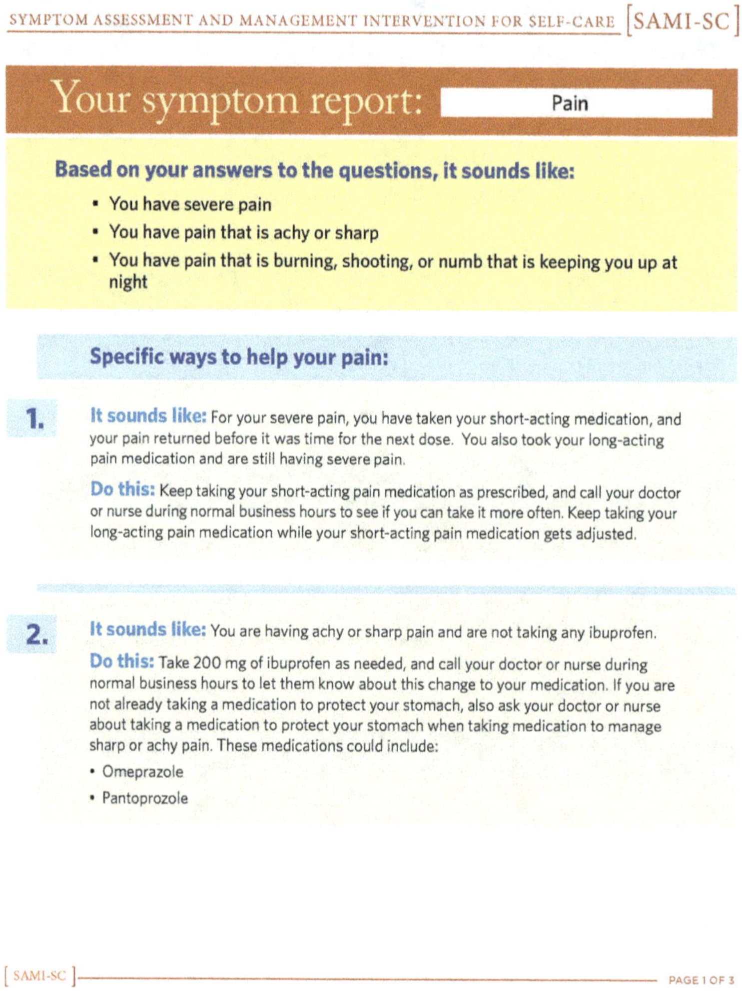
SYMPTOM ASSESSMENT AND MANAGEMENT INTERVENTION FOR SELF-CARE [SAMI-SC]

Your symptom report: Pain

Based on your answers to the questions, it sounds like:

- You have severe pain
- You have pain that is achy or sharp
- You have pain that is burning, shooting, or numb that is keeping you up at night

Specific ways to help your pain:

1. **It sounds like:** For your severe pain, you have taken your short-acting medication, and your pain returned before it was time for the next dose. You also took your long-acting pain medication and are still having severe pain.

   Do this: Keep taking your short-acting pain medication as prescribed, and call your doctor or nurse during normal business hours to see if you can take it more often. Keep taking your long-acting pain medication while your short-acting pain medication gets adjusted.

2. **It sounds like:** You are having achy or sharp pain and are not taking any ibuprofen.

   Do this: Take 200 mg of ibuprofen as needed, and call your doctor or nurse during normal business hours to let them know about this change to your medication. If you are not already taking a medication to protect your stomach, also ask your doctor or nurse about taking a medication to protect your stomach when taking medication to manage sharp or achy pain. These medications could include:

   - Omeprazole
   - Pantoprozole

[SAMI-SC] PAGE 1 OF 3

Fig. 2 First revision for SAMI-Self Care report

vomiting, and three sessions for constipation. With clinicians, we conducted two sessions for pain, three sessions for nausea/vomiting, and one session for constipation. All discussions were audio-recorded and transcribed.

Survey instruments

The Acceptability E-scale measured the acceptability of the CDS program [39]. This scale has been used in adult patients with various types of cancers from medical oncology, radiation oncology and stem cell transplant to measure acceptability of Web-based systems, including computerized symptom and quality of life assessments, patient educational materials and patient-centered decision support. Psychometric testing was conducted in 627 adults with cancer [40, 41]. Cronbach alpha reliability coefficient was 0.75 and factor analysis revealed that the scale was unidimensional [39]. Five-point Likert-type items (1–5; larger number equals higher acceptability and a score of 3 indicates a neutral response) were presented to elicit feedback from both patient/caregiver and clinician participants regarding: 1) understandability of language, 2) helpfulness of suggestions provided for symptom self-management, 3) usefulness of reports, and 4) overall satisfaction with the program. The a priori target for acceptability of SAMI-Self-Care was a mean score of ≥4 on each item since this score indicated a positive acceptability response. In addition to the Acceptability E-scale, participants were asked what other types of information would have been helpful for symptom self-management. The scale took less than 2 min to complete and was written at a 5th grade reading level.

Analysis

Patient/caregiver and clinician demographic data were summarized as descriptive statistics. Acceptability E-scale results were summarized as item means and standard deviations.

Audio-recorded session content was transcribed and reviewed by three study team members (MEC, DFL, MMN), coded inductively, and grouped into common

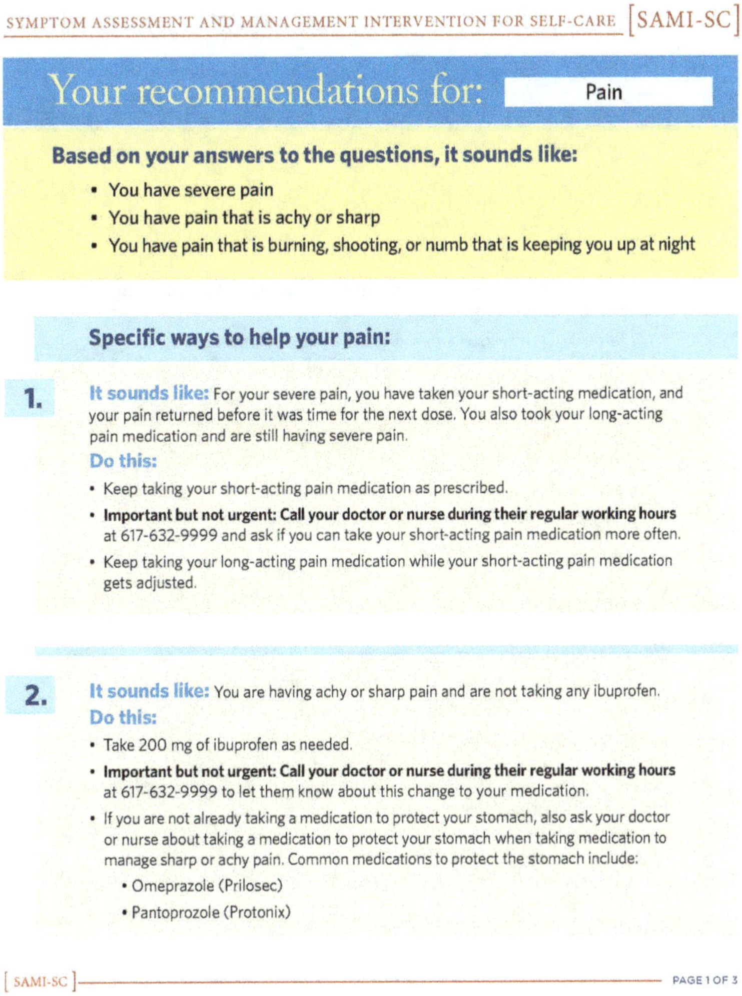

SYMPTOM ASSESSMENT AND MANAGEMENT INTERVENTION FOR SELF-CARE [SAMI-SC]

Your recommendations for: Pain

Based on your answers to the questions, it sounds like:

- You have severe pain
- You have pain that is achy or sharp
- You have pain that is burning, shooting, or numb that is keeping you up at night

Specific ways to help your pain:

1. **It sounds like:** For your severe pain, you have taken your short-acting medication, and your pain returned before it was time for the next dose. You also took your long-acting pain medication and are still having severe pain.

Do this:

- Keep taking your short-acting pain medication as prescribed.
- **Important but not urgent: Call your doctor or nurse during their regular working hours** at 617-632-9999 and ask if you can take your short-acting pain medication more often.
- Keep taking your long-acting pain medication while your short-acting pain medication gets adjusted.

2. **It sounds like:** You are having achy or sharp pain and are not taking any ibuprofen.

Do this:

- Take 200 mg of ibuprofen as needed.
- **Important but not urgent: Call your doctor or nurse during their regular working hours** at 617-632-9999 to let them know about this change to your medication.
- If you are not already taking a medication to protect your stomach, also ask your doctor or nurse about taking a medication to protect your stomach when taking medication to manage sharp or achy pain. Common medications to protect the stomach include:
  - Omeprazole (Prilosec)
  - Pantoprozole (Protonix)

[SAMI-SC] PAGE 1 OF 3

Fig. 3 Second revision for SAMI-Self Care report

responses to identify revisions that needed to be made in the CDS tool. Common responses were then combined and reconciled though discussion. A list of suggested revisions to improve SAMI-Self-Care algorithms and the simulated model was created and ranked based on audio files and notes. Critical revisions were implemented immediately, while other less critical revisions were monitored for repetition. This process was repeated, after each iteration of CDS tool development, until no new responses or suggestions for changes emerged from the usability testing. Phase 2 analyses focused on the revisions that needed to be make to the CDS tool.

Phase 3: Design objectives and barriers to uptake of patient-centered CDS

Once all the data were collected and the usability testing completed, three investigators (MEC, DFL, MMN) reviewed all of the qualitative data in order to identify design objectives and barriers to uptake of the patient-centered CDS program. Eight sessions were needed to organize the data collected from the expert panel, patients, caregivers and clinicians and discuss the themes that were identified through inductive content analysis [42]. These data were then shared and discussed with other members of the research team to generate a final list of design objectives, patient barriers, and clinician concerns to use of the CDS program.

Analyses

Audio-recorded session content was transcribed and reviewed by three study team members (MEC, DFL, MMN), coded, and grouped into themes. Themes were then combined and reconciled though discussion. Inductive analyses of the coded qualitative data for phase 3 focused on interpreting patient barriers to using the CDS program, defining clinician concerns about use of CDS by patients/caregivers, and identifying strategies to overcome the areas of concern. It was noted during the analysis that the themes that emerged from the qualitative data were consistent with the Chronic Care Model

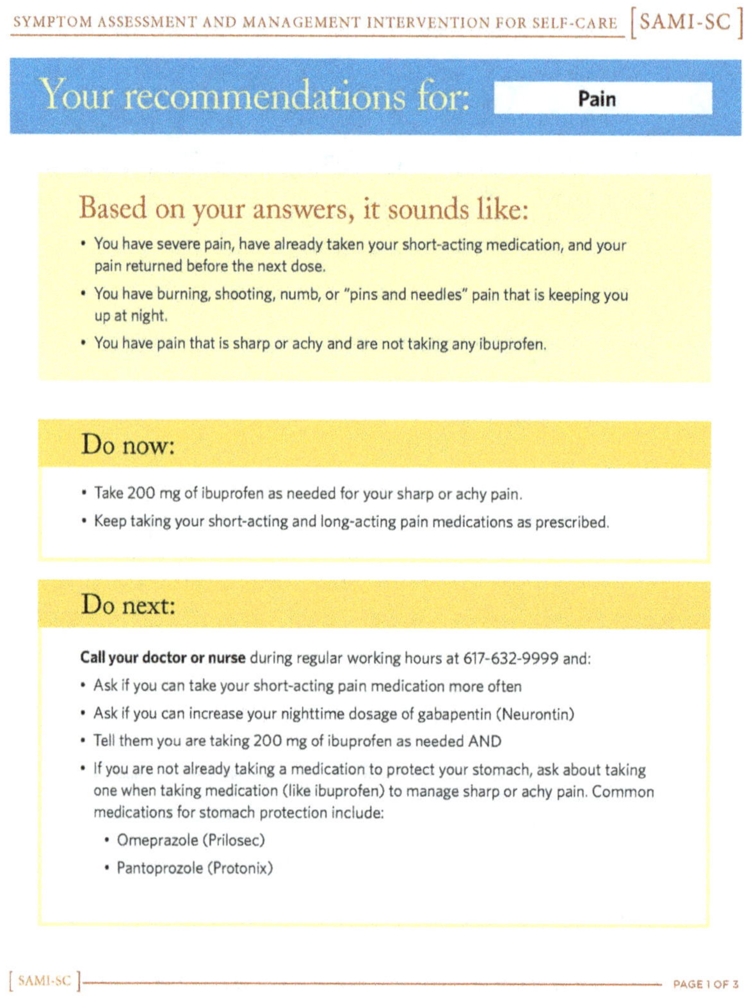

SYMPTOM ASSESSMENT AND MANAGEMENT INTERVENTION FOR SELF-CARE [SAMI-SC]

Your recommendations for: Pain

Based on your answers, it sounds like:

- You have severe pain, have already taken your short-acting medication, and your pain returned before the next dose.
- You have burning, shooting, numb, or "pins and needles" pain that is keeping you up at night.
- You have pain that is sharp or achy and are not taking any ibuprofen.

Do now:

- Take 200 mg of ibuprofen as needed for your sharp or achy pain.
- Keep taking your short-acting and long-acting pain medications as prescribed.

Do next:

Call your doctor or nurse during regular working hours at 617-632-9999 and:

- Ask if you can take your short-acting pain medication more often
- Ask if you can increase your nighttime dosage of gabapentin (Neurontin)
- Tell them you are taking 200 mg of ibuprofen as needed AND
- If you are not already taking a medication to protect your stomach, ask about taking one when taking medication (like ibuprofen) to manage sharp or achy pain. Common medications for stomach protection include:
  - Omeprazole (Prilosec)
  - Pantoprozole (Protonix)

[SAMI-SC] PAGE 1 OF 3

Fig. 4 Third revision for SAMI-Self Care report

[3, 43]. Thus, five design objectives detailed below (in Results) were developed to address these concerns. As a result, content analysis was then used to regroup the themes to fit within the Chronic Care Model.

Results

Phase 1: Rule-based CDS intervention development

Nine potential participants were approached for membership in the expert panel, and all accepted the invitation. Altogether, 16 members of the research team and expert panel contributed to algorithm development. Work sessions were conducted in person and by Web conferencing so that the flow charts could be displayed more easily for discussion. Branching logic was used to develop the algorithms and these were displayed as flow charts that were shared among all team members. Research staff provided support to access current guidelines that were available for the targeted symptoms and to assist with literature reviews. Each work group had someone assigned who was expert in pharmacological, non-pharmacological and self-management approaches so that a comprehensive approach to enable self-management would be embedded into the algorithms.

Once the development of the algorithms and usability testing was completed, a multidisciplinary consensus meeting was held with the expert panel, research team and co-investigators to review, modify and approve the final versions. In order to iteratively improve the program, the expert panel focused on several issues. The primary issue was patient safety. Safety was addressed by identifying potential serious causes of each symptom and directing patients to seek contact with their clinicians. Accordingly, all three algorithms began with the identification of "red flag symptoms" that caused patients a forced exit of the CDS tool and a directive to call a clinician immediately for guidance. A second issue was how to make the tool accessible to patients across a range of health literacies. Our solution was to provide information that patients could elect to review or skip based on their needs. A third issue was how to provide medication-related advice that was aligned with therapies recommended by a patient's clinician. To address this issue, we asked the patient whether the medication we were recommending for the problem (e.g. senna for constipation) was approved by his/her clinician. If it was approved, we inquired whether the patient had taken that medication. If not, the patient was advised to take it. If the patient had not been prescribed the recommended therapy, he or she was advised to contact his/her clinician and inquire if this therapy could be appropriate. The resulting algorithms had a large number of decision nodes ranging from 51 to 257 (moderate and severe pain combined). A decision node is a point in the algorithm where the logic branches into two or more directions. A higher number of decision nodes reflect greater algorithmic complexity [44]. Table 1 provides information about the number of decision nodes and red flag questions that were present within each symptom algorithm. A simple majority vote was taken at the end of the discussion surrounding each symptom algorithm to determine whether agreement was reached regarding modifications and approval. Table 1 provides an overview of the number of red flags that were required for each symptoms and the complexity of the algorithms.

Phase 2: Usability testing

Participant sample

One-hundred-and-three patients were screened to identify the 24 patients and caregivers for study inclusion (Table 2). Twenty-six patients were deemed ineligible by their clinicians due to the incapacitating nature of their condition and 14 did not meet other eligibility criteria or could not be contacted. Seventeen potential subjects declined participation; 22 indicated interest but were unable to attend scheduled sessions or did not respond to scheduling requests. Participating patients and caregivers were predominately Caucasian, almost evenly split between men and women and most had some college level education.

Forty-four clinicians were contacted to identify 13 who participated in focus groups and interviews (Table 3). Of the clinicians who did not participate, 20 did not respond, 2 declined, and 9 indicated interest but were unable to attend scheduled sessions. Clinician participants were predominately female and Caucasian.

Table 1 Number of decision nodes and red flag questions in each symptom algorithm

Symptom	Decisional Nodes	Red Flag Questions
Nausea & Vomiting	54	6
Pain	257	2[a]
Severe Pain	125	
Moderate Pain	122	
Constipation	51	4

[a]Red flag questions are the same for both the moderate and severe pain pathways

Table 2 Cancer Patient and Caregiver Demographics ($N = 24$)

Characteristic	*n*	%
Role		
Patient	15	63
Caregiver	9	37
Gender		
Female	13	54
Age		
Median/Range	55	21–69
< 50	5	21
≥ 50	19	79
Race		
Caucasian	20	83
Black/African American	2	8
Other	2	8
Ethnicity		
Hispanic	4	17
Non-Hispanic	18	75
Did Not Report	2	8
Education		
High School or Less	3	12
Some College or More	21	88
Income		
$49,999 or Less	4	17
$50,000 or More	19	79
Did Not Report	1	4
Cancer Type ($n = 15$)		
Hematologic Malignancies	5	33
Solid Tumor Malignancies	10	67
Types of Solid Tumor		
Breast	1	7
Gastrointestinal	3	20
Genitourinary	1	7
Gynecologic	1	7
Head and Neck	1	7
Neuro-oncology	1	7
Thoracic	2	13
Internet Use to Obtain Health Information		
Never/Rarely	0	0
Sometimes	10	42
Often/Very Often	13	54
Missing	1	4

Focus groups and interviews

Patients and caregivers provided feedback about the visual appeal of the program, especially related to the color scheme, text density, and font size. Participant feedback

Table 3 Oncology Clinician Demographics (N = 13)

Characteristic	n	%
Gender		
Female	11	85
Race		
Caucasian	11	84
Black/African American	1	8
Asian	1	8
Ethnicity		
Non-Hispanic	11	85
Did Not Report	2	15
Training		
Physicians	3	23
Nurse Practitioners	4	31
Physician Assistants	2	15
Registered Nurses	4	31
Cancer Specialty Area		
Hematologic Malignancies	4	31
Solid Tumor Malignancies	9	69
Types of Solid Tumor		
Gastrointestinal	2	15
Genitourinary	1	8
Neuro-oncology	1	8
Head and Neck	1	8
Thoracic	2	15
Radiation Oncology	1	8
General Practice	1	8
Prior Use of Patient-Focused Information Tools		
Never/Rarely	8	61
Sometimes/Often/Very Often	5	39

sought to make the display inviting and easy to read. Some of the issues raised by clinicians who viewed the program were similar to issues identified by patients and their caregivers. For example, clinicians made suggestions about use of language, decreasing the density of text and providing graphic images to enhance understanding. For the most part, patients, caregivers and clinicians had similar comments to enhance the usability of the program. However, clinicians provided additional feedback about the content of the algorithms, and to ensure patient safety. They suggested adding questions at the beginning of the algorithms that would identify potentially dangerous symptoms that needed immediate attention and prompt patients to exit the program and call their clinicians. We also found that clinicians disagreed about what were best practices for self-management in pain management. Some clinicians felt that patients with pain levels of ≥ 9 should not self-manage and call their clinicians immediately, whereas others felt that it was acceptable to use the suggestions and then call their clinicians for refractory pain. Tables 4 and 5 provide an overview of comments provided by participants to improve the usability of the program.

Acceptability surveys

Participants completed surveys regarding the acceptability of SAMI-Self-Care for "nausea/vomiting" and "pain" after each round of system development and viewing the simulated interface. Nine patients and their caregivers completed surveys, four assessing pain and five assessing nausea and vomiting. Two rounds of assessment for usability and acceptability were conducted with patients to reach or surpass the predetermined threshold for acceptability. In general, patients found the system easy to understand and helpful for self-management.

Thirteen clinicians completed surveys, nine assessed pain and three assessed nausea and vomiting, and one assessed constipation. Two rounds of assessment for usability and acceptability were conducted with clinicians. The simulated program for nausea/vomiting and constipation reached and surpassed the threshold for acceptability. However, the helpfulness of suggestions for the pain algorithm was scored lower than our target threshold of 4.0. For the most part, clinicians also viewed the system for pain as usable and helpful. Subsequent discussions revealed that some clinicians felt that patients with a pain score ≥ 9 should contact their clinicians and not pursue self-management. The algorithm was subsequently changed to reflect that patients with severe pain, should contact their clinicians, but time limitations prevented the modified algorithm from being reevaluated.

Phase 3: Design Objectives and Barriers to Patient-centered CDS

Design objectives

From patient, caregiver, and stakeholder feedback, we identified five design objectives that were relevant for the development of algorithm-based patient-centered CDS, which included: ensure patient safety, communicate clinical concepts effectively, promote communication with clinicians, support patient activation, and facilitate navigation (see Table 6). This table includes information about the design objective, specific stakeholder barriers related to this objective, solutions that were identified to address the barrier and changes that were made in the user interface. A discussion surrounding each of these design objectives is found in the following section followed by some barriers to patient-centered CDS that emerged from our findings.

Table 4 Results of Usability Testing for the SAMI-Self-Care CDS Program: Patient Perspectives

Usability Testing Themes	CDS Tool Content*	CDS Tool Component**	Examples
Visual appeal	Comments about introductory pages that had a lot of content	Visual appeal and design	"Some pages seem overwhelming."
Understanding of terminology	Pain severity question	Written content and terminology	"What does 'bearable pain' mean?"
	Medication questions for all symptoms	Written content and terminology	"What does 'able and willing' [to take a medication] mean?"
	Nausea and vomiting question	Written content and terminology	"Position change- does that mean when I lift my head up?"
	Medication questions	Written content and terminology	"Unclear about the word 'dose' in the questions."
	Medication question	Written content and terminology	"Did you take the dose you were due for? Does that mean the dose time already passed or the next dose I am due for?"
	Pain quality question	Written content and terminology	"Define what type of pain you are referring too", is it "pokey pain, electrical current, shock pains burning pains, etc."
	Pain quality question	Written content and terminology	"I wouldn't have categorized numbness as pain...I'm glad it's there."
	Pain severity question	Written content and terminology	"I like 'faces' as part of the pain scale. They make the pain measure more clear."
	Constipation definition	Written content and terminology	"Definitions were too wordy, for example, constipation definition had too much information."
	Pain medication list	Written content and terminology	"I have trouble understanding meaning or relevance to words such as Morphine or Opioids."
	Constipation medication list	Written content and terminology	"Is Senna tea the same as Senna medication?"
	Nausea and vomiting red flag safety questions	Written content and terminology	"What are two glasses of water per day?"
	All symptom medication questions	Written content and terminology	"Need to add a time frame to the question: 'Did you take your medication?'"
	General content related to introduction of program and definition of all symptoms	Written content and terminology	Simplicity of terminology required for some patients with little medical sophistication makes clinical concepts difficult to communicate and can be tedious for more medically sophisticated patients.
	Nausea and vomiting questions	Written content and terminology	"Why are you asking me about acid reflux and then position change? Are they related?"
	Nausea and vomiting red flag safety questions	Written content and terminology	"Why is bone marrow transplant question asked?"
	Pain red flag safety questions	Written content and terminology	Reason for why some questions are asked is not understood, e.g., "Not everyone has back pain."
	Nausea and vomiting questions	Written content and terminology	"Some patients may be getting some agents that aren't considered chemotherapy but the patient thinks they are getting chemo."
	Constipation questions and medication lists	Written content and terminology	"I didn't know that morphine and opioids can cause constipation."
	Pain and nausea and vomiting medication questions	Written content and terminology	"Don't you want to know exact time and date of [a medication] dose?"
	Pain questions and medication list	Written content and terminology	Word "narcotic" brought up negative feelings it was "a scary word."
	Pain question and medication list	Written content and terminology	"I know narcotic is bad for you."
	General comment from bilingual participants	Written content and terminology	"Is this available in Spanish?"

Table 4 Results of Usability Testing for the SAMI-Self-Care CDS Program: Patient Perspectives *(Continued)*

Usability Testing Themes	CDS Tool Content*	CDS Tool Component**	Examples
Format and navigation	Pain and nausea and vomiting medication questions	Format and navigation	"Can we input all the medications we are taking into the system?"
	All symptom assessment questions	Format and navigation Suggestions to improve	"Add checkboxes to make this [the entry of symptoms] easier."
	All symptom questions	Written content and terminology	"Create an option of 'I don't know."
	General comment about iPad functionality	Format and navigation	"Are there instructions for those who are not computer users to know how to use this function?" (Referring to functionality of hovering over a definition for more information.)
	General comment on iPad	Format and navigation	"Use 'back' instead of 'previous.'"
Wording of self-management suggestions	General comment for instructions for call clinicians on report	Written content and terminology	"I don't want to bother my care team."
	General comment for instructions to call clinicians on report	Written content and terminology	"When should I contact my care team?"
	General comment for instructions to call clinicians on report	Written content and terminology	"What should I tell my care team?"
Other			
Patient safety	Pain report suggestions	Written content for report	"Is it safe for me to take this medication?"
	Nausea and vomiting red flag safety questions	Written content for safety questions	"Are we allowed to drink 2 large glasses a liquid per day? Shouldn't we ask the doctor first?"
	Constipation report suggestions	Written content for suggestions	"Is it safe for me to initiate the proposed intervention?"
Resources	Constipation suggestions	Other concerns	"Do I have suggested medications in my home?"
	General comment about iPad	Format and navigation	"Some people will lack the technology to access the system."

* CDS tool content refers to what aspect of the CDS tool that the comment sought to improve (i.e. medication vs. pain severity question)
** CDS tool component refers to what aspect of the CDS tool that the component that the comment sought to improve (i.e. written content vs. visual appeal)

Ensure patient safety

To ensure that the use of SAMI-Self-Care would not overlook a life-threatening condition, we identified a set of screening questions for each symptom that sought to direct patients with potentially dangerous conditions to stop using the algorithm and seek contact with their clinicians. To ensure that the advice provided through SAMI-Self-Care was sound, we derived algorithm logic and recommendations from evidence-based clinical guidelines. When appropriate, we also inquired if a recommended therapy had already been suggested by the patient's clinician. If the therapy had not been suggested, we encouraged the patients to check with their clinician to request approval before initiating a new medication.

Communicate clinical concepts effectively

In order to communicate clinical concepts effectively, we conducted cognitive testing of content with patients to ensure an adequate level of understanding, and we added graphics to support concepts in the text when appropriate. We also designated a section of the display for explanations or lists so that patients who needed more information could easily access it. Formative testing of questions through the cognitive interviewing process helped us to recognize that we needed to make questions as explicit and detailed as possible so patients were not left to speculate about how to respond. Finally, we used established interface development practices for screen appearance, layout, and text fonts to enhance readability [45].

Promote communication with clinicians

To encourage communication with patients' clinicians, we included explicit suggestions regarding when to contact their clinicians and a script for what to say to them. We also advised patients to notify their clinicians within a specified time frame about interventions they may have followed from SAMI-Self-Care.

Table 5 Results of Usability Testing for the SAMI-Self-Care CDS Program: Clinician Perspectives

Usability Testing Themes	CDS Tool Context*	CDS Tool Component**	Examples
Visual appeal	General comment related to the look and feel of the system	Format	"Use larger fonts and colors as a way to distinguish instructions from question."
	Nausea and vomiting	Format	"Give a visual description of what a 16-oz container might look like, e.g., a Poland spring water bottle."
Understanding of terminology	Pain severity question	Written content and preference for terminology	Disapproval of wording, "bearable pain."
	Nausea and vomiting question	Written content	"Clearly indicate what issue is being evaluated, e.g., [for] position change, are we asking about getting up quickly or vertigo?"
	Pain question	Written content	"Add timeframes, e.g., did taking the pain mediation offer you relief after 30 min?"
	Nausea and vomiting	Format	"Add graphics such as [a picture of] fire in the esophagus, which doesn't need a definition."
	All symptoms	Written content and format	"Medication lists might be overwhelming for some patients."
	Pain	Written content	"Offer educational explanation such as risk factors regarding why the patients shouldn't take certain medication, e.g., for ibuprofen explain why stomach protection is needed for those 65 or older."
Format and navigation	Comment about introduction and orientation to the program	Format	"Select a symptom that is bothering the patients the most, and then come back to evaluate other symptoms."
	Nausea and vomiting question	Written content and algorithms. This related to the issue that chemotherapy induced nausea may be more common than position-induced nausea	"Prioritize question order based on frequency of issues experienced by the patients to reduce number of questions patients have to answer and to avoid patients having to answer questions to symptoms majority might not experience."
	Comment to improve the look and feel of the program	Format and navigation	"Try to reduce the number of clicks needed to move the system forward, e.g., they shouldn't have to select the symptom and press next to move forward."
	Provide an introduction to questions so patients will know what to expect and why	Format and navigation	"Tell patients upfront the different symptoms or medications the program will ask about."
	General comment related to sequencing of questions	Format and navigation	"Add skip patterns for those who might have used the system before."
	General comment about sequence of questions	Written content	"Work on lessening redundancy of the questions."
Wording of self-management suggestions	Symptom reports	Written content	"Be clear with instructions regarding communication w/ clinicians."
	Symptom reports for red flag questions.	Written content	"Clearly indicate to the patient to call now, so they do not mistakenly think the report has been automatically sent to their clinician and that someone will follow up."
	Symptom reports	Written content	"Educate the patient on how to use the paging service."
	Symptom reports	Written content	"Don't put 'during normal business hours' because it sounds like we're telling patients to stop bothering us."
	Symptom reports	Written content	"List phone number of clinician on the report or a paging service for after hours."
Other			
Patient safety	All symptoms red flag questions developed for safety	Algorithm content	Identify all red flag/emergency issues.
	Pain red flag safety questions	Algorithm content	"Ask about new or severe pain not just one [or the other] and, [a] 'yes' [response] should mean call your doctor right away."

Table 5 Results of Usability Testing for the SAMI-Self-Care CDS Program: Clinician Perspectives *(Continued)*

Usability Testing Themes	CDS Tool Context*	CDS Tool Component**	Examples
	General comment about reports that are generated for self-management	Written content	Clinicians worried that they may not be informed about patient problems.
	All symptoms red flag questions added	Algorithm content	Clinicians concerned they may miss or overlook critical situations.
	General comment about the report	Written content	"Include notification to patient that they should always call provider with questions."
	General comment	Written content	"Wouldn't want the patient to use the program instead of getting care."
Resources	General concern about use of iPad	Format	Concern that some patients will not have access to computers.
Best care practices	Pain self-management for severe pain	Written content about when to call their clinicians	Lack of consensus among clinicians regarding clinical best practices.
	Nausea and vomiting acid reflux	Algorithm content	Some providers recommend medication like TUMS, but GI doctors may avoid it because it creates acid.
	Pain and nausea and vomiting	Written content wanted more comprehensive lists for medications	Recommended some medications be added on to lists [of medications already included].
	Pain medication question	Written content	"Change dosing criteria for long acting to 8–12 h."
	Pain medication lists	Written content	"Certain medications on the list not used across the board causing worry, e.g., fentanyl or tapentadol."

* CDS tool content refers to what aspect of the CDS tool that the comment sought to improve (i.e. medication vs. pain severity question)

** CDS tool component refers to what aspect of the CDS tool that the component that the comment sought to improve (i.e. written content vs. visual appeal)

Support patient activation

We sought to engage patients by providing personalized and actionable instructions. As appropriate, we asked patients about resource availability and their willingness to follow interventions prior to making recommendations. Through the educational display section, we provided content to help patients understand why certain questions were being asked and why specific recommendations were provided. Helpful features included suggestions for pharmacologic and non-pharmacologic therapies.

Facilitate navigation and use

To expedite SAMI-Self-Care use we identified methods to optimize traversal of the algorithms and minimize the burden of data entry (see Table 6). We included a progress bar for patients to know their position in the process, and we added capabilities to change responses or to pause a session. We also added display content to enable a patient to recognize the context of every interaction through tabs illustrating the symptom being addressed and text clarifying the context of each question. Finally, we ensured that all pathways could be traversed, were unique and not redundant.

Barriers that need to be addressed to promote patient-centered CDS

Barriers to promote patient-centered CDS regarding symptom self-management that emerged appeared to be consistent with the Chronic Care Model so the themes that emerged were reorganized around the components of this model which included: patient safety, cultural competency, care coordination, resource availability, and acceptance of technology.

Barriers pertaining to cultural competency were the most common and included challenges related to unfamiliar terminology, lack of reference to a clinical framework, and unusual health beliefs. Although many of the concerns identified by patients were shared by clinicians, a few items were unique to patients and their caregivers, including expressing uncertainty about some self-management suggestions and whether the actions would be acceptable to their clinicians, expressing negative health beliefs associated with the use of narcotic medications, and not having the suggested medications available at home. There also were concerns about communication with their clinicians, availability of technology in the community, and use of the technology.

Discussion

We developed a simulated algorithm-based CDS program to support symptom self-management among adults with cancer and their caregivers. Our CDS program is more complex than other previously developed programs and provides patents with specific information, tailored to their situation regarding when to call their clinician, what to tell them, and how to self-manage their symptoms. In order to accomplish this task, we have many more decisional nodes than previous patient-

Table 6 Design Objectives for Development of Patient-Centered CDS

Design Principle	Design Principle Details	Examples of Solutions	Change in User Interface
1 Ensure Patient Safety	1a Build algorithm content based on established clinical guidelines	Use of the NCCN guidelines for cancer pain management to guide algorithm content [63]	Based on published best practices, evidence-based content used for developing symptom management algorithms
			Iterative review process of algorithm content and recommendations by multidisciplinary expert panel members
	1b Identify at the beginning of a session potentially serious conditions for which continued use of algorithm could be harmful or life threatening	Additional characteristics of symptoms that suggest potentially dangerous or life threatening conditions identified. e.g., "in pain algorithm, besides enquiring about new or increased pain, adding a question that asksabout cramping or squeezing in chest or stomach".	Questions added that identify severity and trigger "call now" advice.
			CDS updated for immediate exit and to contact clinician if red flag was triggered
		Distinguished nuances between pain symptoms, (e.g. new pain (e.g. fracture) and chronic pain)	Any time red flag is triggered, patient provided with specific suggestions on the screen.
		Disclaimer needed to ensure safety (e.g. "In case of emergency, call your doctor or 911 immediately. Do not use this program for medical emergencies.")	Warning placed on the welcome page of the program.
			Bold font used as a way to capture patients' attention.
		There should be gradation of severity indicating what issues should the patient address first	Visual cues added to the report to help prioritize self-management strategies
			Colors (red-orange-green) and fonts used to ensure patient reviewed specific aspect of the report. e.g. call clinician now
			Report provided at the end can be viewed on the screen or as a printed report
	1c Inquire about appropriateness of recommendations prior to offering advice	Provide guidance on why particular intervention should not be implemented (e.g. taking ibuprofen)	Content modified to provide reasons why a particular intervention would not be permissible (e.g. stomach ulcers)
		Provide language to ensure any questions are directed to care team at all times	Report content updated to contact clinician if uncertainty about concerns on implementing recommendations
2 Communicate Clinical Concepts Effectively	2a Test word selection with intended end-users	Cognitive testing of terms and its interpretation	Modified wording utilized in assessment and recommendations to improve understanding of concepts
	2b Develop explicit, detailed questions	Remove ambiguity of decision points	Added specificity of timeframes to questions to improve meaning (, e.g., "Did taking short acting pain medication give you relief from your pain within 30 min of taking it?")
			Reference specific medications and dosages as appropriate
			Designed explicit decisions points to enable machine processing
	2c Enhance communication with graphics, especially for clinical concepts	Improve system use by reducing content	Added "faces" and word anchors as part of the pain scale
			Created content at a 5th grade reading level
			Inserted images to re-enforce concepts (e.g., stop sign for emer gency, picture to show acid reflux)
	2d Provide lists to enable patient to identify specific items such as medications	Utilization of system could be improved by equipping patients with necessary information	Provided lists of most common medications in defined classes in a designated area of the screen for lookup as needed
			Included generic and brand names of medications for ease of recognition
	2e Provide educational information to promote understanding	Using CDS as a way to reinforce and provide education on why certain questions are being asked	Educational content added in final summary reports customized to their symptoms
			Provided rationale of why certain questions were asked and promoted understanding
		Improve utility by improving layout of content	Used large and "heavier" font size to make text more visible

Table 6 Design Objectives for Development of Patient-Centered CDS *(Continued)*

Design Principle	Design Principle Details	Examples of Solutions	Change in User Interface
	2f Enhance readability with font style, font size, content density, selective highlighting of words		Reduced text density
			Used a plain white background
			Provided bolding to emphasize words
3 Promote Communication with Clinicians	3a Provide explicit instructions for patients regarding contacting clinicians about their concerns	Urgency of establishing clinical contact based on severity of the symptom needed(e.g. call right away vs. waiting 24 h)	Additional features added to generate report immediately on screen if patient triggered any of the emergency "red flag" questions and highlighted the importance of calling clinician NOW.
		Post assessment report that provides guidance on what should be done and when.	Immediate instructions provided to the patient, on calling clinician, onscreen of the program and not just within the report.
			Added explicit language on what patients should say when calling clinician.
		Initial reports lost the message about the importance of communicating with the clinician	Report restructured to reinforce importance of contacting clinicians and keeping them informed of regimen changes. E.g. tell your doctor or nurse you are taking 200 mg of ibuprofen as needed.
		Clearly communicate recommendations	Report modified into sections of: do now, do next and more suggestions, to help streamline and prioritize suggestions for what the patient can do and when
		Lack of specification of which symptoms are available for assessment at beginning of the program	3 symptoms patients can choose in current system listed at the beginning of the program.
			Patients advised to contact clinicians if experiencing symptoms not addressed by the system.
	3b Encourage patients to notify their clinical care team about interventions that they have followed	Reinforce the importance of notifying clinicians about any interventions that have been initiated within the recommendations	Provided instructions about what patients should specifically tell their clinicians about interventions
4 Support Patient Activation	4a Determine what resources are available to the patient	Improve efficiency of the system and utilization by modifying question based on what patients have available to them	Added questions to determine what interventions had already been prescribed
			Inquired if a prescription was already available for a recommended medication as a way to align with current therapy of the patient's care team
	4b Identify health beliefs that may impact interpretation of content and modify content accordingly	Modifying how content is framed	Content modified conveying meaning acceptable by patients. (e.g. pain medication vs. narcotics)
	4c Determine what patients are willing to do prior to making recommendations	Improving look and feel of the system that quickly provides information and allows the patient to take an active role in their care	Provided explicit, detailed instructions that include dosage amounts, frequencies, medication list and lifestyle suggestions
			Prioritized display in patient report to quickly and easily inform the patient on what they should do next
	4d Provide explicit, detailed, actionable instructions to the extent possible		Inquired about what patients were willing to do prior to recommending an intervention, e.g., use of enemas for constipation
	4e Personalize content, e.g., used possessive pronouns such as "my" or "your" where appropriate	Create an opportunity relate to the patient and provide self-management techniques	Changed the text to make it personable and user friendly, e.g., used possessive pronouns such as "my" or "your" where appropriate
5 Facilitate Navigation and Use	5a Designate consistent presentation areas on screen for repeated display of a specific type of information	Make it easy for patients to find information within the site	Posted medical terms with definitions in a specific area on the screen so end user can easily and quickly access information as needed

Table 6 Design Objectives for Development of Patient-Centered CDS *(Continued)*

Design Principle	Design Principle Details	Examples of Solutions	Change in User Interface
			Avoided "pop-ups" because they felt to be interruptive and harder to navigate for a limited computer proficient user
	5b Provide comprehensive set of selection options	Ensure all possible decision points are covered	Guidelines and best practices used for comprehensive coverage to ensure all possible selections covered for every decision node
	5c Streamline data entry	Improve flow and provide feedback quickly	Introduced check boxes to cut down on number of questions required to determine what advice to provide and improved efficiency
	5d Optimize workflow through questions	Inquiring about symptom characteristics at the beginning of the algorithm	Enabled selection of an item on a page to advance to the next page as appropriate
			Directed patients to highly specific interventions
	5e Optimize workflow through questions	Inquiring about symptom characteristics at the beginning of the algorithm	Facilitated patients starting at the appropriate place in the algorithm by inquiring what interventions have already been attempted
			Introduced check boxes to reduce number of question and reduce redundancy
	5f Track progress for patient	Promote efficient workflow	Added progress bar showing numeric value, not just graphic representing progress
			Included "Go Back" function to allow patient to modify earlier responses
	5g Accommodate patient changes and pauses		Offered multiple ways to start over such as: "Back to Start button" as well as tabs with symptom names
			Included "Take a Break" button to allow patient to pause the program and come back to it again
	5h Provide context for all interactions so that patient recognizes where he/she is within an algorithm		Added tabs as a way to indicate to the patient which algorithm they were in
			Provided headers to supply context for each page anchoring the patient on where they are in a given algorithm
	5i Ensure completeness and uniqueness of pathways through algorithm		Provided brief overview of different topics that were covered to orient patients at the beginning of a session
			Re-enforced context and inter-relatedness of questions by showing question and answer from the previous page
			Ensured that questions allow for a single non-redundant, unique pathway for all possible scenarios
			Ensured that every pathway led to advice
	5j Create tools that will function across multiple platforms	Assessed target patient population to determine that 85% of patients had access or knew how to obtain access to computers or smart phones	Created CDS tool design to function on Web, smart phone, or iPad

centered CDS systems [12, 22]. Acceptability testing results among patients were favorable, suggesting that patients found the SAMI-Self Care prototype a satisfactory approach to for symptom self-management. Providing CDS directly to patients may be a valuable tool. Future studies should explore the best modalities for providing access to these tools including the Web, tablet computers, or mobile phones [46]. We anticipate that the SAMI-Self-Care tool could be implemented on a Web-based platform that could be accessible across computers, tablets and smartphones. A link to this content could be inserted in the homepage of a patient's oncology treatment group or sent out directly to patients through electronic mail.

We noted that the acceptability results from clinicians for pain were less favorable than for nausea/vomiting and constipation, and were below our desired threshold of 4.0 for helpfulness of the report and suggestions. This result required obtaining a larger sample size to gather responses about usability testing as compared to other symptoms. In spite of our efforts to adhere to pain guidelines, [47] some clinicians were reluctant to support self-management because they wanted to remain aware of their patients' symptoms and to be directly involved in management. This finding is interesting as implementation of pain guidelines has been a challenge. Evidence suggests that pain management practices have not changed over the last twenty years and many patients with cancer continue to experience severe uncontrolled pain [48, 49]. Further study is needed to understand clinician attitudes toward pain management and barriers to encouraging patient self-care management. One concern that clinicians expressed is that they wanted to be aware of patients who had severe levels of pain. The addition of a system that alerts clinicians when patient symptoms pass a predetermined level of severity would address this concern. Cleeland and colleagues [13] found that automated symptom severity alerts after surgery for lung cancer reduced symptom distress. In a recent study that examined clinician preferences for CDS, the use of an alerting system for increased symptom severity was identified as a desirable component [50].

Our design objectives were specifically developed in this study to support development of effective patient-focused CDS. To date, CDS design objectives have focused on use by clinicians. Thus, even though our CDS system was designed for patients, we sought to include features known to be associated with effective CDS systems for clinicians [35, 36, 51]. The system features identified in our study that were similar to clinician CDS included: graphics to enhance understanding of content; explicit, actionable recommendations provided at the point of decision-making; presentation of advice that cultivated trust by providing an explanation of medical logic if needed [36]. In addition, similar to Bates and colleagues, [35] our Design Objectives focused on streamlining the user interaction by decreasing the number of questions needed to inform the algorithm, targeting anticipated needs with advice in real-time, providing supplemental information as needed but without interruption, and relying on a user-centered iterative design [43]. Ozkaynak and colleagues [52] noted that an important difference between patient and clinician design for CDS is integrating technology into the user's work flow. Designing CDS around clinician work flow is much easier than for patient work flow as clinicians function within a health system, whereas work flow for patients spans multiple health care settings and includes home, routines of daily living and communication with family, clinicians and the health care system [52–55]. The CDS program that was evaluated in this study attempts to bridge the gap between care delivered in health care settings and self-care in the home. There is a need for applications that improve outcomes across settings and patient populations [56]. Future studies are needed to assess the impact of this CDS program on patient outcomes.

Through this process, we identified patient barriers to use of CDS and clinicians' concerns about patients using CDS for self-management. From these barriers and concerns, we derived Design Objectives for CDS for symptom self-management, which included ensuring patient safety, communicating clinical concepts effectively, promoting communication with clinicians, supporting patient activation and facilitating navigation and use. These objectives may be useful to inform the design of CDS systems for symptom self-management of other conditions.

The barriers we identified for CDS for cancer symptom self-management had similarities and differences to barriers associated with self-management in patients with non-malignant conditions [57, 58]. Similar barriers included lack of knowledge, poor communication between patients and clinicians, and logistical issues in obtaining care. However, in contrast to the patients who did not have cancer, the cancer patients did not report barriers related to physical limitations, financial constraints, a need for social and emotional support, or challenges adhering to treatment [57, 58]. Other differences in concerns that we noted between patients with cancer and those with non-malignant conditions were that cancer patients and their caregivers expressed concerns related to ensuring patient safety and negative health beliefs about use of narcotic pain medications. Shumacher and colleagues [59, 60] examined pain management processes among cancer patients and their caregivers and found similar concerns related to ensuring patient safety, especially in the context of narcotic pain medications. Patients and their caregivers had little interaction with clinicians in the home setting and had to master complex tasks related to taking their medications and reported that they felt that they had to be the final safety check.

Limitations

The sample for this study was drawn from one institution using purposive sampling so it is not representative of all cancer patients. All of the patients and their caregivers in this study indicated that they used the Internet for seeking health information at least sometimes. This rate is higher than the 72% of Internet users found in the 2014 Pew Research survey [61]. Our rates for Internet usage may be higher as the majority of our sample had greater than a high school education. Factors associated with lower access of the Internet are older age, lower education and lower income [62]. Another limitation is that the majority of the sample was Caucasian and had higher levels of education. Further testing of this approach in a more diverse group of patients with cancer is warranted. Although the use of a simulated model provided a practical and economical approach to iterative development of the CDS tool, this approach did not allow for real time navigation through the algorithms for patients. This would be the next step in the development process.

Conclusions

The boundaries of health care are expanding and patients and their caregivers often have to self-manage complex cancer care at home. Thus, patient-centered decision support that meets this need is important and timely. Our system provides tailored information that informs patients when to call their clinicians, provides a script about what to tell tem about their symptom and specific suggestions about how the self manage their symptoms at home. Patients and their caregivers rated SAMI-Self-Care as highly acceptable and found the recommendations helpful. The patient-centered CDS design objectives we derived for cancer symptom self-management may be applicable for the self-management of other conditions.

Abbreviations

CDS: Clinical decision support; SAMI-Self-Care: Symptom Assessment and Management Intervention - Self Care

Acknowledgements

We acknowledged the significant contributions of the expert panel in selecting the patient-focused decision-support project and refining the content and design of the decision support tools specified through this project. In addition to the co-authors of this manuscript, members of this expert panel included Annmarie Uliano, Richard Boyajian, MS; Jane Brzozowski, MS; and Drs. Aymen Elfiky, Anne Gross, Joseph Jacobson, Christopher Lathan, and Larry Shulman. We also acknowledge the contributions of the Dana-Farber Harvard Comprehensive Cancer Center Health Communication Core of for their contributions to the design and development of the SAMI-SC prototype. The authors also wish to thank the participants who shared their valuable time and effort. We appreciate the data collection contributions of research coordinator Maribel Melendez and Taylor Hendel for manuscript preparation.

Author contributions

MEC participated in conception of the project, data collection, analyses and interpretation of data, writing and revising the manuscript, final approval of the manuscript and is accountable for the quality of work. JLA participated in conception of the project, analyses and interpretation of data, writing and revising the manuscript, final approval of the manuscript and is accountable for the quality of work. DLB participated in conception of the project, interpretation of data, writing and revising the manuscript, final approval of the manuscript and is accountable for the quality of work. MSR participated in conception of the project, interpretation of data, writing and revising the manuscript, final approval of the manuscript and is accountable for the quality of work. IMB participated in conception of the project, interpretation of data, writing and revising the manuscript, final approval of the manuscript and is accountable for the quality of work. Patient stakeholder, JP, participated in conception of the project, interpretation of data, writing and revising the manuscript, final approval of the manuscript and is accountable for the quality of work. MMN participated in data collection, analyses and interpretation of data, writing and revising the manuscript, final approval of the manuscript and is accountable for the quality of work. DFL participated in conception of the project, analyses and interpretation of data, writing and revising the manuscript, final approval of the manuscript and is accountable for the quality of work. All authors read and approved the final manuscript.

Funding

This work was supported by The Patient Centered Outcomes Research Institute Grant PI-12-001.

Competing interests

The authors declare that they have no competing interests.

Author details

[1]The Phyllis F. Cantor Center, Dana-Farber Cancer Institute, 450 Brookline Avenue, Boston, MA 02115, USA. [2]Department of Psychosocial Oncology and Palliative Care, Dana-Farber Cancer Institute, 450 Brookline Avenue, Boston, MA 02115, USA. [3]The Phyllis F. Cantor Center and the Department of Medicine, Dana-Farber Cancer Institute, 450 Brookline Ave, LW-512, Boston, MA 02115, USA. [4]Lowe Center for Thoracic Oncology, Dana-Farber Cancer Institute, 450 Brookline Avenue, Boston, MA 02115, USA. [5]Klesis Healthcare and Department of Family Medicine, Durham, NC 27705, USA. [6]Department of Family Medicine, Duke University Medical Center, 2100 Erwin Road, Durham, NC 27710, USA.

References

1. Institute of Medicine Committee on Quality of Health Care in A. Crossing the quality chasm: a new health system for the 21st century. Washington (DC): National Academies Press (US) Copyright 2001 by the National Academy of Sciences. All rights reserved; 2001.
2. Patient Self-Management Support Programs: An Evaluation. Final Contract Report [http://www.orau.gov/ahrq/sms_report_08.asp?p=browse_guide]. Accessed Feb 2016.
3. McCorkle R, Ercolano E, Lazenby M, Schulman-Green D, Schilling LS, Lorig K, Wagner EH. Self-management: enabling and empowering patients living with cancer as a chronic illness. CA Cancer J Clin. 2011;61(1):50–62.
4. Schulman-Green D, Bradley EH, Knobf MT, Prigerson H, DiGiovanna MP, McCorkle R. Self-management and transitions in women with advanced breast cancer. J Pain Symptom Manag. 2011;42(4):517–25.
5. Schulman-Green D, Bradley EH, Nicholson NR, Jr., George E, Indeck A, McCorkle R: One step at a time: self-management and transitions among women with ovarian cancer. Oncol Nurs Forum 2012, 39(4):354–360.
6. Bodenheimer T, Lorig K, Holman H, Grumbach K. Patient self-management of chronic disease in primary care. JAMA. 2002;288(19):2469–75.
7. Warsi A, Wang PS, LaValley MP, Avorn J, Solomon DH. Self-management education programs in chronic disease: a systematic review and methodological critique of the literature. Arch Intern Med. 2004;164(15):1641–9.

8. Lorig KR, Sobel DS, Stewart AL, Brown BW Jr, Bandura A, Ritter P, Gonzalez VM, Laurent DD, Holman HR. Evidence suggesting that a chronic disease self-management program can improve health status while reducing hospitalization: a randomized trial. Med Care. 1999;37(1):5–14.
9. McKay HGG, Russell E, Feil EG, Boles SM, Barrera M Jr. Internet-based diabetes self-management and support: initial outcomes from the diabetes network project. Rehabil Psychol. 2002;47(1):31–48.
10. Mooney KH, Beck SL, Friedman RH, Farzanfar R, Wong B. Automated monitoring of symptoms during ambulatory chemotherapy and oncology providers' use of the information: a randomized controlled clinical trial. Support Care Cancer. 2014;22(9):2343–50.
11. Ruland CM, Andersen T, Jeneson A, Moore S, Grimsbo GH, Borosund E, Ellison MC. Effects of an internet support system to assist cancer patients in reducing symptom distress: a randomized controlled trial. Cancer Nurs. 2013;36(1):6–17.
12. Berry DL, Hong F, Halpenny B, Partridge A, Fox E, Fann JR, Wolpin S, Lober WB, Bush N, Parvathaneni U, et al. The electronic self report assessment and intervention for cancer: promoting patient verbal reporting of symptom and quality of life issues in a randomized controlled trial. BMC Cancer. 2014;14:513.
13. Cleeland CS, Wang XS, Shi Q, Mendoza TR, Wright SL, Berry MD, Malveaux D, Shah PK, Gning I, Hofstetter WL, et al. Automated symptom alerts reduce postoperative symptom severity after cancer surgery: a randomized controlled clinical trial. J Clin Oncol Off J Am Soc Clin Oncol. 2011;29(8):994–1000.
14. Barlow J, Wright C, Sheasby J, Turner A, Hainsworth J. Self-management approaches for people with chronic conditions: a review. Patient Educ Couns. 2002;48(2):177–87.
15. Samoocha D, Bruinvels DJ, Elbers NA, Anema JR, van der Beek AJ. Effectiveness of web-based interventions on patient empowerment: a systematic review and meta-analysis. J Med Internet Res. 2010;12(2):e23.
16. Gustafson DH, Hawkins R, McTavish F, Pingree S, Chen WC, Volrathongchai K, Stengle W, Stewart JA, Serlin RC. Internet-based interactive support for Cancer patients: are integrated systems better? J Commun. 2008;58(2):238–57.
17. Marie N, Luckett T, Davidson PM, Lovell M, Lal S. **Optimal patient education for cancer pain: a systematic review and theory-based meta-analysis**. Support Care Cancer. 2013;21(12):3529–37.
18. Yun YH, Lee KS, Kim YW, Park SY, Lee ES, Noh DY, Kim S, Oh JH, Jung SY, Chung KW et al: Web-based tailored education program for disease-free cancer survivors with cancer-related fatigue: a randomized controlled trial. J Clin Oncol Off J Am Soc Clin Oncol 2012, 30(12):1296–1303.
19. Lewis FM, Brandt PA, Cochrane BB, Griffith KA, Grant M, Haase JE, Houldin AD, Post-White J, Zahlis EH, Shands ME. The enhancing connections program: a six-state randomized clinical trial of a cancer parenting program. J Consult Clin Psychol. 2015;83(1):12–23.
20. Ruland CM, Jeneson A, Andersen T, Andersen R, Slaughter L, Bente Schjodt O, Moore SM. Designing tailored internet support to assist cancer patients in illness management. AMIA Annu Symp Proc. 2007;2007:635–9.
21. Osheroff JA, Teich JM, Middleton B, Steen EB, Wright A, Detmer DE. A roadmap for national action on clinical decision support. J Am Med Inform Assoc. 2007;14(2):141–5.
22. Head BA, Keeney C, Studts JL, Khayat M, Bumpous J, Pfeifer M. Feasibility and acceptance of a telehealth intervention to promote symptom management during treatment for head and neck Cancer. J Support Oncol. 2011;9(1):e1–e11.
23. Weaver A, Young AM, Rowntree J, Townsend N, Pearson S, Smith J, Gibson O, Cobern W, Larsen M, Tarassenko L. Application of mobile phone technology for managing chemotherapy-associated side-effects. Ann Oncol. 2007;18(11): 1887–92.
24. Berry DL, Hong F, Halpenny B, Partridge AH, Fann JR, Wolpin S, Lober WB, Bush NE, Parvathaneni U, Back AL, et al. Electronic self-report assessment for cancer and self-care support: results of a multicenter randomized trial. J Clin Oncol Off J Am Soc Clin Oncol. 2014;32(3):199–205.
25. Ruland CM, Maffei RM, Borosund E, Krahn A, Andersen T, Grimsbo GH. Evaluation of different features of an eHealth application for personalized illness management support: cancer patients' use and appraisal of usefulness. Int J Med Inform. 2013;82(7):593–603.
26. Creswell JW, Plano Clark VL. Designing and conducting mixed methods research, 2nd edn. Thousand Oaks: Sage Publications; 2011.
27. Fervers B, Burgers JS, Haugh MC, Latreille J, Mlika-Cabanne N, Paquet L, Coulombe M, Poirier M, Burnand B. Adaptation of clinical guidelines: literature review and proposition for a framework and procedure. Int J Qual Health Care. 2006;18(3):167–76.
28. Amer YS, Elzalabany MM, Omar TI, Ibrahim AG, Dowidar NL. The 'Adapted ADAPTE': an approach to improve utilization of the ADAPTE guideline adaptation resource toolkit in the Alexandria Center for Evidence-Based Clinical Practice Guidelines. J Eval Clin Pract. 2015;21(6):1095–106.
29. Fervers B, Burgers JS, Voellinger R, Brouwers M, Browman GP, Graham ID, Harrison MB, Latreille J, Mlika-Cabane N, Paquet L, et al. Guideline adaptation: an approach to enhance efficiency in guideline development and improve utilisation. BMJ Qual Saf. 2011;20(3):228–36.
30. Ruegg TA. A nurse practitioner-led urgent care center: meeting the needs of the patient with cancer. Clin J Oncol Nurs. 2013;17(4):E52–7.
31. Cooley ME, Lobach DF, Johns E, Halpenny B, Saunders TA, Del Fiol G, Rabin MS, Calarese P, Berenbaum IL, Zaner K, et al. Creating computable algorithms for symptom management in an outpatient thoracic oncology setting. J Pain Symptom Manag. 2013;46(6):911–24. e911
32. Scariot CA, Heemann A, Padovani S. Understanding the collaborative-participatory design. Work (Reading, Mass). 2012;41(Suppl 1):2701–5.
33. Revere D, Dixon BE, Hills R, Williams JL, Grannis SJ. Leveraging health information exchange to improve population health reporting processes: lessons in using a collaborative-participatory design process. EGEMS (Wash, DC). 2014;2(3):1082.
34. Collins D. Pretesting survey instruments: an overview of cognitive methods. Qual Life Res Int J Qual Life Asp Treat Care Rehab. 2003;12(3):229–38.
35. Bates DW, Kuperman GJ, Wang S, Gandhi T, Kittler A, Volk L, Spurr C, Khorasani R, Tanasijevic M, Middleton B. Ten commandments for effective clinical decision support: making the practice of evidence-based medicine a reality. J Am Med Inform Assoc. 2003;10(6):523–30.
36. Kawamoto K, Houlihan CA, Balas EA, Lobach DF. Improving clinical practice using clinical decision support systems: a systematic review of trials to identify features critical to success. BMJ. 2005;330(7494):765.
37. Crabtree BF, Yanoshik MK, Miller WL, O'Connor PJ. Successful focus groups: advancing the state of the art. Thousand Oaks: SAGE Publications, Inc.; 1993.
38. Virzi R. Refining the test phase of usability evaluation: how many subjects is enough? Hum Factors. 1992;34(4):457–68.
39. Tariman JD, Berry DL, Halpenny B, Wolpin S, Schepp K. Validation and testing of the acceptability E-scale for web-based patient-reported outcomes in cancer care. Appl Nurs Res. 2011;24(1):53–8.
40. Berry DL, Halpenny B, Wolpin S, Davison BJ, Ellis WJ, Lober WB, McReynolds J, Wulff J. Development and evaluation of the personal patient profile-prostate (P3P), a web-based decision support system for men newly diagnosed with localized prostate cancer. J Med Internet Res. 2010;12(4):e67.
41. Mullen KH, Berry DL, Zierler BK. Computerized symptom and quality-of-life assessment for patients with cancer part II: acceptability and usability. Oncol Nurs Forum. 2004;31(5):E84–9.
42. Elo S, Kyngas H. The qualitative content analysis process. J Adv Nurs. 2008; 62(1):107–15.
43. Coleman K, Austin BT, Brach C, Wagner EH. Evidence on the chronic care model in the new millennium: thus far, the evidence on the chronic care model is encouraging, but we need better tools to help practices improve their systems. Health affairs (Project Hope). 2009;28(1):75–85.
44. Lobach DF, Johns EB, Halpenny B, Saunders TA, Brzozowski J, Del Fiol G, Berry DL, Braun IM, Finn K, Wolfe J *et al*: Increasing complexity in rule-based clinical decision support: the symptom assessment and management intervention. JMIR Med Inform 2016, 4(4):e36.
45. Johnson CM, Johnson TR, Zhang J. A user-centered framework for redesigning health care interfaces. J Biomed Inform. 2005;38(1):75–87.
46. Mirkovic J, Kaufman DR, Ruland CM. Supporting cancer patients in illness management: usability evaluation of a mobile app. JMIR mHealth and uHealth. 2014;2(3):e33. doi:https://doi.org/10.2196/mhealth.3359.
47. Gordon DB, Dahl JL, Miaskowski C, McCarberg B, Todd KH, Paice JA, Lipman AG, Bookbinder M, Sanders SH, Turk DC, et al. American pain society recommendations for improving the quality of acute and cancer pain management: American pain society quality of care task force. Arch Intern Med. 2005;165(14):1574–80.
48. Isaac T, Stuver SO, Davis RB, Block S, Weeks JC, Berry DL, Weingart SN. Incidence of severe pain in newly diagnosed ambulatory patients with stage IV cancer. Pain Res Manag. 2012, **17**;(5):347–52.
49. Zhao F, Chang VT, Cleeland C, Cleary JF, Mitchell EP, Wagner LI, Fisch MJ. Determinants of pain severity changes in ambulatory patients with cancer: an analysis from eastern cooperative oncology group trial E2Z02.

50. Berry DL, Nayak MM, Abrahm JL, Braun I, Rabin MS, Cooley ME. Clinician perspectives on symptom and quality of life experiences of patients during cancer therapies: implications for eHealth. Psycho-Oncology. 2017;
51. Horsky J, Schiff GD, Johnston D, Mercincavage L, Bell D, Middleton B. Interface design principles for usable decision support: a targeted review of best practices for clinical prescribing interventions. J Biomed Inform. 2012; 45(6):1202–16.
52. Ozkaynak M, Brennan PF, Hanauer DA, Johnson S, Aarts J, Zheng K, Haque SN. Patient-centered care requires a patient-oriented workflow model. J Am Med Inform Assoc. 2013;20(e1):e14–6.
53. Ahern DK, Woods SS, Lightowler MC, Finley SW, Houston TK. Promise of and potential for patient-facing technologies to enable meaningful use. Am J Prev Med. 2011;40(5 Suppl 2):S162–72.
54. Clauser SB, Wagner EH, Aiello Bowles EJ, Tuzzio L, Greene SM. Improving modern cancer care through information technology. Am J Prev Med. 2011; 40(5 Suppl 2):S198–207.
55. Valdez RS, Holden RJ, Novak LL, Veinot TC. Transforming consumer health informatics through a patient work framework: connecting patients to context. J Am Med Inform Assoc. 2015;22(1):2–10.
56. McCoy AB, Wright A, Eysenbach G, Malin BA, Patterson ES, Xu H, Sittig DF. State of the art in clinical informatics: evidence and examples. Yearb Med inform. 2013;8(1):13–9.
57. Bayliss EA, Steiner JF, Fernald DH, Crane LA, Main DS. Descriptions of barriers to self-care by persons with comorbid chronic diseases. Ann Fam Med. 2003;1(1):15–21.
58. Fort MP, Alvarado-Molina N, Pena L, Mendoza Montano C, Murrillo S, Martinez H. Barriers and facilitating factors for disease self-management: a qualitative analysis of perceptions of patients receiving care for type 2 diabetes and/or hypertension in San Jose, Costa Rica and Tuxtla Gutierrez, Mexico. BMC Fam Pract. 2013;14:131.
59. Schumacher KL, Plano Clark VL, West CM, Dodd MJ, Rabow MW, Miaskowski C. Pain medication management processes used by oncology outpatients and family caregivers part II: home and lifestyle contexts. J Pain Symptom Manag. 2014;48(5):784–96.
60. Schumacher KL, Plano Clark VL, West CM, Dodd MJ, Rabow MW, Miaskowski C. Pain medication management processes used by oncology outpatients and family caregivers part I: health systems contexts. J Pain Symptom Manag. 2014;48(5):770–83.
61. Fox S, Duggan M. Health online 2013. Pew Research Center. Internet, Science, and Tech. Internet. 15 Jan 2013. (http://www.pewinternet.org/2013/01/15/health-online-2013/)
62. Smith A, PRCI. Science and technology: technology adoption by lower income populations. San Diego: American Public Human Services Association, IT Solution Management; 2013.
63. NCCN. Clinical practice guidelines in oncology. Adult Cancer Pain. Version 2. 2014 [http://williams.medicine.wisc.edu/pain.pdf

11

Presentation of laboratory test results in patient portals: influence of interface design on risk interpretation and visual search behaviour

Paolo Fraccaro[1,2,3*], Markel Vigo[5], Panagiotis Balatsoukas[7], Sabine N. van der Veer[2,3], Lamiece Hassan[2,3], Richard Williams[1,2,3], Grahame Wood[4], Smeeta Sinha[4], Iain Buchan[6] and Niels Peek[1,2,3]

Abstract

Background: Patient portals are considered valuable instruments for self-management of long term conditions, however, there are concerns over how patients might interpret and act on the clinical information they access. We hypothesized that visual cues improve patients' abilities to correctly interpret laboratory test results presented through patient portals. We also assessed, by applying eye-tracking methods, the relationship between risk interpretation and visual search behaviour.

Methods: We conducted a controlled study with 20 kidney transplant patients. Participants viewed three different graphical presentations in each of low, medium, and high risk clinical scenarios composed of results for 28 laboratory tests. After viewing each clinical scenario, patients were asked how they would have acted in real life if the results were their own, as a proxy of their risk interpretation. They could choose between: 1) Calling their doctor immediately (high interpreted risk); 2) Trying to arrange an appointment within the next 4 weeks (medium interpreted risk); 3) Waiting for the next appointment in 3 months (low interpreted risk). For each presentation, we assessed accuracy of patients' risk interpretation, and employed eye tracking to assess and compare visual search behaviour.

Results: Misinterpretation of risk was common, with 65% of participants underestimating the need for action across all presentations at least once. Participants found it particularly difficult to interpret medium risk clinical scenarios. Participants who consistently understood when action was needed showed a higher visual search efficiency, suggesting a better strategy to cope with information overload that helped them to focus on the laboratory tests most relevant to their condition.

Conclusions: This study confirms patients' difficulties in interpreting laboratories test results, with many patients underestimating the need for action, even when abnormal values were highlighted or grouped together. Our findings raise patient safety concerns and may limit the potential of patient portals to actively involve patients in their own healthcare.

Keywords: User-computer interface [MeSH], Computers/utilization [MeSH], Decision making [MeSH], Personal health record [MeSH], Patient access to records [MeSH], Patient portals, Decision support systems, clinical [MeSH], Personal health records, Patients access to records, Laboratory test results, Computer utilization, Eye tracking

* Correspondence: paolo.fraccaro@manchester.ac.uk
[1]NIHR Greater Manchester Primary Care Patient Safety Translational Research Centre, The University of Manchester, Manchester, UK
[2]Health eResearch Centre, Farr Institute for Health Informatics Research, London, UK
Full list of author information is available at the end of the article

Background

Patient portals are frequently assumed to motivate and involve patients in their own health and care [1–6]. These systems allow patients to book appointments online, view laboratory test results, or communicate with their physicians. Currently, many patient portals are for patients living with long-term conditions [7, 8], where longitudinal follow-ups are complex, and where self-management is a key component [9].

Patients mainly use patient portals to check their laboratory test results [10–14]. Yet, laboratory test results are among the most difficult data for patients to understand [15–18], and there are concerns about the suitability of patient portals to support patients in this task [7, 19]. Misinterpretation of laboratory test results can have adverse effects on patient safety, increase patient anxiety, and reduce self-management efficacy [7, 14, 20]. With the increasing availability of patient portals [21, 22], it is therefore important to understand how patients interact with, and process, laboratory test results to inform the online presentation of this information for accurate risk interpretation and improved user interaction.

It is known that several contextual factors, like a patient's numeracy and health literacy, can influence risk interpretation in the context of online laboratory test results [17, 23], however little is known about the effect of presentation on risk interpretation and interaction with this type of information. Previous studies have reported that patients found it difficult to understand laboratory test results shown in tables [15–17, 23] and graphs [15, 18], even when patients were familiar with the clinical scenarios at hand (i.e. glucose level monitoring for diabetes patients) [17]. A possible explanation for this phenomenon is the way numerical data were presented to patients [24]. Horizontal coloured bars that contextualise the latest value in relation to the standard range have been one of the few alternative presentations that have been implemented to improve risk interpretation of laboratory test results [16, 23]. They outperformed tables in terms of perceived usefulness [16] and decrease perceived urgency of borderline (i.e. low deviance from reference range) laboratory test results [23]. However, so far they have been only tested on static implementations (e.g., not on fully functioning patient portals) and on a limited number of laboratory tests at the same time. More widely, there are new presentation techniques that have been shown to enhance human decision making and information seeking behaviours in other web-based contexts [25–30]. However, these have not been tried in patient portals. For example, grouping (e.g., presenting together items that have similar characteristics) combined with the overview preview metaphor (e.g. where all user interaction happens within the same page) have been proven more effective than tables or list-based presentations in information-seeking and decision-making tasks [28–30]. However, this approach was never tested in the context of online laboratory test results.

We conducted a controlled study in which participants accessed different web-based presentations of laboratory test results across different clinical scenarios. We hypothesized that presentations using colour, which positively influences human cognition for risk interpretation tasks [31], and graphical cues (e.g., horizontal coloured bars and personalised grouping) improve patients' interpretation of laboratory test results presented through patient portals. To investigate whether correct interpretations were associated with specific visual search behaviours, our secondary objective was to assess and compare metrics derived from eye-tracking data including search efficiency and cognitive load.

Methods

Study population

We focused on patients with Chronic Kidney Disease (CKD), for whom there is an online platform, named PatientView [32], that provides access to laboratory results and is available in 90% of renal units in the UK. We included patients who had a kidney transplant (at least 12 months before recruitment). These patients undergo longitudinal follow-up with quarterly visits, including a review of their laboratory test results. This allowed us to obtain a homogeneous group of participants in terms of their experience with and knowledge of the disease. We excluded patients with any visual impairment, to avoid ineffective eye tracking data collection, and patients who did not use the internet in their everyday lives, to ensure a certain level of digital proficiency required to be a potential patient portal user.

We recruited 20 patients from the Renal Transplant Clinic at Salford Royal NHS Foundation Trust (SRFT), which has one of the largest communities of PatientView users in the UK. The study received ethical approval from NHS and local R&D ethical committees (IRAS ID: 183,845). Research nurses from the NIHR Clinical Research Network Portfolio (Study CPMS ID: 20,645) were responsible for approaching eligible patients and collecting signed informed consents of patients willing to participate.

Patient involvement

Increasingly patients are becoming involved as active partners in planning and undertaking research, rather than only as participants or data sources [33]. Throughout the project, we involved three patients from the local CKD patient community (http://gmkin.org.uk/) as collaborators, of whom two had experience of using PatientView. Initially, these patient collaborators participated in a workshop with researchers, during which they provided insights on their perceived importance and relevance of monitoring laboratory test results in CKD, and the role of PatientView in such tasks. During the workshop the patient collaborators also commented on preliminary visual presentations that we had prepared based on the literature discussed in the background and suggested additional features that might support them in interpreting their laboratory results on PatientView. After the workshop the patient collaborators were involved via email, providing comments on visual presentations and the study protocol. One patient collaborator also pilot-tested our data collection procedure and commented on our interpretation of the results.

The continuous involvement of patient collaborators allowed us to design a more realistic, relevant and acceptable experiment. Furthermore, two of our patient collaborators were experienced PatientView users, often interacting with other fellow patients in the local CKD patient community on this topic. Therefore, their advice and feedback was extremely important while developing our visual presentations.

Controlled study design

The study followed a "3 × 3" repeated measures, within-subjects design where each participant used, in a random order, three different presentations of web-based laboratory test results to complete the same simulated task in three different clinical scenarios. These were designed by a nephrologist at SRFT to reflect:

- *High risk clinical scenarios:* characterised as life threatening situations that required immediate action; creatinine and estimated Glomerular Filtration Rate (eGFR) (i.e. the main indicators of kidney function [34]), as well as potassium (associated with higher mortality in kidney patients [35]) strongly deviated from the standard range.
- *Medium risk clinical scenarios:* identified by abnormal creatinine and eGFR, but normal potassium and stable conditions; no urgent action was necessary, however further tests were required within 4 weeks;
- *Low risk clinical scenarios:* characterised by normal creatinine, eGFR and potassium; not requiring any action until the next scheduled appointment.

In addition to creatinine, eGFR and potassium each scenario included 25 laboratory test results with different deviances from the standard range in relation to the reflected risk (i.e. higher risk scenarios had more concomitant abnormal values).

There was no previous training or time limit for performing the task. Participants could decide to stop exploring the laboratory test results whenever they felt ready to reply to the follow up questions.

The controlled study was conducted at the Interaction Analysis and Modelling laboratory of the University of Manchester, and each patient participated individually. All participants performed the tasks using a desktop computer with a 17-in. screen with an embedded eye tracker (Tobii T60), which permits a 60-Hz sampling rate, 0.5 degrees gaze point accuracy, and free head motion.

Presentations

We implemented three presentations of laboratory test results (see Fig. 1 and Additional file 1: Figure S1-S9 for details). In developing these presentations, we aimed at maintaining similar amount of textual information, but showing it through different formats and visual cues to enhance patient interpretation. These were chosen based on review of the literature and patient collaborators' feedback on preliminary prototypes.

The *Baseline presentation* was based directly on, and very similar to, the current PatientView [32] interface, which uses tiles to show the latest available laboratory test results. Each tile reports information on the value of a laboratory test, its unit, the date of the test, data source, and standard range. By clicking on a tile the user can access previous results (i.e. longitudinal information), with the possibility of comparing it with another test within the same graph. This feature can be particularly useful in the context of CKD, where the use of some medications improves renal function but can also negatively affect the functioning of other organs. This would be reflected by abnormal values in laboratory test results.

The comparison presentations were based on the Baseline presentation, but provided different visual cues, colours and tools to show normal and abnormal values. Chronic patients have an increased risk of having test results falling slightly outside the reference range, with only those with high deviance from the population reference range likely to be clinically relevant [36]. Therefore, the second presentation (*Contextualised presentation*) used horizontal coloured bars that contextualise the latest value in relation to the standard range in each tile [16, 23, 37], which, as already said in the background, have outperformed tables in terms of perceived usefulness [16] and decrease perceived urgency of borderline (i.e. low deviance from reference range) laboratory test results [23]. The third presentation (*Grouped presentation*) aimed at helping patients in identifying abnormal results, and made use of personalised grouping (i.e. dynamically grouping the tiles in "Outside the standard range", "No standard range available", and "Inside the standard range") and the aforementioned overview-preview metaphor [28–30]. Both the Contextualised and Grouped presentation graphs reported personalised statistics for the selected test [38–40] and used colours, showing the area inside the standard range in green and the remaining area in red

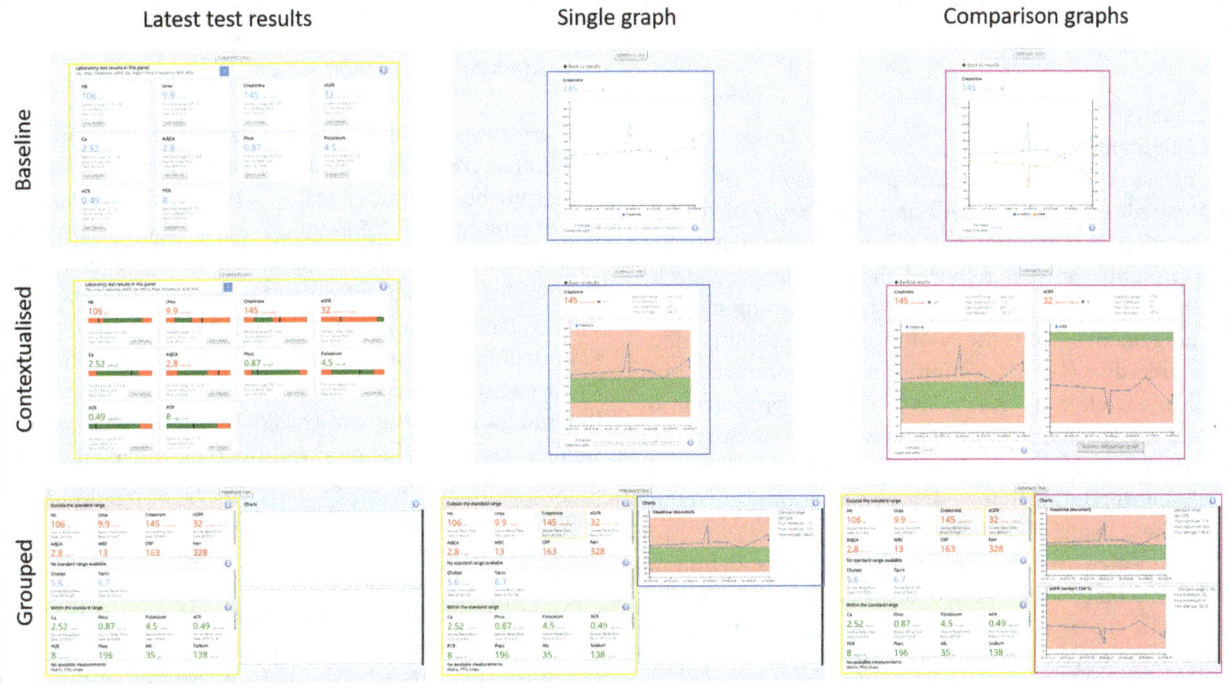

Fig. 1 Latest test results overview and longitudinal detailed information for one or two tests at the same time across the three presentations. Coloured rectangles represent the different areas of interest (AoIs) we defined across the three presentations (yellow: latest test results; blue: single graph; purple: comparison graphs)

[41]. We applied the same approach to colour the latest laboratory test results in the tiles in both presentations. This had the aim of drawing patient's attention on laboratory test results that might require more careful review (i.e. the ones in red), as well as visually filtering out those ones that were normal (i.e. the ones in green).

All plots within the same scenario displayed the same time period to avoid the well-known difficulties with scale changes [42]. Particularly, each plot displayed the period from the earliest to the latest laboratory test result available, which for each scenarios was between 1 and 2 years. Furthermore, in order to make the task as realistic as possible (i.e. pretending to have just received some results from the clinic), all results were shifted towards the day the experiment was carried out.

Since the purpose of the experiment was to expose patients to three very different types of scenario, keeping fixed ranges for each laboratory test as suggested by Zikmund-Fisher et al. [23] would have been detrimental for our purpose. That is, predefined value ranges specific to the type of clinical scenario (i.e. low, medium and high risk) might have revealed the pattern shown in the data. Therefore, we dynamically tailored the value ranges shown in the plots, for all three presentations, and horizontal coloured bars, for the Contextualised presentation. Specifically, the range of values shown always included the minimum and maximum value of the longitudinal series of results for each laboratory test. If the minimum or maximum fell inside the laboratory test reference range, they were replaced by lower and upper reference range limit, respectively. To ensure that the within and outside reference range areas were always clearly displayed, an offset was added to the minimum and maximum of the value range.

Data collection

At the beginning of the experiment each participant was asked to complete four questionnaires: demographics (age, gender, education, years since transplant, frequency of internet usage, and frequency of PatientView use); Subjective Numeracy Scale (SNC) [43] on a 1–6 scale; self-reported health literacy on a 0–4 scale based on Chew et al. [44], with lower scores indicating better health literacy; and graph literacy, calculated as % of correct answers on the questionnaire from Galesic et al. [45].

After exploring each presentation of laboratory test results, participants were asked to respond to a question about their behavioural intentions in relation to what they saw, which we used as a proxy of their risk interpretation. Particularly, patients were asked what they would do in real life if the results they had just explored were their own. They could choose between: 1) Calling their doctor immediately (high interpreted risk); 2) Trying to arrange an appointment within the next 4 weeks (medium interpreted risk); 3) Waiting for the next appointment in 3 months (low interpreted risk).

Data analysis

Risk interpretation

To assess the effect of the presentations (Baseline, Contextualised and Grouped) on the accuracy of risk interpretation, we created a 3 × 3 confusion matrix for each presentation that reported the judgments made by patients versus our gold standard (i.e. nephrologists' clinical judgement). From the confusion matrices, we calculated precision (i.e. proportion of correct interpretations of all interpretations as risk X), recall (i.e. proportion of correct interpretations on clinical scenarios with risk X) and accuracy (i.e. proportion of correct interpretations of all interpretations) for each presentation, and compared these using chi-squared tests.

We repeated the analysis with a secondary definition of the outcome, which aimed at investigating a situation in which, from a safety perspective, a misjudgement could have serious consequences. We evaluated the presentation's performance in terms of patients correctly identifying the need for action (i.e. at least medium interpreted risk in medium and high risk clinical scenarios). To evaluate whether performance was driven by single patients (i.e. there were some patients that misinterpreted most of the information), we counted the mistakes that each patient made. We distinguished between: patients underestimating the need for action (i.e. low interpreted risk in medium or high risk scenarios); and patients over-estimating the need for action and asking for help when not needed (i.e. interpreted medium or high risk in low risk clinical scenarios).

Visual search behaviour

To investigate whether correct interpretations were related to specific visual search behaviours, our secondary objective was to evaluate differences (if any) in eye-tracking data between patients who consistently identified the need for action and those who did not in at least one occasion. We collected the following metrics:

- Fixation count: a fixation is a stable gaze on screen lasting between 40 and 500 ms. We collected the number of fixations lasting at least 180 ms [46], because higher thresholds are considered to be more reliable when the stimuli include graphical content [47]. Fixation count is an indicator of visual search efficiency [48].
- Average fixation duration: we computed the average fixation duration, as an indicator of task difficulty and cognitive load whereby longer fixation durations indicate more challenging tasks [48].
- Dwell time: this metric, which is the aggregated fixation duration, is typically an indicator of attention and interest [48].

There were three AoIs in each presentation (see Additional file 1: Figure S1): 1) tiles showing the latest values for all laboratory tests; 2) the graph showing detailed longitudinal information for a single laboratory test; 3) the graphs comparing detailed longitudinal information for two laboratory tests. At first sight, due to their clear demarcations, the natural unit for defining AoIs would have been each single tile. However, their small size would have resulted in unreliable data because the precision of the eye-tracker is compromised with smaller AoIs. What is more, all the tiles convey the same functionality so the added value of treating them independently would have been negligible. Consequently we defined larger AoIs that grouped widgets with the same appearance and functionality.

Overall differences in fixation count and dwell time were assessed with a mixed ANOVA, including patient group (i.e. patients who did not underestimate the need for action versus the others) and the within subject factors (i.e. presentation, clinical scenario and specific AoIs). We also assessed differences in fixation durations with a mixed ANOVA, this time not accounting for the specific AoI in the within-subject factors. This choice was mandated by the low frequency with which participants looked at some AoIs, therefore limiting our statistical power in assessing differences. To account for the skewedness and non-normality of residuals introduced by count and bounded data, we ran the mixed ANOVAs on the log-transformed eye fixation counts, eye fixation duration, and dwell time, rather than on the raw data.

Eye-tracking data were extracted using the Tobii Studio (version 3.4.0). All data analyses were performed in R version 3.3.1 [49].

Results

Patient characteristics

Table 1 reports the characteristics of the 20 patients who participated in the study. The majority were male, had at least a college education and used the internet for more than 5 h per week. Frequency of PatientView use was balanced within our study population, with 11 participants who were regular users (i.e. quarterly use) and the remaining nine using it less than twice per year.

Data analysis

Risk interpretation

Table 2 shows the confusion matrices and performance measures (precision and recall) for all presentations across the clinical scenarios (i.e. low, medium and high risk). In most cases, patients correctly interpreted low

Table 1 Patients' characteristics

Parameters		Values
Number of patients		20
Gender	Female, n (%)	4 (20)
	Male, n (%)	16 (80)
Age in years, mean (SD)		51.8 (10.3)
Years since kidney transplant, mean (SD)		10.7 (8.7)
Subjective Numeracy Scale[a], mean (SD)		4 (0.8)
Health literacy[b], mean (SD)		0.5 (0.6)
Graph literacy[c] score, mean (SD)		73.5 (11.3)
Education	Lower than GCSE, n (%)	1 (5)
	GCSE, n (%)	7 (35)
	A-level/College, n (%)	5 (25)
	Higher education/University degree, n (%)	7 (35)
Internet use	Less than one hour per week, n (%)	1 (5)
	One to five hours per week, n (%)	5 (25)
	Five to 10 h per week, n (%)	5 (25)
	More than 10 h per week, n (%)	9 (45)
PatientView use	Never used, n (%)	3 (15)
	No more than once per year, n (%)	5 (25)
	Twice per year, n (%)	1 (5)
	Quarterly, n (%)	11 (55)

Abbreviations: SD Standard deviation, *SNC* Subjective Numeracy Scale, *GCSE* General Certificate of Secondary Education
[a]On a 1–6 scale [43]
[b]On a 0–4 scale, with values close to 0 indicating better self-reported health literacy [44]
[c]Percentage [45]

and high risk clinical scenarios across all the presentations, while medium risk clinical scenarios were often confused with low risk ones. For each presentation, at least two patients misinterpreted high risk clinical scenarios as low risk ones. The precision scores of the interpreted risks were similar for the Baseline and Contextualised presentations, and ranged from 0.33 to 0.69 and from 0.38 to 0.70, respectively. For the Grouped presentation performance was lower, and ranged between 0.28 and 0.58. Likewise, recall scores for the Baseline and Contextualised presentations were similar, and ranged from 0.30 to 0.70. The only main difference was observed for high risk clinical scenarios, where recall was 0.70 for the Contextualised presentation and 0.55 for the Baseline. Again, a drop in performance was noticed for the Grouped presentation. Overall accuracy was 0.55 for the Contextualised presentation, 0.52 for the Baseline presentation and 0.45 for the Grouped presentation. These differences were not statistically significant, with all *P*-values in pairwise comparisons greater than 0.350.

In addition, we calculated confusion matrices to compare situations in which an action was needed (i.e. scenarios with at least medium risk) versus those that did not require any action (i.e. low risk clinical scenarios) (see Table 3). For scenarios where an action was needed, the three presentations performed similarly with a precision around 0.8 and a recall around 0.7. However, in about 50% of the scenarios where patients interpreted that no action was needed, this was not in line with the gold standard. We did not find statistically significant differences between the different presentations, with *P*-values greater than 0.700 in pairwise comparisons.

Additional file 1: Table S1 shows the number of times patients underestimated or overestimated the need for action across all presentations and clinical scenarios. Thirteen patients (65%) underestimated the need for action at least once, of whom seven (35%) misinterpreted at least half of the scenarios requiring an action. Fourteen patients (70%) overestimated the need for action at least once. Individual patient characteristics are reported in Additional file 1: Table S2 and S3.

Visual search behaviour

We were not able to track eye movements for two participants, resulting in 18 patients being included in the

Table 2 Confusion matrix of the interpreted risk by patients versus the risk of clinical scenarios as assessed by nephrologists (gold standard), and performance (i.e. precision and recall) for each presentation

Presentation	Interpreted risk by participants	Clinical scenarios (gold standard)			Performance	
		Low risk	Medium risk	High risk	Precision	Recall
Baseline	Low	14	10	2	0.54	0.70
	Medium	5	6	7	0.33	0.30
	High	1	4	11	0.69	0.55
Contextualised	Low	13	9	2	0.54	0.65
	Medium	6	6	4	0.38	0.30
	High	1	5	14	0.70	0.70
Grouped	Low	11	9	3	0.48	0.55
	Medium	7	5	6	0.28	0.25
	High	2	6	11	0.58	0.55

Table 3 Confusion matrix of the interpreted risk by patients versus the gold standard (nephrologists judgement) and performance (i.e. precision and recall) for clinical scenarios where an action was needed (i.e. at least medium risk) and those where no action was needed (i.e. low risk)

Presentation	Interpreted risk by participants	Clinical scenarios (gold standard)		Performance	
		Action needed	No action needed	Precision	Recall
Baseline	Action needed	28	6	0.82	0.70
	No action needed	12	14	0.54	0.70
Contextualised	Action needed	29	7	0.81	0.72
	No action needed	11	13	0.54	0.65
Grouped	Action needed	28	9	0.76	0.70
	No action needed	12	11	0.48	0.55

eye tracking data analysis. Encountering difficult eye-tracking circumstances in about 10% of participants is not uncommon in eye tracking studies [50]. This can be related to participant's characteristics like glasses, particular shapes of eye-lids or very small pupils [50].

Overall, we observed 5071 eye fixations across all patients and clinical tasks on any of the three AoIs, with an overall time of 1416 s (23.6 min) and a mean fixation duration of 0.279 s (Standard Deviation [SD], 0.129 s). The median total eye fixation count per patient across the nine tasks was 255 (Inter Quartile Interval [IQI], 108–422), while the median total dwell time was 75 s (IQI, 29–120 s).

Of the patients for whom we could track eye movements, eleven underestimated the need for action at least once, while seven consistently understood when an action was needed. Figure 2 shows their eye fixation counts across the different presentations, scenarios, and AOIs, with medians ranging between 0 and 25 eye fixations. No statistically significant differences were found among the different presentations in the mixed ANOVA ($P = 0.247$), with median fixation count that was 22 (IQI, 6–46), 20 (IQI, 8–43), and 21 (IQI, 6–44) for the Baseline, Contextualised and Grouped presentation, respectively. Also no significant differences were found between the different clinical scenarios ($P = 0.842$), for which we observed an overall median of 18 (IQI, 7–48) fixations for low risk clinical scenarios, 23 (IQI, 6–39) fixations for medium risk clinical scenarios, and 21 (IQI, 5–45) fixations for high risk clinical scenarios. Conversely, different patterns were found for the different AoIs, with a P-value below 0.001 in the mixed ANOVA. Particularly, patients mostly looked at the AoI containing the summary of the latest test results, with a median of 13 fixations (IQI, 4–26) against 3 (IQI, 0–13) and 0 (IQI, 0–0) for the single graph and comparison graphs AoIs respectively. The latter was mainly looked at in the Grouped presentation. This was confirmed by the mixed ANOVA test that found a statistically significant result for the interaction term between presentation and the specific AoI ($P < 0.001$). In terms of the main difference between the two groups of patients, we found that patients who never underestimated the need for action required fewer eye fixations to make a decision, with overall median fixation counts of 11 (IQI, 2–28) and 32 (IQI, 13–58). This was shown also by the mixed ANOVA, where the term referring to patient's group was statistically significant ($P = 0.021$). Similar results were found for dwell time (see Additional file 1: Figure S10).

Eye fixation durations are shown in Fig. 3, with medians between 0.202 and 0.313 s. We did not find differences in eye fixation durations between the different presentations ($P = 0.186$), which had median fixation duration values between 0.260 (IQI, 0.245–0.275) seconds for the Contextualised presentation and 0.268 (IQI, 0.243–0.294) for the Baseline presentation. Also no difference was found across patient groups for the different tasks ($P = 0.357$), with a median of 0.268 (IQI, 0.246–0.287) seconds for patients who underestimated the need for action and 0.259 (IQI, 0.218–0.303) seconds for those who did not. The only statistically significant difference we found was between low, medium, and high risk clinical scenarios ($P = 0.028$). Median values were 0.255 (IQI, 0.231–0.275), 0.272 (IQI, 0.246–0.298) and 0.266 (IQI, 0.246–0.289) seconds, respectively. This is not surprising, as lower eye fixation durations reflect less cognitive demand, which is expected for low risk clinical scenarios. Although not statistically significant (P of interaction term equal to 0.161), it is interesting to highlight how the two groups of patients showed different cognitive loads in relation to the risk presented. Particularly, for low and high risk clinical scenarios, patients who did not underestimate the risk had lower median values across the three presentations. While the opposite was observed for medium risk clinical scenarios.

Discussion

We conducted a controlled study to investigate whether presentations using colours and graphical cues (e.g., horizontal coloured bars and personalised grouping) improve patients' abilities to correctly interpret laboratory test results presented through patient portals.

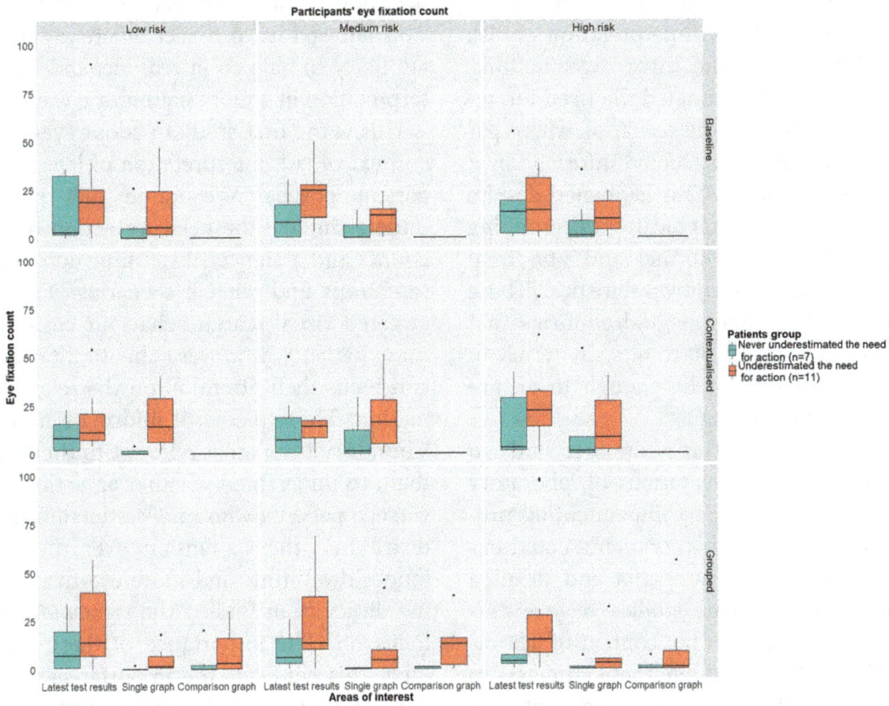

Fig. 2 Fixation count on the different areas of interest across the presentations and clinical scenarios for patients who never underestimated the need for action ($n = 7$) and those who did ($n = 11$). To facilitate comprehension four measurements pertaining to the 99th percentile (i.e. fixation count greater than 100) were excluded from this graph

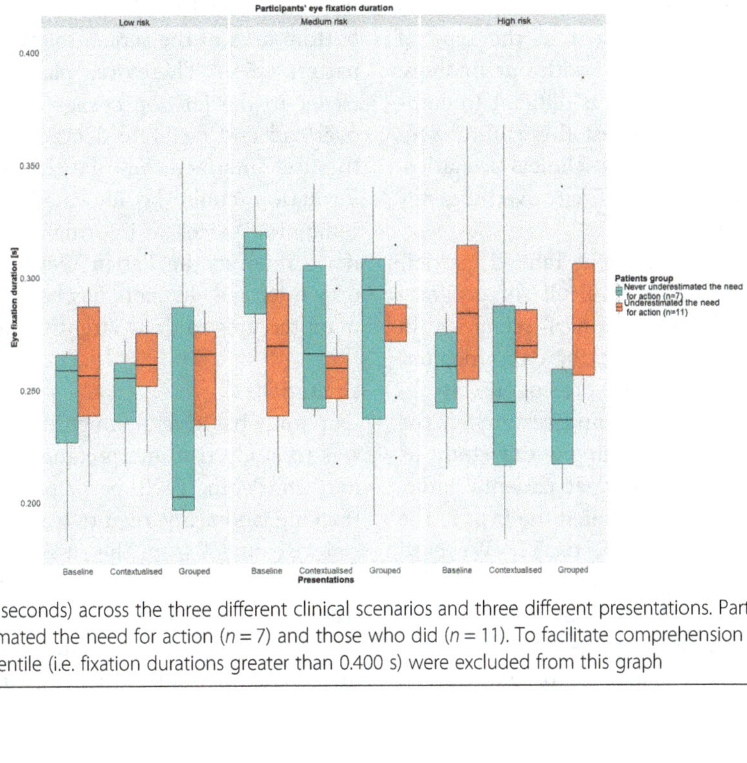

Fig. 3 Fixation duration (in seconds) across the three different clinical scenarios and three different presentations. Participants are stratified by those who never underestimated the need for action ($n = 7$) and those who did ($n = 11$). To facilitate comprehension two measurements pertaining to the 99th percentile (i.e. fixation durations greater than 0.400 s) were excluded from this graph

We found no influence of presentation on the accuracy of risk interpretation, with misinterpretation of risk being consistently high across the three presentations. Notably, 65% of patients underestimated the need for action at least once, and in 50% of the scenarios where patients decided not to act on the presented information it would have been better to do so. This happened despite the presentation of visual and graphical cues; grouping of laboratory test results with normal and abnormal readings; and personalised descriptive statistics. These findings raise patient safety concerns and confirms that the presentation of laboratory test results, in terms of interface design alone, might not be enough to ensure the accuracy of risk interpretation [19].

To the best of our knowledge this is the first study to assess the effect of different presentations of laboratory test results on risk interpretation by implementing presentations of different systems where patients could explore a broad panel of laboratory results and detailed longitudinal information. Previous studies have examined how patients interpret risk in the context of laboratory test results [15–17, 23, 51]. While these studies also found that patients had difficulties in interpreting risk correctly, only two made comparisons between different presentations of laboratory test results [16, 23]. Particularly, Brewer et al. [16] and Zikmund-Fisher et al. [23] compared a tabular format to horizontal coloured bars. In line with our results, Brewer et al. [16] did not find significant improvement in recall. Conversely, Zikmund-Fisher et al. [23] found improvements in terms of understanding the level of urgency of near-normal laboratory test results when using coloured bars instead of a tabular format. They also found that high risk clinical scenarios were perceived as urgent, independent of the type of presentation used, which is consistent with our findings. Their finding on near-normal results is difficult to compare to our results as we did not test this clinical scenario: conversely to our medium risk clinical scenarios, their aim was to decrease the level of perceived urgency rather than prompt an action.

As shown by the confusion matrix in Table 2, participants in our study found it more difficult to recognise medium risk than low or high risk clinical scenarios. In addition, as displayed by the eye tracking data, medium risk clinical scenarios seemed to be more cognitively demanding even for those who never underestimated the need for action. This is a unique finding of our study, as most of previous studies that looked at patients' interpretation of laboratory test results limited the task to the identification of abnormal values [15, 16, 52]. We used an approach similar to Zikmund-Fisher et al. [17, 23] who evaluated participants' behavioural intentions in relation to interpretation of laboratory test results. The difference in our study was the explicit use of participant's behavioural intentions as a proxy of their interpreted risk. This allowed us to reflect different clinical scenarios that are likely to happen in real life, and evaluate patients' interpretation in a more naturalistic way.

This is the first study to adopt eye-tracking data in the context of risk interpretation of laboratory test results in patient portals. We found that patients who never underestimated the need for action had less eye-fixation counts and a shorter dwell time across the different presentations and clinical scenarios. This suggests a more targeted visual search behaviour consistently adopted by these patients, who were able to filter the data on-screen and focus their attention on the relevant pieces of information. These pieces of information are likely to be the laboratory tests most relevant to their condition, helping them to understand whether an action was needed. Conversely, patients who underestimated the need for action distributed their attention over the different AoIs for longer dwell time and more eye-fixation counts suggesting difficulty in finding the right piece of information to focus on. The importance of these results are twofold. First, this confirms the importance of patient education (i.e. teaching which laboratory tests are more important and when they should act) prior to the use of patient portals [53]. Second, from an interface design perspective, further highlighting the pieces of information that are most relevant for patients and filtering those that are less relevant might enhance patients' interpretation. Without making dramatic changes to the PatientView interface we used for our study, this could be achieved by taking advantage of reading patterns on the Web and placing the most relevant information accordingly: attention decreases from left to right and from the top to the bottom area of the screen following an F-shaped reading pattern [54]. Therefore, placing relevant information closer to the left-top corner would remove information overload and facilitate decision-making. If the layout of the user interface could be altered, the most relevant information could be allocated a larger area than the remaining pieces of information shown (e.g. larger tiles if we refer to the PatientView interface), as size of the user interface elements has been proved to be one of the main features to draw attention on Web pages [55].

Limitations

Our study has several limitations. First, since our objective was to study risk interpretation and visual search behaviour in depth, each participant had to visit our eye-tracking laboratory, requiring a substantial time and financial investment from the research team. Due to research resource limitations, it was not possible to perform the study with a larger cohort of patients. This limited our statistical power to investigate the association between risk interpretation and patient characteristics (i.e. health literacy, numeracy and graph literacy), which have previously been shown to be relevant in the context of laboratory test result interpretation [17, 23]. Furthermore, although the population we selected was homogeneous in terms of their experience with monitoring their laboratory test results (i.e. all having quarterly tests after the kidney transplant), the small sample size limits the generalisability of our findings. However, our study still provides important insight on the risk interpretation and visual search behaviours of patients accessing laboratory test results on patient portals, and it should be considered as complementary, rather than alternative, to other studies that had larger populations, but studied risk interpretation in less depth (e.g. using static prototypes or surveys). Second, patients were given fictitious clinical scenarios to assess risk, in which they might have been less cautious because of the simulation nature of the study. Observing patients' interpretation of data from their own laboratory test results could simulate a more naturalistic research environment and strengthen the applicability of our results in clinical practice. Finally, since the study was performed in a laboratory setting where participants knew they were observed and studied, participants' behaviours might have been different than their behaviours in real life as consequence (i.e. Hawthorne effect).

Conclusions

This study confirmed patients' difficulties in interpreting laboratory test results, with many patients underestimating the need for action even when abnormal values were highlighted using colours and graphical cues. Participants who consistently understood when action was needed showed a higher visual search efficiency, suggesting a better strategy to cope with information overload, enabling them to focus on the laboratory tests most relevant to their condition. Our findings raise concerns over the limitations of patient portals in supporting self-care and possible safety risks.

Additional file

Additional file 1: Figures S1-S9 that show details of the three Presentations, highlighting the three areas of interest under study; **Table S1** that reports a contingency table for the number of patients who underestimated and overestimated the need for action; **Tables S2** and **S3** that show the characteristics of patients who underestimated and overestimated the need for actions and those who did not; **Figure S10** that shows participant's dwell time on the different areas of interest across the different presentations and clinical scenarios, stratified by patients who underestimated the need for action and those who did not. (DOCX 2455 kb)

Abbreviations

AoI: Area of interest; CKD: Chronic Kidney Disease; eGFR: estimated Glomerular Filtration Rate; IQI: Interquartile interval; SD: Standard deviation; SNC: Subjective Numeracy Scale; SRFT: Salford Royal NHS Foundation Trust

Acknowledgements

We thank: the NIHR Clinical Research Network Portfolio for the support in the recruitment of participants; and Mr. Rob Finnigan, patient representative of the Greater Manchester Kidney Information Network, for the valuable collaboration provided throughout the project.

Funding

This work is supported by the NIHR Greater Manchester Primary Care Safety Translational Research Centre and by the MRC Health eResearch Centre grant MR/K006665/1. The views expressed are those of the authors and not necessarily those of the NHS, the NIHR or the Department of Health.

Authors' contributions

PF, IB and NP developed the idea of the project. PF, PB, SS, and NP designed the study. PF and LH took care of all aspects regarding Patient Involvement. GW and SS created the clinical scenarios used in the experiments. PF and RW developed the prototypes used during the experiments. PF scheduled experiments with patients, collected and analysed all data. PF, MV, PB, and NP wrote the manuscript. SV and IB critically edited the manuscript. All authors approved the manuscript.

Competing interests

The authors declare that they have no competing interests.

Author details

[1]NIHR Greater Manchester Primary Care Patient Safety Translational Research Centre, The University of Manchester, Manchester, UK. [2]Health eResearch Centre, Farr Institute for Health Informatics Research, London, UK. [3]Centre for Health Informatics, Division of Informatics, Imaging and Data Science, The University of Manchester, Manchester, UK. [4]Renal Clinic, Salford Royal NHS Trust, Salford, UK. [5]School of Computer Science, The University of Manchester, Manchester, UK. [6]Microsoft Healthcare, Microsoft Research, Cambridge, UK. [7]Centre for Health Informatics, City University, London, UK.

References

1. Pearce C, Bainbridge M. A personally controlled electronic health record for Australia. J Am Med Inform Assoc. 2014;21:707–13. doi:https://doi.org/10.1136/amiajnl-2013-002068.
2. Institute of Medicine (USA). Achieve Meaningful use - Stage 2. http://www.webcitation.org/6qBAzdht7.
3. Urowitz S, Wiljer D, Apatu E, Eysenbach G, Delenardo C, Harth T, et al. Is Canada ready for patient accessible electronic health records? A national scan BMC Med Inform Decis Mak. 2008;8:33. doi:https://doi.org/10.1186/1472-6947-8-33.
4. Pagliari C, Shand T, Fisher B. Embedding online patient record access in UK primary care: a survey of stakeholder experiences. JRSM Short Rep. 2012;3:34. doi:https://doi.org/10.1258/shorts.2012.012009.
5. Fisher B. Patients' access to their electronic record: offer patients access as soon as you can. Br J Gen Pract. 2013;63:e423–5. doi:https://doi.org/10.3399/bjgp13X668384.

6. Adler-Milstein J, Sarma N, Woskie LR, Jha AK. A comparison of how four countries use health IT to support care for people with chronic conditions. Health Aff (Millwood). 2014;33:1559–66. doi:https://doi.org/10.1377/hlthaff.2014.0424.
7. Kruse CS, Argueta DA, Lopez L, Nair A. Patient and provider attitudes toward the use of patient portals for the Management of Chronic Disease: a systematic review. J Med Internet Res. 2015;17:e40. doi: https://doi.org/10.2196/jmir.3703.
8. Price M, Bellwood P, Kitson N, Davies I, Weber J, Lau F. Conditions potentially sensitive to a personal health record (PHR) intervention, a systematic review. BMC Med Inform Decis Mak. 2015;15:1–12. doi:https://doi.org/10.1186/s12911-015-0159-1.
9. Bayliss EA, Ellis JL, Steiner JF. Barriers to self-management and quality-of-life outcomes in seniors with multimorbidities. Ann Fam Med. 2007;5:395–402. doi:https://doi.org/10.1370/afm.722.
10. Cimino JJ, Patel VL, Kushniruk AW. The patient clinical information system (PatCIS): technical solutions for and experience with giving patients access to their electronic medical records. Int J Med Inform. 2002;68:113–27. doi:https://doi.org/10.1016/S1386-5056(02)00070-9.
11. Shah SGS, Fittonb R, Hannanc A, Fisherd B, Younga T, Barnette J. Accessing personal medical records online: a means to what ends? Int J Med Inform. 2015;84:111–8. doi:https://doi.org/10.1016/j.ijmedinf.2014.10.005.
12. Bhavnani V, Fisher B, Winfield M, Seed P. How patients use access to their electronic GP record–a quantitative study. Fam Pract. 2011;28:188–94. doi:https://doi.org/10.1093/fampra/cmq092.
13. Phelps GR, Taylor J, Simpson K, Samuel J, Turner NA. Patients' continuing use of an online health record: a quantitative evaluation of 14,000 patient years of access data. J Med Internet Res. 2014;16:e241. doi:https://doi.org/10.2196/jmir.3371.
14. Young MJ, Scheinberg E, Bursztajn H. Direct-to-patient laboratory test reporting: balancing access with effective clinical communication. JAMA. 2014;312:127–8. doi:https://doi.org/10.1001/jama.2014.5823.
15. Taha J, Sharit J, Czaja SJ. Usability of an electronic personal health record (PHR) among a diverse group of adults. In: Proceedings of the human factors and ergonomics society. USA: University of Miami, Miller School of Medicine; 2014. p. 619–23. doi:https://doi.org/10.1177/1541931214581132.
16. Brewer NT, Gilkey MB, Lillie SE, Hesse BW, Sheridan SL. Tables or bar graphs? Presenting test results in electronic medical records. Med Decis Mak. 2012;32:545–53. https://www.ncbi.nlm.nih.gov/pmc/articles/PMC3770735/.
17. Zikmund-Fisher BJ, Exe NL, Witteman HO. Numeracy and literacy independently predict patients' ability to identify out-of-range test results. J Med Internet Res. 2014;16:e187. doi:https://doi.org/10.2196/jmir.3241.
18. Britto MT, Jimison HB, Munafo JK, Wissman J, Rogers ML, Hersh W. Usability testing finds problems for novice users of pediatric portals. J Am Med Inform Assoc. 2009;16:660–9. https://www.ncbi.nlm.nih.gov/pubmed/19567793.
19. O'Kane M, Freedman D, Zikmund-Fisher BJ. Can patients use test results effectively if they have direct access? BMJ Br Med J. 2015;350:h673. http://www.bmj.com/content/350/bmj.h673.
20. Fagerlin A, Zikmund-Fisher BJ, Ubel PA. Helping patients decide: ten steps to better risk communication. JNCI J Natl Cancer Inst. 2011;103:1436–43. doi:https://doi.org/10.1093/jnci/djr318.
21. Simborg DW, Detmer DE, Berner ES. The wave has finally broken: now what? J Am Med Inform Assoc. 2013;20:e21–5. doi:https://doi.org/10.1136/amiajnl-2012-001508.
22. Iacobucci G. Patients promised online access to their medical records by 2018. BMJ. 2015;2015:351. http://www.bmj.com/content/351/bmj.h4740.
23. Zikmund-Fisher BJ, Scherer AM, Witteman HO, Solomon JB, Exe NL, Tarini BA, et al. Graphics help patients distinguish between urgent and non-urgent deviations in laboratory test results. J Am Med Informatics Assoc. 2016; http://jamia.oxfordjournals.org/content/early/2016/12/30/jamia.ocw169.
24. Reyna VF, Nelson WL, Han PK, Dieckmann NF. How numeracy influences risk comprehension and medical decision making. Psychol Bull. 2009;135:943–73. doi:https://doi.org/10.1037/a0017327.
25. Klimov D, Shahar Y. A framework for intelligent visualization of multiple time-oriented medical records. AMIA Annu Symp Proc. 2005;2005:405–9. https://www.ncbi.nlm.nih.gov/pmc/articles/PMC1560450/.
26. Gotz D, Sun J, Cao N, Ebadollahi S. Visual cluster analysis in support of clinical decision intelligence. AMIA Annu Symp Proc. 2011;2011:481–90. https://www.ncbi.nlm.nih.gov/pmc/articles/PMC3243281/.
27. Wang TD, Wongsuphasawat K, Plaisant C, Shneiderman B. Visual information seeking in multiple electronic health records: design recommendations and a process model. In: Proceedings of the 1st ACM international health informatics symposium. New York: ACM; 2010. p. 46–55. doi:https://doi.org/10.1145/1882992.1883001.
28. Kules B, Shneiderman B. Users can change their web search tactics: design guidelines for categorized overviews. Inf Process Manag. 2008;44:463–84. doi:https://doi.org/10.1016/j.ipm.2007.07.014.
29. Dumais S, Cutrell E, Chen H. Optimizing search by showing results in context. In: Proceedings of the SIGCHI conference on human factors in computing systems. New York: ACM; 2001. p. 277–84. doi:https://doi.org/10.1145/365024.365116.
30. Greene S, Marchionini G, Plaisant C, Shneiderman B. Previews and overviews in digital libraries: designing surrogates to support visual information seeking. J Am Soc Inf Sci. 2000;51:380–93. doi:https://doi.org/10.1002/(SICI)1097-4571(2000)51:4<380::AID-ASI7>3.0.CO;2-5.
31. Hill S, Spink J, Cadilhac D, Edwards A, Kaufman C, Rogers S, et al. Absolute risk representation in cardiovascular disease prevention: comprehension and preferences of health care consumers and general practitioners involved in a focus group study. BMC Public Health. 2010;10:108. doi:https://doi.org/10.1186/1471-2458-10-108.
32. Bartlett C, Simpson K, Turner AN. Patient access to complex chronic disease records on the internet. BMC Med Inform Decis Mak. 2012;12:87. doi:https://doi.org/10.1186/1472-6947-12-87.
33. Staniszewska S. Patient and public involvement in health services and health research: a brief overview of evidence, policy and activity. J Res Nurs. 2009;14:295–8. doi:https://doi.org/10.1177/1744987109106811.
34. Radhakrishnan J, Remuzzi G, Saran R, Williams DE, Rios-Burrows N, Powe N, et al. Taming the chronic kidney disease epidemic: a global view of surveillance efforts. Kidney Int. 2014;86:246–50. doi:https://doi.org/10.1038/ki.2014.190.
35. Luo J, Brunelli SM, Jensen DE, Yang A. Association between serum potassium and outcomes in patients with reduced kidney function. Clin J Am Soc Nephrol. 2016;11:90–100. http://cjasn.asnjournals.org/content/11/1/90.
36. Smellie WSA. When is "abnormal" abnormal? Dealing with the slightly out of range laboratory result. J Clin Pathol. 2006;59:1005–7. doi:https://doi.org/10.1136/jcp.2005.035048.
37. Elder NC, Barney K. "But what does it mean for me?" primary care patients' communication preferences for test results notification. Jt Comm J Qual Patient Saf. 2012;38:168–76. http://www.ncbi.nlm.nih.gov/pubmed/22533129. Accessed 24 Nov 2014.
38. Johnson CM, Shaw RJ. A usability problem: conveying health risks to consumers on the internet. AMIA Annu Symp Proc. 2012;2012:427–35. https://www.ncbi.nlm.nih.gov/pmc/articles/PMC3540473/.
39. Rothman AJ, Kiviniemi MT. Treating people with information: an analysis and review of approaches to communicating health risk information. JNCI Monogr. 1999;1999:44–51. http://jncimono.oxfordjournals.org/content/1999/25/44.
40. Ahmed H, Naik G, Willoughby H, Edwards AGK. Communicating risk. BMJ. 2012;344:e3996. http://www.bmj.com/content/344/bmj.e3996.
41. Andry F, Naval G, Nicholson D, Lee M, Kosoy I, Puzankov L. Data visualization in a personal health record using rich internet application graphic components. In: HEALTHINF 2009 - proceedings of the 2nd international conference on health informatics. San Mateo: InterComponentWare Inc.; 2009. p. 111–6. http://fandry.net/pub/ANDRY_ET_AL_HealthINF09.pdf.
42. Zikmund-Fisher BJ, Fagerlin A, Ubel PA. What's time got to do with it? Inattention to duration in interpretation of survival graphs. Risk Anal. 2005;25:589–95. doi:https://doi.org/10.1111/j.1539-6924.2005.00626.x.
43. Fagerlin A, Zikmund-Fisher BJ, Ubel PA, Jankovic A, Derry HA, Smith DM. Measuring numeracy without a math test: development of the subjective numeracy scale. Med Decis Mak. 2007;27:672–80. http://mdm.sagepub.com/content/27/5/672.
44. Chew L, Griffin J, Partin M, Noorbaloochi S, Grill J, Snyder A, et al. Validation of screening questions for limited health literacy in a large VA outpatient population. J Gen Intern Med. 2008;23:561–6. doi:https://doi.org/10.1007/s11606-008-0520-5.
45. Galesic M, Garcia-Retamero R. Graph literacy: a cross-cultural comparison. Med Decis Mak. 2011;31:444–57. http://journals.sagepub.com/doi/abs/10.1177/0272989X10373805.
46. Rayner K. Eye movements and attention in reading, scene perception, and visual search. Q J Exp Psychol. 2009;62:1457–506. doi:https://doi.org/10.1080/17470210902816461.
47. Bai X, Rayner K, Shen D, Yan G. Cognitive and cultural influences on eye movements. Psychology Press; 2008.
48. Ehmke C, Wilson S. Identifying web usability problems from eye-tracking data. In: Proceedings of the 21st British HCI group annual conference on people and computers: HCI...But not as we know it, vol. Volume 1. Swinton:

British Computer Society; 2007. p. 119–28. https://dl.acm.org/citation.cfm?id=1531311.
49. R Development Core Team. R: a language and environment for statistical computing. Vienna, Austria; 2011. http://www.webcitation.org/6qB8vSvjo.
50. Matos R. Designing eye tracking experiments to measure human behavior. 2010. http://www.webcitation.org/6qB95Hc4m.
51. Segall N, Saville JG, L'Engle P, Carlson B, Wright MC, Schulman K, et al. Usability evaluation of a personal health record. AMIA Annu Symp Proc. 2011;2011:1233–42. https://www.ncbi.nlm.nih.gov/pmc/articles/PMC3243224/. Accessed 21 Oct 2014.
52. Segall N, Saville JG, L'Engle P, Carlson B, Wright MC, Schulman K, et al. Usability evaluation of a personal health record. AMIA Annu Symp Proc. 2011;2011: 1233–42. https://www.ncbi.nlm.nih.gov/pmc/articles/PMC3243224/.
53. Otte-Trojel T, de Bont A, Rundall TG, van de Klundert J. What do we know about developing patient portals? A systematic literature review. J Am Med Informatics Assoc. 2015; http://jamia.oxfordjournals.org/content/early/2015/09/01/jamia.ocv114.
54. Jakob N. F-shaped pattern for reading web content. Alertbox Curr issues web usability. 2006.
55. Buscher G, Cutrell E, Morris MR. What do you see when You'Re surfing?: using eye tracking to predict salient regions of web pages. In: Proceedings of the SIGCHI conference on human factors in computing systems. New York: ACM; 2009. p. 21–30. doi:https://doi.org/10.1145/1518701.1518705.

12

Development of a personalized diagnostic model for kidney stone disease tailored to acute care by integrating large clinical, demographics and laboratory data: the diagnostic acute care algorithm - kidney stones (DACA-KS)

Zhaoyi Chen[1*], Victoria Y. Bird[2], Rupam Ruchi[3], Mark S. Segal[3], Jiang Bian[4], Saeed R. Khan[5], Marie-Carmelle Elie[6] and Mattia Prosperi[1]

Abstract

Background: Kidney stone (KS) disease has high, increasing prevalence in the United States and poses a massive economic burden. Diagnostics algorithms of KS only use a few variables with a limited sensitivity and specificity. In this study, we tested a big data approach to infer and validate a 'multi-domain' personalized diagnostic acute care algorithm for KS (DACA-KS), merging demographic, vital signs, clinical, and laboratory information.

Methods: We utilized a large, single-center database of patients admitted to acute care units in a large tertiary care hospital. Patients diagnosed with KS were compared to groups of patients with acute abdominal/flank/groin pain, genitourinary diseases, and other conditions. We analyzed multiple information domains (several thousands of variables) using a collection of statistical and machine learning models with feature selectors. We compared sensitivity, specificity and area under the receiver operating characteristic (AUROC) of our approach with the STONE score, using cross-validation.

Results: Thirty eight thousand five hundred and ninety-seven distinct adult patients were admitted to critical care between 2001 and 2012, of which 217 were diagnosed with KS, and 7446 with acute pain (non-KS). The multi-domain approach using logistic regression yielded an AUROC of 0.86 and a sensitivity/specificity of 0.81/0.82 in cross-validation. Increase in performance was obtained by fitting a super-learner, at the price of lower interpretability. We discussed in detail comorbidity and lab marker variables independently associated with KS (e.g. blood chloride, candidiasis, sleep disorders).

Conclusions: Although external validation is warranted, DACA-KS could be integrated into electronic health systems; the algorithm has the potential used as an effective tool to help nurses and healthcare personnel during triage or clinicians making a diagnosis, streamlining patients' management in acute care.

Keywords: Diagnostic algorithm, Kidney stones, Big data analysis

* Correspondence: zhaoyi@ufl.edu
[1]Department of Epidemiology, College of Public Health and Health Professions & College of Medicine, University of Florida, 2004 Mowry Road, PO Box 100231, Gainesville, Florida 32610-0231, USA
Full list of author information is available at the end of the article

Background

Kidney stone (KS) disease prevalence has increased in the United States from 5.2% (6.3% males and 4.1% females) in 1994 to 8.8% (10.6% males and 7.1% females) in 2012 [1]. Since it is one of the costliest urologic diseases in the United States, an increase in prevalence poses a huge economic burden on society. The cost of diagnosis, treatment and prevention of KS disease in 2007 was estimated to be ~$4 billion and, due to population growth alone, is projected to increase by more than $780 million by 2030 [2, 3]. The presence of KS also places the individuals at increased risk of development of chronic kidney disease. In a prospective cohort study, those who had KS was associated with a 50–67% higher risk of developing chronic kidney disease as compared to those who did not have, KS group also had twice the risk of developing end-stage renal disease [4].

The emergency department (ED) is a common place where patient with KS are evaluated and diagnosed. During the past two decades, a significant increase in ED visits with stone-related symptoms has been observed [5], with over 1.3 million individuals per year presenting to the ED with KS in the United States. The clinical presentation to the ED with KS commonly involves acute back, flank or groin pain, nausea, vomiting and sometimes blood in urine. The workup may include initial lab tests such as complete blood count with differential, comprehensive metabolic panel, and urine analysis; but often these tests are not promptly measured or are inappropriately interpreted [5].

A cross-sectional analysis of the 2007–2010 National Health and Nutrition Examination Survey (NHANES) dataset suggests that obesity, diabetes, and gout all have a significant positive association with kidney stone history [1]. Results from the Nurses' Health Study, a large population-based longitudinal study (years 2001–2012) demonstrated that high body-mass index (BMI), cholelithiasis, diabetes and specific dietary factors are associated with a higher risk of KS formation in females [6]. In 2014, a clinical prediction score -named STONE- was derived and validated in retrospective and prospective cohorts [7]. The STONE score includes five variables: male sex, short duration of pain, non-black race, presence of nausea or vomiting, and microscopic hematuria. The STONE score was also externally validated and showed good validity in patients with flank pain [8]. An updated STONE-PLUS score, augmented by point-of-care limited ultrasonography assessing hydronephrosis, was recently released and tested prospectively on an ED population sample, with only a moderate improvement in risk stratification [9]. As KS disease is multifactorial in nature, we hypothesized that an approach incorporating laboratory data and additional clinical characteristics would dramatically improve a KS diagnostic model, leading to earlier diagnosis and a better understanding of its complex etiology. In addition, this approach could reduce the number of unnecessary radiographic testing i.e. CT scans, in the acute care setting.

In this study, we tested a big data approach, merging demographic, vital signs, clinical, and laboratory information, to infer and validate a 'multi-domain' personalized diagnostic score for KS. We utilized a large, single-center database of patients admitted to ED and other intensive/acute care units in a large tertiary care hospital (over 58,000 admissions with majority admitted through ED). We analyzed the information domains individually (e.g. only comorbidities, or only lab tests), together, and compared our approach with the STONE score. A number of statistical and machine learning models were fit and compared to optimize performance. Using this multi-domain integration approach our goal was to significantly improve the sensitivity and specificity of KS diagnosis in acute settings.

Methods

Study population

The study population comprised individuals admitted to critical care units at the Beth Israel Deaconess Medical Center in Boston, Massachusetts, United States, between 2001 and 2012. Data are stored electronically in the Medical Information Mart for Intensive Care (MIMIC-III) database, which is available to the public upon request, upon Collaborative Institutional Training Initiative (CITI) training, and license agreement for full download and research [10]. MIMIC-III includes information on: demographics; clinical diagnoses and procedures encoded with the International Classification of Diseases ver. 9 (ICD-9) ontology; vital sign measurements made at the bedside (~ 1 data point per hour); laboratory test results; medications; caregiver notes; imaging reports; mortality (both in- and out-of-hospital).

This is a secondary data analysis. We used the MIMIC-III ver. 1.4, released on September 2nd, 2016. Our study included patients aged 18 years and older, divided into four groups based on the ICD-9 diagnoses during hospitalization: (a) KS cases (ICD-9592, including sub-codes 592.0, 592.1, 592.9); (b) patients diagnosed with genitourinary diseases (GUD) except KS (any ICD-9 code in the intervals 580–591 or 593–599), e.g. patients with nephritis, nephrotic syndrome, nephrosis; (c) patients admitted to acute care with other conditions (OTH) who did not have any KS or GUD diagnosed (any ICD-9 code not including 580–599) to represent a general patient population; (d) patients admitted with acute localized pain (ALP) of abdominal (ICD-9 code: 789.0), back (ICD-9 code: 724.2), flank, or groin (identified through patients' electronic chart record). In addition to ICD-9 codes, we also examined recorded charted events on ALP from the dataset. Patients with both KS and GUD codes were put into the KS group. Each patient was associated to a covariate vector of demographic info, vital signs, clinical diagnoses, procedures, medicaments, and laboratory tests performed during hospitalization.

Statistical analysis

Descriptive analysis was used to assess demographic characteristics (e.g. gender, age, insurance status, and religion), vital signs (e.g. BMI, blood pressure), laboratory tests (e.g. creatinine), and distribution of ICD-9 diagnoses at admission and during hospitalization. We also calculated the Charlson Comorbidity Index (CCI) using Deyo's algorithm [11], and the estimated glomerular filtration rate (eGFR) using the CKD-EPI (Chronic Kidney Disease Epidemiology Collaboration) equation equation [12].

Due to a low frequency of KS, we included only ICD-9 diagnostic codes that were occurred in less than 5 counts of the KS group, and lab tests that performed in at least 50% of the KS formers. Missing values were imputed via population median/mode. Univariate analysis was conducted to assess differences between KS and GUD/OTH/ALP groups on demographics, ICD-9 diagnoses, and lab tests, using Student's t-test, Wilcoxon rank test, or chi-square test, where appropriate. Significance *p*-values were adjusted using False Discover Rate (FDR) correction [13].

In order to infer a KS diagnostic score, we fitted a collection of multivariable logistic regression models with the GUD, OTH or ALP as negative examples, using different input covariate domains. Specifically, we evaluated seven models: (a) demographic variables and vital signs (including blood pressure, heart rate and body temperature) (b) CCI, plus demographic variables; (c) eGFR alone; (d) ICD-9 diagnosis (top-25 as selected by the univariate filter, i.e. the top-25 variables that were differently distributed between KS and other groups), plus demographic variables; (e) laboratory tests (top-25 as selected by the univariate filter), plus demographic variables; (f) ICD-9 diagnosis and laboratory tests (top-50 as selected by the univariate filter), plus all other variables included in models (a) to (e); (g) stepwise (forward-backward) selection of model (f); (h) STONE model. Note that ICD-9 codes used to define the GUD were not used as input covariates to any of the models, except for the STONE model where hematuria (ICD-9 code 599.7) is a covariate. Also, the duration of pain to presentation in the STONE score could not be precisely ascertained from our data; we used ICD-9 codes in the 338 s family plus codes 780.96 and 789.0, excluding chronic pain entries, using a weight of 2 (the STONE score a < 6 h pain is weighted 3 and 6–24 h pain is weighted 1, but duration of pain was not available in our data set). In addition to ICD-9 codes, we also used charted events to identify pain events. For nausea/vomiting we used ICD-9787.0 codes. In a sensitivity analysis, we also evaluated the contribution of GUD codes to overall performance of models (d) to (g).

Model comparison, evaluation, and selection were carried out using a 10-fold cross-validation framework [14], comparing performance index (see below) distributions from the repeated sampling folds using Bengio and Nadeau's correction to the Student's t-test [15].however, th.

In addition to logistic regression, we also fit a number of machine learning techniques on the full variable set as in model (f). In details: (i) a *decision tree* by means of the C4.5 algorithms [16]; (ii) *LogitBoost* algorithm in conjunction to logistic regression [17]; (iii) a *random forest* (optimizing number of trees up to 1000) [18]; (iv) a *super learner* stacking all the above methods plus a single-rule linear model, internally optimized via 5-fold cross-validation [19]. Given the high class imbalance, in addition to the standard model fit, we also used the synthetic minority over-sampling technique (SMOTE) internally to the cross-validation [20]. The univariate feature selection for these machine learning algorithms was done internally within the cross-validation setting.

The performance and discriminative ability of models was assessed using sensitivity (true positive rate), specificity (true negative rate), and the area under the receiver operating characteristic (AUROC), which is the expectation that a uniformly drawn random positive case is ranked before a uniformly drawn random negative (an area of 100% represents a perfect test; an area of 50% represents a worthless test) [21]. The optimal sensitivity/specificity cutoff was chosen based on the maximal of the Youden's J statistic [22]. All statistical analyses were conducted using SAS software ver. 9.4 (SAS Institute Inc., Cary, NC, USA) and Weka ver. 3.9 [23].

Results

There were 38,597 distinct adult patients (> 18-year-old) in the MIMIC-III database admitted to critical care units between June 2001 to October 2012 (90% from emergency room admission, 8% elective surgery, and 2% urgent care services), of which 217 were diagnosed with KS, 14,391 with GUD, 23,931 as OTH who did not have any GUD nor KS, and 7446 as ALP with abdominal, back, flank, groin pain.

Table 1 summarizes population characteristics among the three groups. There was an excess of females in the KS group as compared to other three groups (45.2% vs. 54.3%, 58.1% and 52.4%, respectively, $p < 0.05$). Most sample population were admitted through emergency or urgent (84.2%). The distribution of race was similar between KS and GUD, but comparing to OTH and ALP, KS had a higher proportion of white (76.5% vs. 71.1%

Table 1 Characteristics of the study population ($n = 38{,}597$), stratified by outcome group

	kidney stones (KS)	other genitourinary diseases (GUD)		other conditions (OTH)		acute localized pain (ALP)	
	% (N)	% (N)	*p*-value	% (N)	*p*-value	% (N)	*p*-value
Total	217	14,391		23,931		7446	
Gender							
Male	45.2% (98)	54.3% (7816)	0.0072	58.1% (13895)	0.0001	52.4% (3902)	0.04
Ethnicity							
White	76.5% (166)	72.0% (10359)	0.34	71.1% (17007)	0.0008	72.7% (5413)	0.04
Black	10.6% (23)	10.4% (1493)		6.0% (1445)		7.4% (549)	
Hispanic	3.2% (7)	2.9% (416)		3.5% (833)		3.1% (231)	
Asian	1.4% (3)	2.5% (358)		2.3% (555)		1.7% (124)	
Other	8.3% (18)	12.2% (1765)		17.1% (4091)		15.2% (1129)	
Insurance							
Medicare/Medicaid/Government	67.3% (146)	77.6% (11164)	0.0002	57.8% (13837)	0.0094	64.7% (4814)	0.48
Self pay/Private	32.3% (70)	21.7% (3130)		40.4% (9671)		34.4% (2560)	
Missing	0.5% (1)	0.7% (97)		1.8% (423)		1.0% (72)	
Admission type							
Elective	9.2% (20)	8.2% (1176)	0.92	20.2% (4841)	< 0.0001	16.0% (1193)	0.01
Emergency	89.4% (194)	89.6% (12895)		76.9% (18406)		80.7% (6005)	
Urgent	1.4% (3)	2.2% (320)		2.9% (684)		3.3% (248)	
	Median (IQR)	Median (IQR)		Median (IQR)		Median (IQR)	
Age	67 (56–77)	72 (59–82)	< 0.0001	62 (50–75)	0.0049	64 (51–77)	0.083
BMI	29.1 (28.3–30.5)	27.5 (26.9–27.6)	0.15	27.2 (27.2–27.2)	0.0023	27.0 (26.9–27.1)	< 0.0001
Charlson Index	1 (0–2)	2 (1–4)	< 0.0001	1 (0–2)	0.74	1 (0–3)	0.12
eGFR	50.8 (33.4, 81.9)	38.9 (22.5, 62.3)	0.0013	82.5 (59.1, 98.7)	< 0.0001	65.1 (37.3, 93.9)	< 0.0001
STONE	4 (2–4)	2 (2–4)	< 0.0001	2 (2–4)	< 0.0001	4 (2–4)	0.46

and 72.7%) and black African American (10.6% vs 6.0% and 7.4%, $p = 0.008$). The median eGFR in KS was 65.3, lower than in OTH (93.1, $p = 0.0013$) and ALP (77.3, $p < 0.0001$), but higher than GUD (49.3, $p < 0.0001$). The median (IQR) STONE score in KS formers was 4, higher than in GUD (2, $p < 0.0001$) or in OTH (2, $p < 0.0001$), but not different from ALP (4, $p = 0.46$). Figure 1 shows the comparison of the distributions of age categories by gender, CCI and BMI in the three groups of KS, GUD and OTH. The highest rates of KS were seen in the age group 71–80 for both males (30%) and females (23%), and the rates of KS increased significantly after 50 years-of-age in males, while in females a steady increase was observed after 30 years-of-age with a leveling off after 70 years. As for BMI, KS had the highest overall distribution (median 29.1) among all four groups (median of GUD, OTH and ALP: 27.5, 27.2, 27.0), it also had the highest proportion of obese (17% vs 11% in GUD, 9% in OTH and 2% in ALP, all p-values < 0.05).

Figure 2 shows the most frequent ICD-9 diagnoses in all four groups of KS, GUD, OTH and ALP, collating the top-10 frequencies of each group. Essential hypertension (45.8%), disorders of fluid, electrolyte, and acid-base balance (44%), and septicemia (41.7%) were most frequently diagnosed conditions among KS patients. Some of these high frequency comorbidities also had different distribution in KS compared to other groups. For example, rates of septicemia and certain adverse effects (including anaphylaxis, unspecified medication adverse effects, unspecified allergy, etc.) in KS were higher than in GUD, OTH or ALP (18%, 36% and 23% higher respectively). The proportion of essential hypertension was 10% higher in KS than GUD or ALP but was similar to the rate in OTH; heart failure and hypertensive renal disease had much lower rates (14% and 16% less respectively) in KS than in GUD, but the rates were higher in KSF comparing to OTH (8% and 10% higher).

When looking at the STONE variables, we found that hematuria was positively associated with KS (7.4% vs. 4.6% in GUD, $p = 0.051$, and vs. 1.1% in OTH, $p < 0.0001$, and vs. 1.5% in ALP, $p < 0.0001$); 98.6% of KS formers had experienced pain while 53.1% of GUD and 57.6% of OTH had pain events (both $p < 0.0001$); 0.92% of KS formers had vomiting

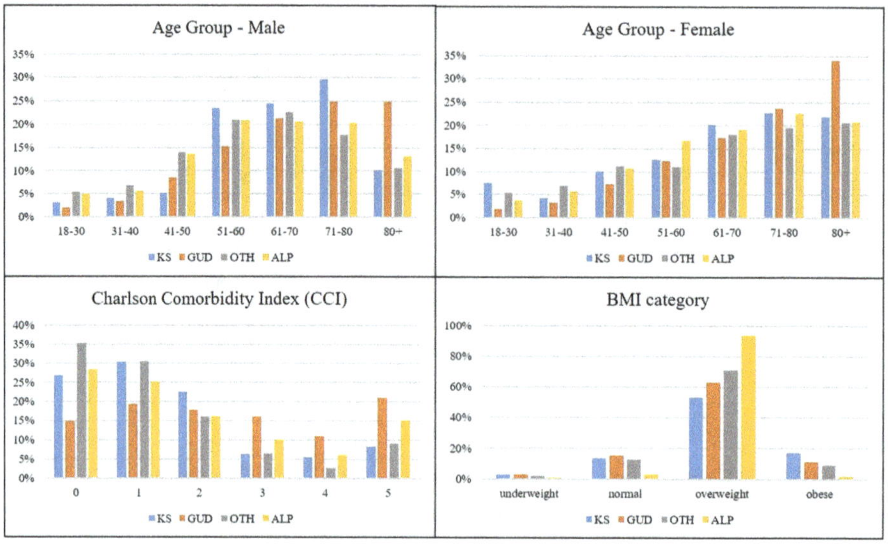

Fig. 1 Distributions of age categories by gender, CCI and BMI in KS, GUD, OTH and ALP groups

and 0.46% had nausea recorded, and the percentages of vomiting and nausea in KS were slightly higher than in other three groups. Hydronephrosis (variable from STONE-PLUS) was also positively associated with KS (35.94% vs. 1.54% in GUD, $p < 0.0001$ and vs. 0% in OTH, $p < 0.0001$).

Next, we performed univariate analysis of ICD-9 diagnosis and lab tests comparing KS with GUD/OTH/ALP. A total of 940 distinct three-letter ICD-9 codes were identified in the whole study population; after code filtering based on low frequency (< 5 cases in KS), 83 variables remained. For laboratory tests, a total of 754 entries were found, further condensed to 637 by manual inspection of physicians, and reduced to 69 after frequency filtering. The frequencies of missing values of these included lab tests ranges from 0 to 45%, 66.0% and 45.2% in GUD, OTH and ALP respectively, with the majority of them have less than 50% of missing.

Table 2 shows frequencies of the top ICD-9 diagnosis identified through univariate analysis, selecting those with an FDR-adjusted p-value below 0.1 (up to the top-25). Overall, 7 ICD-9 were differentially distributed

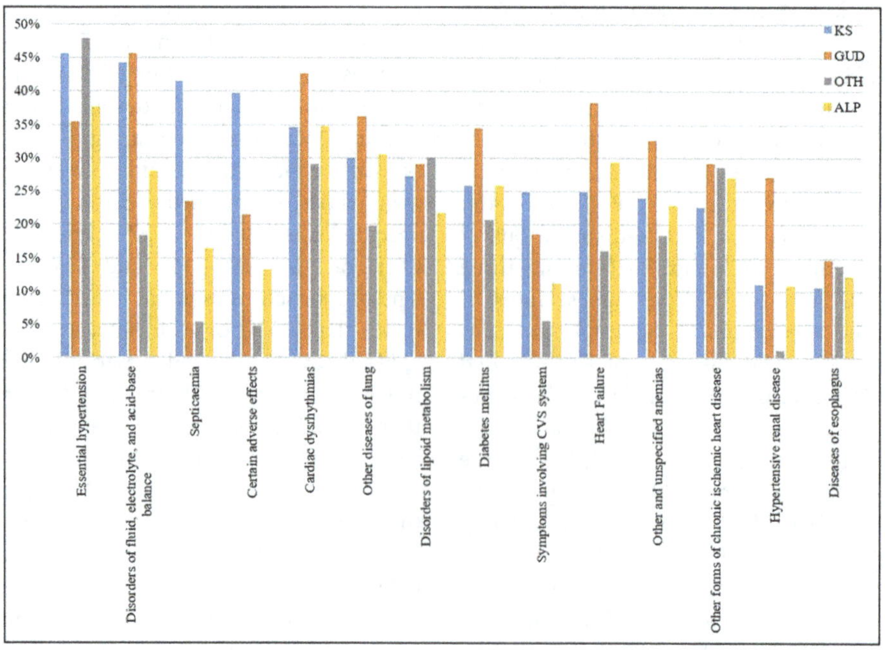

Fig. 2 Prevalence of the top-10 most frequent ICD-9 diagnoses in KS, GUD, OTH and ALP groups

Table 2 Top-ranked ICD-9 diagnoses differentially associated with KS vs. GUD / OTH / ALP

ICD-9 code	Condition	frequency in kidney stones (KS)	other genitourinary diseases (GUD)		other conditions (OTH)		acute localized pain (ALP)	
			frequency	*p*-value*	frequency	*p*-value*	frequency	*p*-value*
401	Essential hypertension	45.6% (99)	35.4% (5101)	0.02	48.5% (11447)	0.63	37.6% (2797)	0.0224
276	Disorders of fluid, electrolyte, and acid-base balance	43.8% (95)	45.6% (6565)	0.78	18.3% (4375)	< 0.0001	27.9% (2047)	< 0.0001
38	Septicaemia	41.5% (90)	23.4% (3361)	< 0.0001	5.4% (1297)	< 0.0001	16.3% (1216)	< 0.0001
995	Certain adverse effects	39.6% (86)	21.4% (3078)	< 0.0001	4.8% (1159)	< 0.0001	13.2% (983)	< 0.0001
785	Symptoms involving cardiovascular system	24.9% (54)	18.5% (2664)	0.09	5.7% (1353)	< 0.0001	11.1% (827)	< 0.0001
428	Heart failure	24.9% (54)	38.3% (5508)	0.00	16.2% (3867)	0.002	29.3% (2185)	0.1945
41	Other bacteria infections	21.2% (46)	16.3% (2350)	0.14	3.1% (752)	< 0.0001	7.5% (559)	< 0.0001
287	Purpura and other hemorrhagic conditions	12.9% (28)	11.7% (1680)	0.76	5.1% (1211)	< 0.0001	7.9% (589)	0.0293
790	Nonspecific findings on examination of blood	12.0% (26)	9.8% (1413)	0.54	5.2% (1243)	< 0.0001	6.0% (449)	0.0019
403	Hypertensive renal disease	11.1% (24)	27.0% (3892)	< 0.0001	1.2% (278)	< 0.0001	10.8% (805)	0.9642
278	Obesity and other hyperalimentation	10.1% (22)	6.0% (863)	0.08	4.7% (1121)	0.001	4.2% (315)	0.0003
311	Depressive disorder, not elsewhere classified	10.1% (22)	7.7% (1104)	0.77	5.9% (1403)	0.01	4.7% (351)	0.0015
300	Neurotic disorders	9.2% (20)	5.68% (817)	0.08	5.71% (1366)	0.03	4.0% (295)	0.0003
327	Sleep disorders	9.2% (20)	5.4% (778)	0.09	3.5% (843)	< 0.0001	2.9% (212)	< 0.0001
112	Candidiasis	8.8% (19)	4.3% (619)	0.02	2.0% (479)	< 0.0001	4.0% (298)	0.0023
416	Chronic pulmonary heart disease	7.8% (17)	6.9% (989)	0.77	3.4% (809)	0.001	4.3% (317)	0.0365
799	Decreased libido and other ill-defined conditions	7.4% (16)	4.7% (668)	0.19	2.4% (569)	< 0.0001	2.5% (186)	< 0.0001
788	Symptoms involving urinary system	7.4% (16)	5.7% (820)	0.77	3.0% (712)	0.001	3.1% (229)	0.0019
288	Diseases of white blood cells	6.0% (13)	4.7% (674)	0.77	2.6% (629)	0.001	2.0% (148)	0.0004
574	Cholelithiasis	5.5% (12)	2.9% (419)	0.11	1.6% (392)	< 0.0001	3.1% (230)	0.0558
570	Acute and subacute necrosis of liver	4.1% (9)	5.0% (717)	0.76	0.8% (184)	< 0.0001	3.1% (228)	0.4404
345	Epilepsy	3.7% (8)	3.4% (491)	0.87	2.9% (688)	0.48	1.5% (111)	0.0345
346	Migraine	2.8% (6)	0.79% (113)	0.02	1.32% (316)	0.11	0.8% (57)	0.0052

* first 25 ICD-9 codes or those with a false discovery rate-adjusted p-value< 0.05 are shown

between KS and GUD at the 5% FDR level, while 25 of them were found different between KS and OTH or ALP at the same significance level. Out of the 69 lab tests performed in more than half of KS patients, 43, 50, and 25 showed a significant (5% FDR level) mean or distribution location shift between KS vs. GUD, KSF vs. OTH, and KSF vs. ALP, respectively. The top-25 lab tests rank is shown in Table 3.

In order to derive a multi-domain diagnostic model of KS diagnosis, we fitted different logistic models on selected covariate input domains, as specified in the Methods section, and compared against the STONE. Table 4 summarizes the performance indices for models (a) through (h), showing average (st.dev.) AUROC, sensitivity, specificity across 10-fold cross-validation runs (i.e. results obtained on the test data), along with the best Youden's J. Figure 3 (top panels) shows the ROC curves for each model, also obtained by averaging the 10 tests sets, for the KS vs.)GUD, KS vs. OTH, and KS vs. ALP data samples. Overall, model (f), i.e. the top-ranked ICD-9 diagnosis and laboratory tests plus demographic variables, and model (g), i.e. the stepwise selection of features included in model (f), showed the best performance, with AUROCs ~ 80%. All other models were significantly less performant (adjusted $p < 0.05$) than these two. Following cross-validated AUROC ranking, the second best-performing models were those with top-ranked ICD-9 codes (d), laboratory tests (e), CCI (b), eGFR (c), and demographics alone (a).

Notably, models using top-ranked ICD-9 diagnostic codes showed high sensitivity and moderate specificity, while models using top lab tests showed moderate sensitivity and high specificity, while both high sensitivity and high specificity were achieved in the multi-domain models. The STONE model (h) yielded relatively low AUROC (62% for KS vs. GUD, 64% for KS vs. OTH, and 61% for KS vs. ALP).

When we added the ICD-9 code for hematuria and other GUD codes to the set of input variables for models (f) and (g), performance increased significantly: For KS

Table 3 Top-ranked laboratory tests differentially associated with KS vs. GUD / OTH / ALP

Lab test item	kidney stones (KS)		other genitourinary diseases (GUD)			other conditions (OTH)			acute localized pain (ALP)		
	mean	Median (IQR)	Mean	Median (IQR)	*p*-value*	Mean	Median (IQR)	*p*-value*	Mean	Median (IQR)	*p*-value*
Urine											
White Blood Cells (WBC) (#/hpf)	5.5	4.9 (3.1, 6.2)	3.0	2.2 (1.7, 2.9)	< 0.0001	1.5	1.5 (1.5, 1.5)	< 0.0001	2.1	1.2 (1.2, 2.2)	< 0.0001
Red Blood Cells (RBC) (#hpf)	5.8	4.5 (3.3, 6.2)	3.4	2.4 (1.7, 3.3)	< 0.0001	1.9	1.4 (1.4, 1.4)	< 0.0001	2.7	1.4 (1.4, 2.4)	< 0.0001
Creatinine (mg/dL)	80.0	73.0 (73.0, 73.0)	84.7	78.0 (70.5, 86.0)	0.03	77.9	75.0 (75.0, 75.0)	0.03	81.9	75.0 (75.0, 78.0)	0.03
Protein (mg/dL)	4.0	4.0 (3.4, 4.2)	3.9	3.8 (3.4, 4.0)	0.03	3.5	3.4 (3.4, 3.4)	< 0.0001	3.7	3.4 (3.4, 3.8)	< 0.0001
pH	6.0	6.0 (5.5, 6.5)	5.8	5.7 (5.2, 6.2)	< 0.0001	6.0	6.0 (5.5, 6.5)	0.86	6.0	6.0 (5.4, 6.5)	0.17
Blood											
Bands	4.5	3.0 (2.0, 3.8)	2.5	1.3 (1.0, 1.9)	< 0.0001	1.5	0.8 (0.8, 0.8)	< 0.0001	2.3	0.8 (0.5, 2.0)	< 0.0001
Potassium (mEq/L)	4.1	4.0 (3.9, 4.1)	4.3	4.2 (4.0, 4.4)	< 0.0001	4.1	4.1 (3.9, 4.2)	0.09	4.2	4.1 (3.9, 4.3)	< 0.0001
Lipase (U/L)	67.1	28.0 (26.0, 33.0)	62.6	35.0 (30.0, 42.0)	0.03	44.9	31.0 (31.0, 31.0)	0.05	65.4	31.0 (27.0, 45.0)	0.03
Magnesium (mEq/L)	2.0	2.0 (1.8, 2.1)	2.1	2.0 (1.9, 2.2)	< 0.0001	2.0	2.0 (1.9, 2.1)	0.03	2.0	2.0 (1.9, 2.1)	0.01
Glucose (mg/dl)	146.0	137.3 (137.3, 137.3)	143.6	134.0 (127.2, 141.0)	0.03	139.5	133.3 (127.6, 139.7)	0.03	141.0	133.3 (124.2, 145.3)	0.03
Creatine Kinase, MB Isoenzyme (ng/mL)	8.5	4.4 (4.0, 5.0)	0.0	5 (4.0, 6.8)	0.03	11.5	5.0 (5.0, 5.0)	0.32	11.9	5 (4.7, 6)	0.03
Red Cell Distribution Width (RDW) (%)	14.9	14.5 (13.7, 15.7)	15.7	15.3 (14.2, 16.7)	< 0.0001	14.5	14.1 (13.4, 15.2)	0.001	15.3	15.0 (13.92, 16.3)	0.005
Total CO_2 (mEq/L)	24.0	24.0 (22.0, 25.5)	24.8	24.8 (22.7, 26.9)	0.03	25.9	25.8 (24.7, 27.0)	< 0.0001	25.7	25.8 (23.8, 27.4)	< 0.0001
Red Blood Cells (cells/mcL)	3.7	3.6 (3.3, 4.0)	3.5	3.4 (3.2, 3.8)	< 0.0001	3.7	3.7 (3.3, 4.1)	0.09	3.6	3.5 (3.3, 3.8)	0.01
Chloride (mEq/L)	102.6	102.4 (101.3, 103.7)	101.9	102.0 (100.5, 103.3)	0.001	101.9	102.0 (100.5, 103.0)	< 0.0001	101.8	101.9 (100.7, 103.0)	< 0.0001
Urea Nitrogen (mg/dL)	25.7	20.8 (14.1, 30.7)	34.5	29.5 (19.5, 44.4)	< 0.0001	17.8	15.8 (12.0, 21.0)	< 0.0001	25.7	20.1 (13.8, 32.3)	0.95
Creatinine (mg/dL)	1.4	1.1 (0.8, 1.6)	1.9	1.4 (1.0, 2.1)	0.003	0.9	0.8 (0.7, 1.0)	< 0.0001	1.3	0.9 (0.7, 1.4)	0.80
Albumin (g/dL)	3.3	3.2 (2.9, 3.6)	3.1	3.1 (2.8, 3.5)	0.002	3.5	3.5 (3.3, 3.7)	< 0.0001	3.2	3.3 (2.8, 2.6)	0.31
Phosphate (mg/dL)	3.3	3.2 (2.8, 3.7)	3.7	3.5 (3.1, 4.1)	< 0.0001	3.3	3.3 (2.9, 3.6)	0.60	3.5	3.4 (3.0, 3.9)	< 0.0001
Oxygen Saturation (mm Hg)	90.1	92.0 (92.0, 92.0)	90.3	92.1 (90.4, 93.8)	0.78	93.4	95.3 (95.3, 95.3)	< 0.0001	91.5	95.0 (90.3, 95.6)	0.02
Base Excess (mEq)	−1.6	−1.4 (−2.7, −0.3)	−1.0	−0.6 (−2.5, 0.9)	0.15	0.1	0.1 (−0.6, 1.0)	< 0.0001	−0.2	0.1 (−1.6, 1.4)	< 0.0001
pH	7.4	7.4 (7.4, 7.4)	7.4	7.4 (0.3, 7.4)	0.44	7.4	7.4 (7.4, 7.4)	< 0.0001	7.4	7.4 (7.3, 7.4)	0.001
pO2 (kPa)	4.8	4.8 (4.6, 4.9)	4.8	4.8 (4.6, 5.0)	0.79	5.1	5.1 (4.9, 5.3)	< 0.0001	4.9	4.9 (4.7, 5.1)	0.001
Bicarbonate (mEq/L)	24.6	24.8 (22.6, 26.5)	24.7	24.8 (22.5, 26.9)	0.78	25.8	25.8 (24.2, 27.4)	< 0.0001	25.5	25.5 (23.6, 27.2)	0.001
Lactate Dehydrogenase (LD) (IU/L)	291.9	237.3 (230.9, 250.0)	399.4	268.0 (230.3, 320.0)	0.08	272.4	235.7 (235.7, 235.7)	0.03	330.4	235.7 (226, 301)	0.29

* first 25 lab items or those with a false discovery rate-adjusted p-value< 0.1 are shown

Table 4 Comparison of prediction performance of different models, using 10-fold cross validation

Model/Outcome		AUC	Sensitivity	Specificity	J
kidney stones (KS) vs. other genitourinary diseases (GUD)					
(a)	Demographic	0.63 (0.02)	0.69	0.51	0.20
(b)	Charlson's comorbidity index	0.69 (0.02)	0.69	0.62	0.31
(c)	eGFR	0.62 (0.02)	0.65	0.56	0.21
(d)	ICD	0.74 (0.02)	0.75	0.63	0.38
(e)	Labs	0.76 (0.02)	0.67	0.74	0.41
(f)	All	0.81 (0.02)	0.75	0.76	0.51
(g)	All (Stepwise)	0.80 (0.02)	0.76	0.71	0.47
(h)	STONE	0.62 (0.02)	0.55	0.64	0.19
KS vs. other conditions (OTH)					
(a)	Demographic	0.65 (0.02)	0.64	0.62	0.27
(b)	CCI	0.65 (0.02)	0.68	0.57	0.25
(c)	eGFR	0.71 (0.02)	0.59	0.75	0.35
(d)	ICD	0.82 (0.02)	0.68	0.87	0.55
(e)	Labs	0.90 (0.01)	0.81	0.87	0.68
(f)	All	0.92 (0.01)	0.90	0.80	0.70
(g)	All (Stepwise)	0.92 (0.01)	0.90	0.81	0.71
(h)	STONE	0.64 (0.02)	0.62	0.65	0.27
KS vs. acute localized pain (ALP)					
(a)	Demographic	0.60 (0.02)	0.71	0.47	0.18
(b)	Charlson's comorbidity index	0.62 (0.02)	0.60	0.61	0.21
(c)	eGFR	0.57 (0.02)	0.59	0.44	0.15
(d)	ICD	0.77 (0.02)	0.74	0.69	0.43
(e)	Labs	0.85 (0.02)	0.66	0.90	0.56
(f)	All	0.88 (0.01)	0.78	0.85	0.63
(g)	All (Stepwise)	0.86 (0.01)	0.81	0.82	0.63
(h)	STONE	0.61 (0.02)	0.58	0.60	0.18

vs. GUD, model (g) achieved AUROC of 88% ($p < 0.0001$ w.r.t. models with non GUD-specific ICD-9 codes) with sensitivity of 77% and specificity of 87%; for KS vs. OTH, model (g) achieved AUROC of 98% ($p < 0.0001$), with sensitivity of 88% and specificity of 98%; for KS vs. ALP, model (g) achieved AUROC of 87% ($p < 0.0001$), with sensitivity of 81% and specificity of 82%. Model (f) had very similar performance (not shown). However, these GUD variables were measured concurrently with KS, so we did not include them in our final prediction model, but it could be used as input if these GUD variables happened in one's history to improve the predictivity and performance of the models.

When we applied the machine learning techniques, using the same cross-validation settings, for the comparison between KS and GUD or OTH, we did not observe a substantial increase in performance indices with the usage of the LogitBoost selector in alternative to the stepwise, but an increased performance was observed for KS vs. ALP ($p < 0.0001$). The variables selected by the LogitBoost were concordant with the variables selected from stepwise logistic regression model (g), although the LogitBoost tended to select a few more. The decision tree showed a peculiar behavior as compared to the logistic regression, with increased sensitivity at higher specificity but then lower plateau. The random forest showed higher (almost perfect) AUROC and sensitivity/specificity (significant below the 0.0001 level with respect to the logistic regression and decision tree) and the super learner was comparable to the random forest. In fact, the highest weight of the super learner was that of the random forest, followed by the decision tree, a single rule, and the LogitBoost. The bottom panels of Fig. 3 show the cross-validated ROC curves corresponding to KS vs. GUD, KS vs. OTH, and KS vs. ALP. The decision tree for KS vs. ALP is depicted in Fig. 4. Using the SMOTE, performance results for all models were lower but ranking similar (not shown).

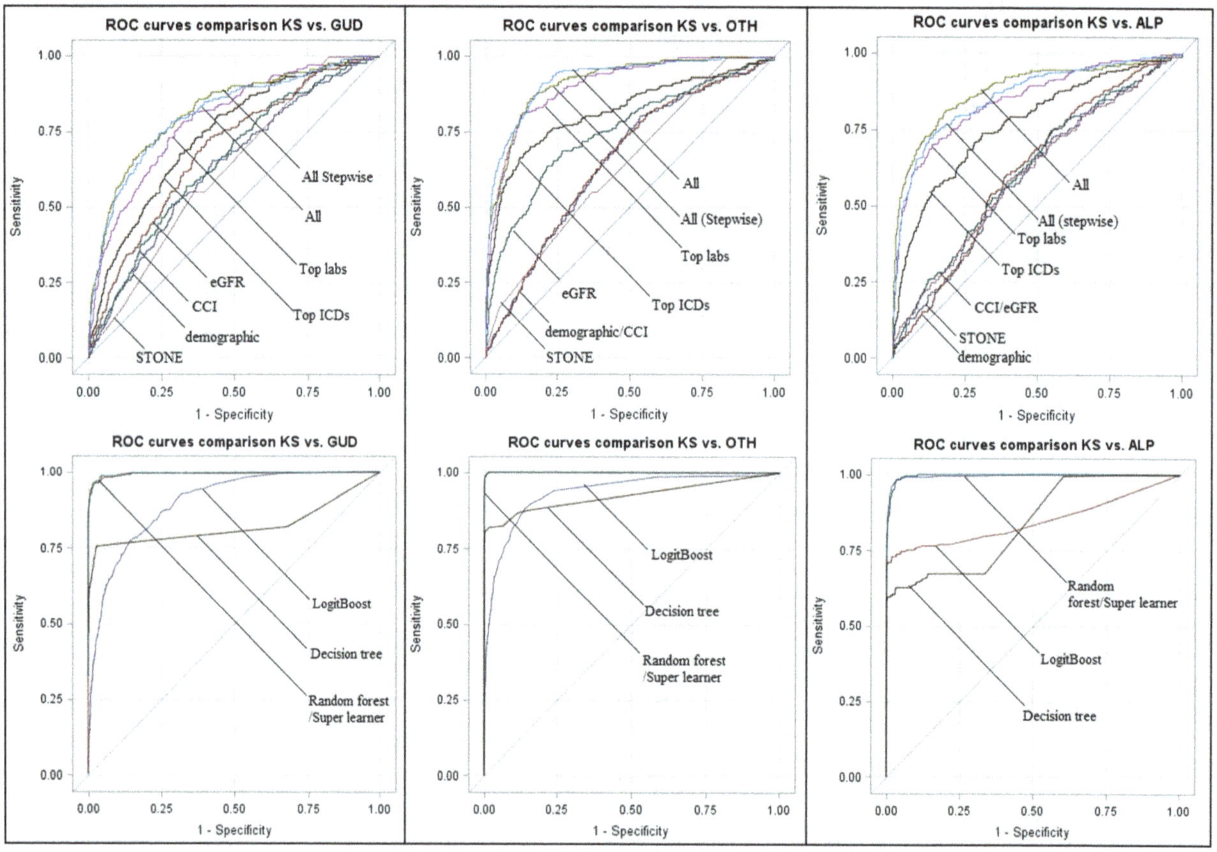

Fig. 3 Model comparison via AUROC. Legend: Left panels: kidney stone (KS) formers vs. other genitourinary diseases (GUD); middle panels: KS vs. other non-genitourinary (OTH) conditions; right panels: KS vs. acute localized pain (ALP) in the abdomen, back, flank, or groin. Top panels: logistic regression models upon stepwise feature selection, fit on selected input domains; Bottom panels: comparison of machine learning techniques on the full input set. Curves shown are averaged over 10-fold cross-validation, i.e. using the test sets

The final model of choice was the stepwise-selected model (g), because in conjunction with optimal performance, it included fewer variables than model (f) (15 variables for each comparison vs. 50 variables in model (f)). Table 5 displays the final model (with odds ratios and confidence intervals) which we name as the Diagnostic Acute Care Algorithm for Kidney Stones (DACA-KS). The stepwise regression for KS vs. GUD yielded a few nonspecific predictors (e.g. nonspecific findings on examination of blood (ICD-9: 790), Other complications of procedures (ICD-9:998)) which were removed without loss in performance. In addition, although random forest and super learner showed better performance, given the high class imbalance we have in the sample population, we cannot sure about the generalizability of these models in different dataset, so we focused more on interpretability especially when the logistic regression model had good performance as well. In fact, the SMOTE performance estimates of the super learner as well as of the random forest are lower.

Discussion

In this large sample of individuals admitted to acute care between 2000 and 2012, we aimed to infer a multi-domain, personalized, diagnostic algorithm risk assessment for KS disease. With a robust model collection and selection framework, under cross-validation settings, we demonstrated that the integrated model improves both specificity and sensitivity as compared to a single domain model. Also, it includes more extensive parameters compared to the STONE score. The STONE score utilizes presentations of KS-related symptoms (pain, hematuria, nausea/vomiting) and two demographic predictors (gender and race). In our sample population, only a small proportion of (KS) patients had hematuria and nausea/vomiting present or recorded. Our study evaluated thousands of potential predictors among the different domains, comparing relative proportions and shifts in distributions between KS formers and the GUD, OTH and ALP groups, our model can make personalized prediction for each individual based on his/her parameters from different domains. The features used in our final models are usually routinely tested in critical care

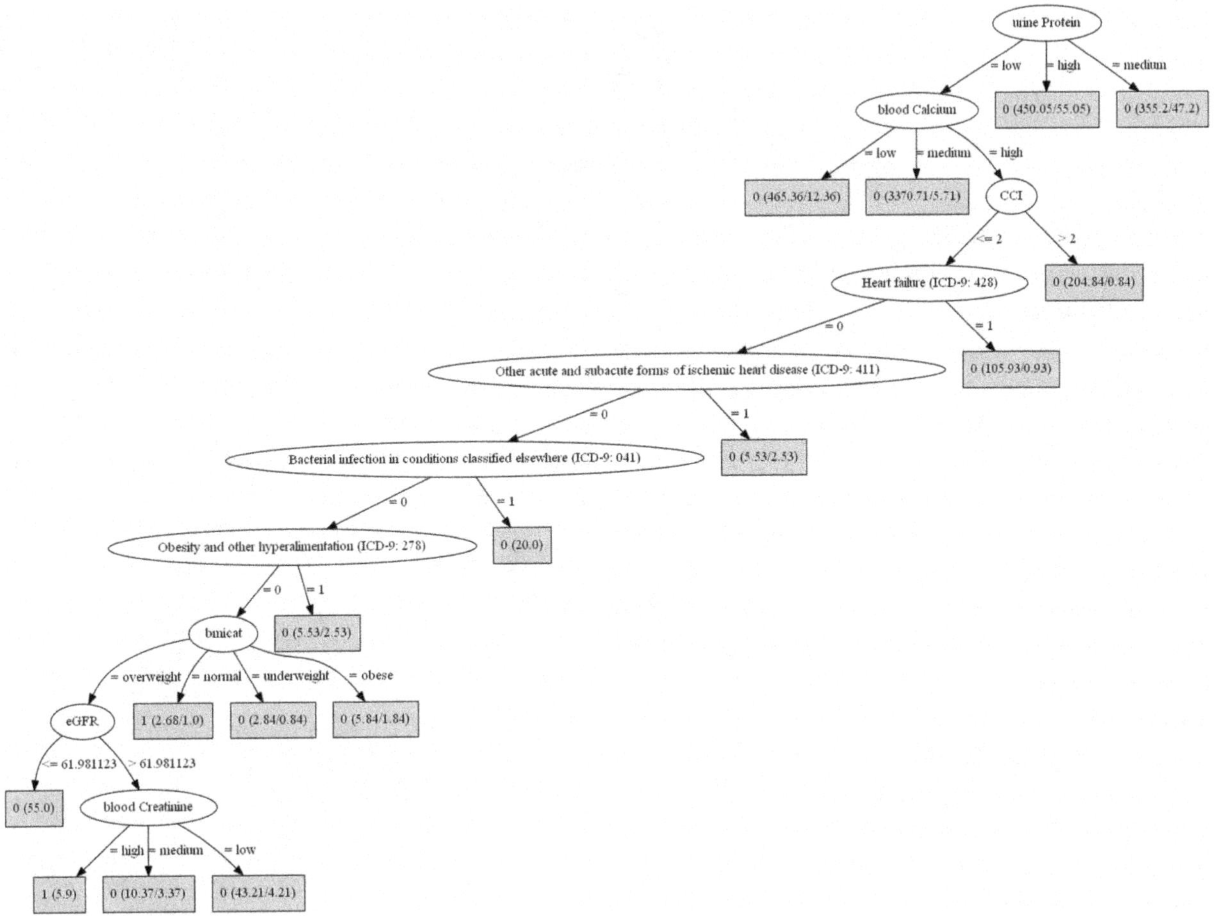

Fig. 4 Decision tree for the diagnosis of KS patients vs. ALP patientsLegend: Each leaf node contains the predicted class (1 if KS, 0 if ALP) and the numbers between parentheses indicate total number of instances (first number) reaching the leaf, and the number of those instances that are misclassified (second number).

unit, or tested at admission, therefore, all information to implement our model should be available in an ICU setting, and can be easily adapted to different clinical settings by adding or removing features. We report a series of novel findings in KS that are significantly different than GUD, OTH and ALP populations and which could aid in the triage of patients when they present to the ED or are admitted/transferred into critical care. A number of these variables are worth of discussion in detail.

In our study cohort, we found that KS peaked at the 7th decade of age; with variation of prevalence at different age groups between both genders, overall, we found a higher prevalence of females in this cohort. KS prevalence was the highest in non-Hispanic whites, similarly to other studies [1]. Lower rates of private insurance coverage were found in KS (comparing with OTH), which suggests that socio-economic status may contribute to risk factors associated with KS. Previous studies showed that lower income [1] and lower coverage of private insurance [24] are associated with higher risk of KS [25].

In our population, KS formers had the highest prevalence of obesity when compared to the GUD/OTH/ALP groups, and our final multivariate model suggested that patients with obesity are two times more likely to be diagnosed with KS comparing with GUD or ALP patients.

We found that KS, OTH and ALP were a healthier cohort with lower CCI and higher eGFR when compared to the GUD. Previous studies have demonstrated that KS formers have higher risk of developing chronic kidney diseases [4, 26]; in fact, in our study we found a tendency to a decreased eGFR in KS with respect to OTH/ALP groups, and this points to the necessity of monitoring and management of KS to prevent progression into chronic kidney disease.

The most common diagnosis associated with ED visits was hypertension, and its prevalence was higher in patients with KS comparing to GUD and ALP. Disorders of fluids, electrolytes, and acid-base balance was also frequently found in KS and GUD, but not in the diagnosis in the OTH/ALP group. A meta-analysis found that

Table 5 The Diagnostic Acute Care Algorithm - Kidney Stones (DACA-KS)

Items	Kidney Stones vs. Other Genitourinary Diseases		Kidney Stones vs. Other Conditions		Kidney Stones vs. Acute Localized Pain	
	OR (95% CI)	*p*-value	OR (95% CI)	*p*-value	OR (95% CI)	*p*-value
Insurance	1.70 (1.25, 2.32)	0.001				
Charlson Comorbidity Index	0.81 (0.75, 0.88)	< 0.0001	0.91 (0.84, 0.97)	0.01	0.88 (0.82, 0.94)	0.001
Certain adverse effects (ICD-9: 995)	2.93 (2.14, 4.00)	< 0.0001	6.33 (4.47, 8.96)	< 0.0001		
Hypertensive renal disease (ICD-9: 403)	0.55 (0.34, 0.89)	0.01	5.37 (2.96, 9.77)	< 0.0001		
Obesity and other hyperalimentation (ICD-9: 278)	2.06 (1.28, 3.32)	0.003			2.18 (1.25, 3.82)	0.04
Candidiasis (ICD-9: 112)	2.37 (1.39, 4.06)	0.002				
Decreased libido and other ill-defined conditions (ICD-9: 799)	2.30 (1.35, 3.93)	0.002	1.98 (1.08, 3.64)	0.03	3.40 (1.85, 6.27)	0.001
urine white blood cells (WBC)	1.13 (1.10, 1.16)	< 0.0001	1.26 (1.22, 1.30)	< 0.0001	1.15 (1.11, 1.19)	< 0.0001
urine pH	1.45 (1.20, 1.74)	< 0.0001				
urine protein	1.26 (1.01, 1.57)	0.04	2.19 (1.78, 2.69)	< 0.0001	1.99 (1.61, 2.45)	< 0.0001
blood Magnesium	0.17 (0.08, 0.35)	< 0.0001				
blood Chloride	3.97 (2.06, 7.65)	< 0.0001	5.05 (2.02, 12.59)	0.001	2.67 (1.01, 7.03)	0.05
blood Albumin	1.78 (1.37, 2.32)	< 0.0001				
blood red blood cells (RBC)	1.60 (1.22, 2.10)	0.001	1.49 (1.11, 1.99)	0.01	1.77 (1.24, 2.52)	0.002
Disorders of fluid, electrolyte, and acid-base balance (ICD-9: 276)			1.70 (1.23, 2.37)	0.002		
Other bacteria infections (ICD-9: 041)			5.47 (3.60, 8.31)	< 0.0001	2.67 (1.81, 3.93)	0.01
Sleep disorders (ICD-9: 327)			3.06 (1.76, 5.31)	< 0.0001	3.29 (1.80, 6.02)	0.001
Chronic pulmonary heart disease (ICD-9: 416)			2.07 (1.13, 3.79)	0.02		
Acute and subacute necrosis of liver (ICD-9: 570)			3.14 (1.38, 7.14)	0.01		
blood pO_2			0.52 (0.36, 0.76)	0.001		
Neurotic disorders (ICD-9: 300)					2.28 (1.34, 3.88)	0.03
Hyperplasia of prostate (ICD-9: 600)					2.88 (1.48, 5.60)	0.02
blood CO2					0.70 (0.61, 0.80)	< 0.0001
blood phosphate					0.60 (0.47, 0.76)	< 0.0001
urine bands					1.15 (1.07, 1.24)	0.002
urine RDW					0.79 (0.71, 0.88)	< 0.0001

increasing water intake was associated with significantly reduced risk of kidney stones and it was dose dependent for each increase of 500 ml of water [27]. For KS formers, the single most significant preventive measure is increasing fluid intake. In the GUD population, disorders of fluids and electrolytes are a well-known entity. In addition, diseases of acid base and electrolytes such as renal tubular acidosis (RTA) and partial RTA, which may present with hyperchloremic acidosis, hypokalemia, and normal or minimally reduced GFR [28], also have a higher prevalence of KS [29]. Interestingly, in our KS cohort we found higher levels of serum chloride and lower levels of serum bicarbonate, lower serum potassium levels, and elevated urine protein comparing to the GUD/OTH/ALP groups, Additional research efforts may be able to fully elucidate the significance of these findings.

We found that purpura and other hemorrhagic conditions were higher in the KS population when compared to the OTH/ALP population but there was no significant difference when compared to the GUD group.

The distribution of serum lipase and creatinine kinase MB isoenzyme were significantly lower in KS as compared to the GUD and OTH/ALP groups. Renal handling of lipase involves removal of lipase from serum by glomerular filtration of lipase with nearly complete absorption of free oxalate in the bowel lumen [30]. Disorders of lipid metabolism have been associated with the metabolic syndrome and obesity [31]. Lower levels of lipase in the KS group needs to be further elucidated as there have not been previous reports of this finding. Creatinine kinase MB (CK-MB) is an enzyme that is elevated in renal disease and it may be elevated even in the absence of myocardial injury; however, the significance of its elevation is controversial [32]. Further investigation is warranted to unveil both the role of low lipase and CK-MB isoenzyme in KS formers.

A set of neurologic findings in our study demonstrated that migraine headaches were higher in KS and OTH compared to GUD/ALP. Sleep disorder, neurotic disorder, and depression disorder were also higher in KS patients. Migraine headache medications such as Topamax promote an (RTA)-like phenomenon [33]. Sleep disorders and fatigue have been associated with migraine headaches [34]. In our analysis, sleep disturbances and low libido were correlated with the diagnosis of KS when compared to GUD, OTH and ALP. Low libido due to low testosterone could be correlated with poor sleep quality, since a normal circadian rhythm/cycle is necessary for central effects on normal testosterone production [35]. Low testosterone levels not only associated with low libido but also have been related with KS, Otunctermur et al. showed that male KS patients had lower testosterone levels, although the potential causal relationship were not confirmed [36].

Perhaps the most important finding and among high morbidity and mortality conditions, septicemia and candidiasis were found to have a high correlation with KS formers only. Reyner et al. [37] reported that of patients presenting to the ED with urosepsis, one-tenth presented with anatomic urinary obstruction, and that mortality was higher in this group, occurring in almost one-third of cases. Early imaging is suggested in this group of patients, due to suspected anatomic obstruction and need for immediate intervention to avoid mortality. Our data confirms this finding of a higher rate of urosepsis in KS patients when compared to other groups. This suggests that, as part of an algorithm to identify patients with KS, a high index of suspicion should trigger immediate action with early imaging to identify anatomic urinary obstruction in septic patients to prevent mortalities. In addition, the presence of candidiasis was found to have a higher association a KS diagnosis. Candidiasis is a fungal infection that can vary in presentation-from local to systemic and invasive, it may be found among debilitated, elderly and inpatients with indwelling urethral catheters [38], combining with our findings, patients presenting to the ED with candiduria may be considered for immediate imaging to identify any potential anatomic obstruction of the urinary tract. Interestingly, some variables in the model were not directly associated with risk of kidney stone: comparing to OTH patients, KS patients were more likely to have chronic pulmonary heart disease or acute and subacute necrosis of liver. These conditions might be associated with certain KS prognostic outcomes. Future studies the help further the understandings of these associations are needed.

There are several limitations of our study. First, we analyzed a sample from a single site, without external validation; the characteristics of patients in the KS, GUD, OTH and ALP are different and there may be a selection bias which we did not adjust for. In addition, many potentially useful lab tests were dropped because of low frequency in the KS group; other relevant lab predictors for KS may be found outside those routinely measured in people being triaged at the ED based on admission's symptoms. Second, there was a high-class imbalance, for which the power of the study can be affected, as well as the derivation of a diagnostic model, even though we tried to address in part this issue using the SMOTE technique. Third, when using logistic regression, we did not consider interactions among variables (considering only two-ways interactions would have produced n^2 variables, and we would have needed to use more efficient libraries, with parallel or cloud computing), therefore the model assumed a linear relationship. Ensemble methods, i.e. the random forest and the super learner, achieved almost perfect performance, but the result was not confirmed with the SMOTE class rebalancing, and this warrants further external validation using the TRIPOD protocol [39]. Even though we used nested cross-validation for parameter optimization, there may have been overfitting. Fourth, we acknowledge a subpar calculation of the STONE score because we could not assess the duration of pain, and the small number of subjects with vomiting and nausea in our sample indicating there may be under-reporting during data collection. Due to the cross-sectional nature of this study, we cannot determine the causality of the predictors for KS formation, but even using longitudinal database with variables only from earlier data, the causality of the predictors is still unable to be confirmed. Future studies may help address these limitations and help designing early-risk diagnostic models applicable to the general population.

Despite these limitations, our study provided a compact and high-performance diagnostic model for diagnosis of KS.

Conclusions

DACA-KS could be integrated into electronic health systems; the algorithm has the potential used as an effective tool to help nurses and healthcare personnel during triage or clinicians making a diagnosis, streamlining patients' management in acute care. As we enter the era of precision medicine, we envision a family of DACA- models for many other conditions in addition to KS, derived in the same way from big integrated biomedical data bases.

Abbreviations
ALP: Acute localized pain; AUROC: Area under the receiver operating characteristics; BMI: Body mass index; CCI: Charlson Comorbidity Index; DACA: Diagnostic acute care algorithm; ED: Emergency department; eGFR: Estimated glomerular filtration rate; GUD: Genitourinary diseases; KS: Kidney stones; OTH: Other conditions; SMOTE: Synthetic Minority Over-sampling Technique

Acknowledgements
We would like to thank MIT Lab for Computational Physiology for making the MIMIC database available for research use.

Funding
This work was supported by the UFHCC/IOA Cancer-Aging Collaborative Grant Program, the funding body has no roles in the design of the study and collection, analysis, and interpretation of data and in writing the manuscript.

Authors' contributions
ZC designed the study, carried out the analysis, revised the results, drafted and revised the manuscript. MP designed the study, carried out the analysis, revised the results, drafted and revised the manuscript and gave final approval for submission. VYB, RR, MSS, JB, SRK and MCE revised the manuscript and gave relevant intellectual contribution. All authors read and approved the final manuscript.

Competing interests
Jiang Bian and Mattia Prosperi are Associate Editors for BMC Medical Informatics and Decision Making.

Author details
[1]Department of Epidemiology, College of Public Health and Health Professions & College of Medicine, University of Florida, 2004 Mowry Road, PO Box 100231, Gainesville, Florida 32610-0231, USA. [2]Department of Urology, University of Florida, Gainesville, Florida, USA. [3]Division of Nephrology, Hypertension, & Renal Transplantation, University of Florida, Gainesville, Florida, USA. [4]Department of Health Outcomes and Biomedical Informatics, University of Florida, Gainesville, Florida, USA. [5]Department of Pathology, Immunology, and Laboratory Medicine, Gainesville, Florida, USA. [6]Department of Emergency Medicine, University of Florida, Gainesville, Florida, USA.

References
1. Scales CD Jr, Smith AC, Hanley JM, Saigal CS. urologic diseases in America project. Prevalence of kidney stones in the United States. Eur Urol. 2012 Jul; 62(1):160–5.
2. Antonelli JA, Maalouf NM, Pearle MS, Lotan Y. Use of the National Health and nutrition examination survey to calculate the impact of obesity and diabetes on cost and prevalence of urolithiasis in 2030. Eur Urol. 2014 Oct; 66(4):724–9.
3. Morgan MS, Pearle MS. Medical management of renal stones. BMJ. 2016 Mar 14;352:i52.
4. Rule AD, Bergstralh EJ, Melton LJ 3rd, Li X, Weaver AL, Lieske JC. Kidney stones and the risk for chronic kidney disease. Clin J Am Soc Nephrol. 2009 Apr;4(4):804–11.
5. Graham A, Luber S, Wolfson AB. Urolithiasis in the emergency department. Emerg Med Clin North Am. 2011 Aug;29(3):519–38.
6. Prochaska ML, Taylor EN, Curhan GC. Insights into nephrolithiasis from the nurses' health studies. Am J Public Health. 2016 Sep;106(9):1638–43.
7. Moore CL, Bomann S, Daniels B, Luty S, Molinaro A, Singh D, Gross CP. Derivation and validation of a clinical prediction rule for uncomplicated ureteral STONE--the STONE score: retrospective and prospective observational cohort studies. BMJ. 2014 Mar 26;348:g2191.
8. Hernandez N, Song Y, Noble VE, Eisner BH. Predicting ureteral stones in emergency department patients with flank pain: an external validation of the STONE score. World J Urol. 2016 Oct;34(10):1443–6.
9. Daniels B, Gross CP, Molinaro A, Singh D, Luty S, Jessey R, Moore CL. STONE PLUS: Evaluation of emergency department patients with suspected renal colic, using a clinical prediction tool combined with point-of-care limited ultrasonography. Ann Emerg Med. 2016 Apr;67(4):439–48.
10. Johnson AE, Pollard TJ, Shen L, Lehman LW, Feng M, Ghassemi M, Moody B, Szolovits P, Celi LA, Mark RG. MIMIC-III, a freely accessible critical care database. Sci Data. 2016 May 24;3:160035.
11. Deyo RA, Cherkin DC, Ciol MA. Adapting a clinical comorbidity index for use with ICD-9-CM administrative databases. J Clin Epidemiol. 1992 Jun;45(6):613–9.
12. Levey AS, Stevens LA, Schmid CH, Zhang YL, Castro AF 3rd, Feldman HI, et al. A new equation to estimate glomerular filtration rate. Ann Intern Med. 2009;150(9):604–12.
13. Benjamini Y, Heller R. False discovery rates for spatial signals. JASA. 2007 Dec;102(480):1272–81.
14. Hastie T, Tibshirani R, Friedman J. The elements of statistical learning: data mining, inference, and prediction. Second edition. New York: Springer; 2009.
15. Nadeau C, Bengio Y. Inference for the generalization error. Mach Learn. 2003;52:239.
16. Quinlan, J. R. C4.5: Programs for Machine Learning. Morgan Kaufmann Publishers, 1993.
17. Friedman J, Hastie T, Tibshirani R. Additive logistic regression: a statistical view of boosting. Ann Stat. 2000;28(2):337–407.
18. Breiman, L. Random Forests Machine Learning 2001, 45: 5–32.
19. van der Laan MJ, Polley EC, Hubbard AE. Super learner. Stat Appl Genet Mol Biol. 2007;6: Article25.
20. Chawla NV, Bowyer KW, Hall LO, Kegelmeyer W. SMOTE: synthetic minority over-sampling technique. J Artif Intell Res. 2002;16:321–57.
21. Fawcett T. An introduction to ROC analysis. Pattern Recogn Lett. 2006;27: 861–74.
22. Schisterman EF, Perkins NJ, Liu A, Bondell H. Optimal cut-point and its corresponding Youden index to discriminate individuals using pooled blood samples. Epidemiology. 2005 Jan;16(1):73–81.
23. Frank E, Hall MA, Witten IH. The WEKA Workbench. Online Appendix for "Data Mining: Practical Machine Learning Tools and Techniques", Morgan Kaufmann, Fourth Edition, 2016.
24. Watnick S, Weiner DE, Shaffer R, Inrig J, Moe S, Mehrotra R. Dialysis advisory Group of the American Society of nephrology. Comparing mandated health care reforms: the affordable care act, accountable care organizations, and the Medicare ESRD program. Clin J Am Soc Nephrol. 2012 Sep;7(9):1535–43.
25. Scales CD Jr, Lin L, Saigal CS, Bennett CJ, Ponce NA, Mangione CM, Litwin MS. NIDDK urologic diseases in America project. Emergency department revisits for patients with kidney stones in California. Acad Emerg Med. 2015 Apr;22(4):468–74.
26. Sands JM, Layton HE. The physiology of urinary concentration: an update. Semin Nephrol. 2009 May;29(3):178–95.
27. Shang W, Li L, Ren Y, Ge Q, Ku M, Ge S, Xu G. History of kidney stones and risk of chronic kidney disease: a meta-analysis. PeerJ. 2017;5:e2907.
28. Xu C, Zhang C, Wang XL, Liu TZ, Zeng XT, Li S, Duan XW. Self-fluid Management in Prevention of kidney stones: a PRISMA-compliant systematic review and dose-response meta-analysis of observational studies. Medicine (Baltimore). 2015 Jul;94(27):e1042.
29. Buckalew VM Jr. Nephrolithiasis in renal tubular acidosis. J Urol. 1989 Mar; 141(3 Pt 2):731–7.
30. Junge W, Mályusz M, Ehrens HJ. The role of the kidney in the elimination of pancreatic lipase and amylase from blood. J Clin Chem Clin Biochem. 1985 Jul;23(7):387–92.
31. Mead JR, Irvine SA, Ramji DP. Lipoprotein lipase: structure, function, regulation, and role in disease. J Mol Med (Berl). 2002 Dec;80(12):753–69.
32. Jeremias A, Albirini A, Ziada KM, Chew DP, Brener SJ, Topol EJ, Ellis SG. Prognostic significance of creatine kinase-MB elevation after percutaneous coronary intervention in patients with chronic renal dysfunction. Am Heart J. 2002 Jun;143(6):1040–5.
33. Welch BJ, Graybeal D, Moe OW, Maalouf NM, Sakhaee K. Biochemical and stone-risk profiles with topiramate treatment. Am J Kidney Dis. 2006 Oct; 48(4):555–63.

34. Lucchesi C, Baldacci F, Cafalli M, Dini E, Giampietri L, Siciliano G, Gori S. Fatigue, sleep-wake pattern, depressive and anxiety symptoms and body-mass index: analysis in a sample of episodic and chronic migraine patients. Neurol Sci. 2016 Jun;37(6):987–9.
35. Pakzad R, Safiri S. Poor sleep quality predicts Hypogonadal symptoms and sexual dysfunction in male non-standard shift workers: methodological issues to avoid prediction fallacy. Urology. 2017 Jan;23
36. Otunctemur A, Ozbek E, Cakir SS, Dursun M, Polat EC, Ozcan L, Besiroglu H. Urolithiasis is associated with low serum testosterone levels in men. Arch Ital Urol Androl. 2015 Mar 31;87(1):83–6.
37. Reyner K, Heffner AC, Karvetski CH. Urinary obstruction is an important complicating factor in patients with septic shock due to urinary infection. Am J Emerg Med. 2016 Apr;34(4):694–6.
38. Pfaller MA, Diekema DJ. Epidemiology of invasive candidiasis: a persistent public health problem. Clin Microbiol Rev. 2007 Jan;20(1):133–63.
39. Moons KG, Altman DG, Reitsma JB, Ioannidis JP, Macaskill P, Steyerberg EW, Vickers AJ, Ransohoff DF, Collins GS. Transparent reporting of a multivariable prediction model for individual prognosis or diagnosis (TRIPOD): explanation and elaboration. Ann Intern Med. 2015 Jan 6;162(1):W1–73.

13

A rank weighted classification for plasma proteomic profiles based on case-based reasoning

Amy M. Kwon

Abstract

Background: It is a challenge to precisely classify plasma proteomic profiles into their clinical status based solely on their patterns even though distinct patterns of plasma proteomic profiles are regarded as potential to be a biomarker because the profiles have large within-subject variances.

Methods: The present study proposes a rank-based weighted CBR classifier (RWCBR). We hypothesized that a CBR classifier is advantageous when individual patterns are specific and do not follow the general patterns like proteomic profiles, and robust feature weights can enhance the performance of the CBR classifier. To validate RWCBR, we conducted numerical experiments, which predict the clinical status of the 70 subjects using plasma proteomic profiles by comparing the performances to previous approaches.

Results: According to the numerical experiment, SVM maintained the highest minimum values of Precision and Recall, but RWCBR showed highest average value in all information indices, and it maintained the smallest standard deviation in F-1 score and G-measure.

Conclusions: RWCBR approach showed potential as a robust classifier in predicting the clinical status of the subjects for plasma proteomic profiles.

Keywords: Case-based reasoning, Plasma proteomic profiles, Classification, Rank

Background

Case-based reasoning (CBR) is an artificial intelligent approach based on an inference technique that is said to be the most effective method to construct an expert system [1]. When a target case occurs, CBR is mainly performed according to the following four procedures: retrieving, reusing, revising and retaining [2, 3]. It solves a target problem by revising the solution with the previous cases in similar situations retrieved from the case-base, and the target case is retained in the case-base for the next problem once the problem is solved. Thus, up-to-date case-base is always maintained in CBR system. The CBR system has been applied in many learning or problem-solving techniques of real-world applications. In particular, the prediction techniques based on CBR can be more appropriate in bio-medical field than other fields because CBR has less risk of overfitting in prediction, and medical cases can't be often explained by general patterns of the case-base. It is important to classify the plasma proteomic profiles solely depending on their shapes because their distinct patterns of profiles are regarded as a potential biomarker according to clinical status [4]. However, plasma proteomic profiles may be a typical example not following the general patterns which lead to poor accuracies in prediction by classification methods based on overall means of similarity due to large within-subject variance, and there is no gold standard to analyze the plasma proteomic profiles yet. The present study conducts a CBR based classification method with the plasma proteomic profiles which does not make decision for classification depending on the overall mean. However, CBR often also shows lower prediction performance compared to other learning techniques. Previous studies proposed some methods to improve the performance of CBR. Those studies were primarily focused on either weight optimization

Correspondence: amykwon@korea.ac.kr
Big Data Science, Division of Economics & Statistics, College of Public Policy, Korea University, Sejong, Korea

methods [5–9] or feature (or subset) selection methods [10, 11], and one study proposed a hybrid generic approach to optimize the both with the number of neighbor cases to compute in the case retrieval procedure of CBR [12]. The meaningful set of features is often predetermined by experts in bio-medical fields, and the most similar case may result in the best accuracy in prediction when output values of each feature are wide-spread like plasma proteomic profiles. If that is the case, a proper weight optimization may only enhance the prediction performance of CBR. The weights are optimized either subjectively or objectively. Subject weights are typically allocated according to the preference scores or information of experts such as Delphi method [5]. Objective weights can be allocated by entropy method [7], statistical method [8] or they can be optimized while proceeding algorithms such as generic algorithm (GA) [12] or neural-net (NN) [6]. Among these approaches, NN needs a large number of inter-connected neurons to allocate weights, so small or moderate-size samples may not attain a standard structure of NN [9]. GA is also criticized due to premature convergence or low reliability [9]. A weight by a statistical method was allocated by the proportion of Wald's statistics [8] which is obtained by assuming asymptotically normal distributions of parameters. The present study proposes a non-parametric weight allocation method without using normality assumption. We investigate the accuracy of a CBR based classification with plasma proteomic profiles to diagnose cervical cancer, and observe the enhancement of the prediction performance of the CBR classifier by allocating feature weights. To validate our approach, we also conduct previous weight allocation methods for the CBR classifier together with the plasma proteomic profiles. The paper is organized as follows. After introduction, section 2 briefly describes the CBR system and reviews previous studies. Section 3 presents the proposed method using Rank, and section 4 describes our data schemes and empirical results. At last, the conclusion and further research are discussed in section 5.

Methods

The CBR classifier with plasma proteomic profiles

The general problem-solving process by the CBR classifier is described in Fig. 1. The CBR classifier describes a target problem using old experiences, and finds a solution of the problem by retrieving similar cases stored in the case-base to the target problem where the case-base is the specific knowledge base of past experiences. The case is typically retrieved by learning techniques for the CBR classifier, and the most common technique is *k*-nearest neighbor (NN). The original CBR classifier uses 1-NN which retrieves the most similar case from the case-base to the target problem. The problem is adapted from the retrieved cases, and is revised. Once the problem is solved, the cases are retained. The CBR classifier with plasma proteomic profiles maintained the same scheme. The problem is to identify the class of a target case by comparing the pattern of the target case with those in the case-base where the case-base consists of trained samples with their class-labels. The case is retrieved from the case-base by *k*-nearest neighbor (NN) to solve the problem, and the target case as well as the retrieved case are stored in the case-base once the class of the target case is determined.

Prior studies for weight optimization

The original classifier assesses the similarity of a target case with cases in the case-base under the assumption that all features are equally likely important. However, it may be practical to think of the relative importance among the features, so some researches differently allocated the weights on features considering the relative importance. Since different weights for the attributes

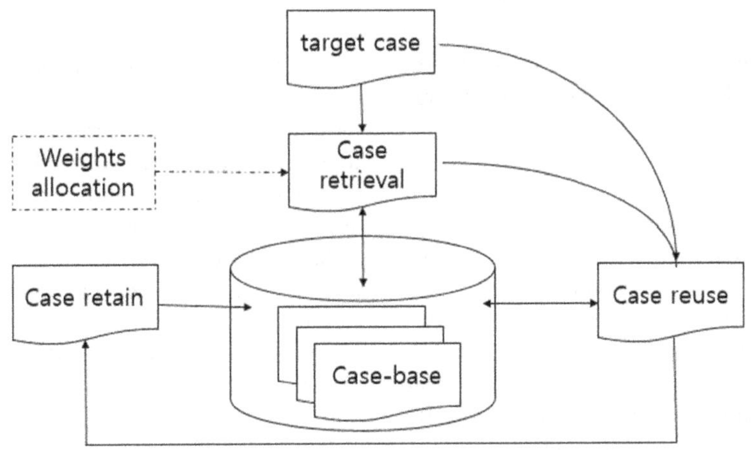

Fig. 1 Problem solving process of CBR Classifier. The CBR classifier finds the solution of the problem by retrieving similar cases stored in the case-base to the target problem as described

can vary the distribution of the overall similarities among the cases, the retrieved cases by the CBR classifier can be different depending on the altered distribution of the similarities. Regarding that matter, the weight allocation or optimization is closely related with the performance of the CBR classifier. In particular, the weight allocation or optimization techniques have gained attention as a way to enhance the performance of the CBR classifier in previous studies.

DELPHI method is one of the most common approaches to allocate feature weights to the CBR classifier. DELPHI method directly reflects experts' opinions about the features as the corresponding weights like Gu et al. [13] or Chang et al. [5], so the weights can be changed by the point of view of the subjects. Alternatively, weights have been objectively allocated using information gain or entropy. Cardie and Howe [14] first selected a set of relevant features using a decision tree, and assigned the weights with information gain to the feature which was chosen by the tree. Ahn and Kim [12] encoded feature weights with numbers from 0 to 7 which represented the relative importance of the features. These numbers were processed as 3-bit binary numbers and transformed into floating decimal numbers (x_f) for weights. Zhao et al. [7] used information entropy for feature weights to select suppliers. They computed the average regression coefficients to seek the integrated average index of each supplier, and calculated both the information gain in ID3 of the decision tree and the entropy. These values were later standardized as the numbers in the range of [0,1] for weights. Besides, Liang et al. [8] optimized feature weights by a statistical approach. They fitted features with binary logistic regression, and computed the Wald statistics of parameter estimates for the features. Then, the statistics are standardized by dividing them by the sum of all the statistics before they are allocated to the features as the weights. Suitable weights may vary depending upon problems we encountered. Prior studies about the weight optimization or allocation methods are summarized in Table 1.

Table 1 Prior studies about the weight optimization methods

Authors	Year	Methods	Weights
Cardie & Howe [14]	(1997)	Information gain	G(f) [a]
Ahn & Kim [12]	(2009)	Relative importance [0-7]	$\frac{x_f}{\sum_{f=1}^{m} x_f}$
Gu et al. [13]	(2010)	Delphi method	–
Chang et al. [5]	(2011)	Delphi method	–
Zhao et al. [7]	(2011)	Entropy method	$\frac{entropy_f}{\sum_{f=1}^{m} entropy_f}$
Liang et al. [8]	(2012)	Logistic regression	$\frac{Wald_f}{\sum_{f=1}^{m} Wald_f}$

[a] indicates information gain of the f-th feature, and entropy is defined as $-\sum_i p_i \cdot \log_2 p_i$

Rank-based weight optimization

Distance functions and problem setting

A typical similarity or dissimilarity measure is a distance metric, and it is crucial to learn a good distance metric to represent the similarity or dissimilarity in feature space although there are considerable researches on distance metrics [15–17]. Some researches have been focused on the comparison of their impacts on the performance in classification with known public database [18, 19]. However, no single similarity or dissimilarity showed dominantly superior to the others in all methods in their studies [18, 19]. Most classifiers try to use a distance metric that keeps data points close if the class labels are the same while keeps distance from the data points if the class labels are different. The goal of the CBR classifier is to predict a class label of a target case of $\vec{x}_0$ by retrieving the most similar case from the case-base using the proper distance metric. Let $\chi = \{\vec{x}_1, \cdots, \vec{x}_n\}$ be a collection of n data points in the case-base with the known class labels of $C = \{c_1, \cdots, c_n\}$ where $\vec{x}_i \in R^m$ and $c_i \in \{1, \cdots, K\}$. The CBR classifier typically adapts the k-NN approach to retrieve the similar cases to the target case with a given k. The k-NN approach assumes that the class conditional probability in the nearest neighbors to $\vec{x}_0, N(\vec{x}_0)$, is constant, and tries to maintain consistency in predicting class labels for $\vec{x}_0$ by obtaining its neighborhood as follows where I(·) is an indicator function.

$$p(j|\vec{x}_0) = \frac{\sum_{i=1}^{n} I(\vec{x}_i \in N(\vec{x}_0)) I(c_i = j)}{\sum_{i=1}^{n} I(\vec{x}_i \in N(\vec{x}_0))} \qquad (1)$$

The global distance between the target case and any case in the case-base is computed by summing up the local distances to determine the nearest neighbors for the target case on Eq. (1). The local distance is computed for each feature between the target case and any case in the case-base by the pre-defined local distance metric, and the types of local distance metric do not have to be the same among the features. Euclidean distance metric is typically used to compute the physical distance between the two data points, but it suffers in the case that vectors of data points aren't linearly distributed like default measurements of proteomic profiles. On the contrary, Fre'chet distance metric is known to be useful to measure the distance between the data points when the vectors of those data points lie on the non-linear curve [20]. According to the characteristics of the feature types, the distance metric consists of either Euclidean distance metric or Fre'chet distance metric for the present study. Euclidean distance metric and Fre'chet distance metric are defined for the feature, f, as follows where $\vec{x}_i^{(f)}$ and $\vec{x}_0^{(f)}$ are sub-vectors of any data point in the case-base and the target case consisting of the feature, f, respectively.

$$d_f\left(\vec{x}_i^{(f)}, \vec{x}_0^{(f)}\right) = \left(\vec{x}_i^{(f)} - \vec{x}_0^{(f)}\right)^T \left(\vec{x}_i^{(f)} - \vec{x}_0^{(f)}\right) \quad (2)$$

$$d_f\left(\vec{x}_i^{(f)}, \vec{x}_0^{(f)}\right) = \inf_{\alpha,\beta} \max_{t' \in [0,1]} d\left(\vec{x}_i^{(f)}(\alpha(t')), \vec{x}_0^{(f)}(\beta(t'))\right) \quad (3)$$

Conversion to rank-order information

Plasma proteomic profiles have the large within-subject variance. Although the class labels are the same, the profiles can be distributed over a considerable extent as well as they are not following the general pattern. We determined the proximity of the cases using the global similarity based on rank-order information of the distances [21] instead of using the distance itself to enhance robustness in predicting the class label of the target case in the present study. The similarity is computed as follows where N′ is the number of cases having a unique ranking-order in the case-base and ω_f is an unknown weight for a feature of *f*.

$$S(\vec{x}_i, \vec{x}_0) = \sum_{f=1}^{m} \omega f \cdot \left[\frac{N' - \operatorname{rank}\left(d_f\left(\vec{x}_i^f, \vec{x}_0^f\right)\right)}{N' - 1}\right] \quad (4)$$

According to Eq. (4), the higher the rank, the greater the similarity between the *i*-th case and the target case.

Weight optimization

Every feature is equally likely important to the original CBR classifier. Since the original CBR classifier often showed lower predictability, there have been some researches to improve the predictability by assigning different weights to the features according to their relative importance. In the same line of thoughts, we adopted the different weights to the feature in calculating the similarity, and optimized the weights according to the objective function from Wilcoxon's rank sum test statistics. The ability of the objective function is mainly influenced by the feature weights, and the weights are determined to maximize the ability of the objective function to differentiate the cases having different class labels. Wilcoxon's rank sum test is a non-parametric test to assess the difference of the mean ranks for two samples, and it is known to be useful when outliers exist in the observations compared to the parametric tests. The similarity is regarded as a function of ranks in the present study because the similarity is computed according to the corresponding rank-order information of the distances for features between the target case and any case in the case-base. Thus, the weights can be naturally allocated to the features in the similarity measure maintaining the same property from the objective function based on Wilcoxon's rank sum statistics. The objective function for the present study can be summarized as follows where n_1 is the number of cases having the class label of 1 when the class labels are denoted as either 0 or 1 and the number of classes, J, is set to 2.

$$\begin{aligned} &\arg\ \max_{\omega_f : f=1,\cdots,m} && \sum_{f=1}^{m} \omega_f \cdot r_f \\ &\text{where} && r_f = \sum_{i=1}^{n_1} \operatorname{rank}\left(d_f\left(\vec{x}_i^{(f)}, \vec{x}_0^{(0)}\right)\right) - \frac{n_1 \cdot (n_1+1)}{2} \\ &\text{constraint to} && \begin{cases} 0 \le \omega_f \le 1 \\ \sum_{f=1}^{m} \omega_f = 1 \end{cases} \end{aligned} \quad (5)$$

On Eq. (5), as the probability increases that the two groups of the cases are truly drawn from the population-cases having the different class labels, the corresponding feature weight of ω_f becomes large because the resulted statistics, *W*, is large. The significance of the test statistics is directly represented by the magnitude of the corresponding *p*-value, so the feature weights can be computed using the magnitudes of *p*-values from the test statistics as follows.

$$\omega_f = \frac{1 - p(|W| \ge r_f)}{\sum_{f=1}^{m} 1 - p(|W| \ge r_f)} \quad (6)$$

where *W* denotes the test statistics of the Wilcoxon's rank sum test. The feature weights from Eq. (6) are used to compute the similarity of Eq. (4).

Application and experiments

Data description The proteomic profiles were obtained from the blood plasma samples which were collected from recruited subjects at the University of Louisville, KY, USA. Total 70 female subjects were recruited for this study, and 50% of those subjects were diagnosed with cervical carcinoma while the others are healthy controls, without any known diseases. The study protocol was approved by the institutional review board of the University of Louisville, and informed consent forms were voluntarily signed by the participants. The origin of the data can be referred to [22], and the secondary data was used for the study. The default output measurement of the proteomic profiles was the excess heat capacity (ΔC_p), which were recorded at the different temperatures from 45 to 90 °C by incrementally adding 1 °C to the previous measuring temperature. The proteomic profiles were preprocessed prior to the analysis. The excess heat capacity (ΔC_p) as the default measurement is a vector of real numbers of length 451 and it typically shows one or two peaks on the range of temperatures during the experiment. We newly extracted 5 features from the pre-processed data besides the excess heat capacity. The feature information is summarized in Table 2. The class information for each proteomic profile was labeled as either 'control' or 'cancer' according to the clinical status of the corresponding subject. On Table 2, PEAK1 and PEAK2 indicate those peaks, and T1 and T2 are temperatures that those peaks occur at where {PEAK1, PEAK2, T1, T2} were estimated by Gaussian kernel regression from the excess heat capacity patterns. IND indicates a set of 451 individual measurement of the excess heat capacity, and IR is a binary value indicating the initial directional tendency of the excess heat capacity as the temperature increases. IR is 1 if the directional tendency is positive, 0 otherwise.

Numerical experiments The purpose of the numerical experiments is to study the performance of the CBR classifier in prediction with the plasma proteomic profiles by comparing with the previous approaches. In particular, we observed whether the rank-based feature weights enhance the performance of the CBR classifier with proteomic profiles or not. As reference methods, two common machine learning methods, *k*-NN (*k* -NN) and support vector machine (SVM), a statistical approach using the composite coefficient [23], and three CBR approaches weighted by different allocation methods in previous studies [7, 8] were conducted to validate the performance of the proposed CBR approach for the present study. The number of neighbors for *k* -NN was 5 which was determined by cross-validation (CV) with training samples, and SVM was conducted based on the radial basis kernel.

The statistical model was introduced to show the difference of the plasma proteomic profiles between two groups having different clinical status using a composite coefficient which was a weighted product of an average probability being in the same group of the reference sample and Pearson's correlation coefficient. In the present study, this model was conducted with the default setting of the composite coefficient as in the literature [23]. Namely, the reference set was composed with the cases in the 'control' class for this model, and the weight factor of the composite coefficient was set to 1 as described in the literature. This classification model is abbreviated as (SCUCC) indicating statistically classified using the composite coefficient for the experiments as a reference method. Among the CBR approaches, the first model is a classical CBR approach (CLCBR), which gives attributes equal-weights and uses *1*-NN for the case retrieval. This model would be the base model to examine the effect of the CBR classifiers having different weights on features. ETCBR and LWCBR are the weighted CBR approaches. The feature weights were allocated with standardized entropy value in ETCBR [7]. In the present study, IR is Berno'ulli and the other features are assumed as normal distribution. The computed entropy was standardized by dividing each entropy by the sum of all entropy values prior to allocation, and 1-NN was used for the case retrieval. LWCBR indicates a weighted CBR approach from logistic regression model. This model adopted standardized Wald statistics of the regression coefficients for feature weights by fitting the observation with binary logistic regression. Namely, the Wald statistics were divided by the sum of the all statistics before they were allocated to the features [8], and also used 1-NN for the case retrieval. Logistic regression is a typical parametric approach and Wald statistics are derived from the regression coefficients under the asymptotic normal assumption, so this model can be a good reference to observe the performance of the proposed feature weights. The proposed CBR approach is abbreviated as RWCBR indicating a rank-weighted CBR approach. As described in the above sections, the feature weights

Table 2 Description of the features

Features (Abbreviation)	Type	Contents
Initial Response (IR)	Binary number	0: decreasing 1: increasing
Temperature 1 (T1)	Real number	Range [45 - 55]
Temperature 2 (T2)	Real number	Range [56 - 90]
Maximum Peak at T1 (PEAK1)	Real number	Range [0 - ∞]
Maximum Peak at T2 (PEAK2)	Real number	Range [0 - ∞]
A set of individual ΔC_p (IND)	A vector of real numbers	Range [0 - ∞]

were computed from Wilcoxon's rank sum test and the most similar case was retrieved as the other CBR approaches.

The data set of proteomic profiles consists of the predefined features on Table 2 with 70 subjects, and the class labels are fully given with the number of classes as two. The data set was randomly partitioned into five equal-sized subsets for 5-fold CV. At each fold, a subset was selected as a test set, and the other four subsets became a training set where the proportion of the cases were equally distributed from the two classes during the experiments. The feature weights for the ETCBR, LWCBR and RWCBR were estimated with the training set, and the optimized weights were allocated to the features in the test set.

Results

Each fold has the same size of cases in the test set and the training set as 14 and 56, respectively during the experiments. The estimated feature weights by ETCBR, LWCBR and RWCBR at each fold are summarized in Table 3. The performances of the seven different models were evaluated at each fold in terms of Precision, Recall, F-1 score, [24, 25] and G-measure [25]. The estimated weights in Table 3 were allocated to the features when the CBR classifiers retrieved the most similar case from the case-base by ETCBR, LWCBR and RWCBR. The information indices of Precision, Recall, F-1 score and G-measure are defined as follows.

Table 3 Estimated feature weights

Fold	Model	IR	PEAK1	PEAK2	T1	T2	IND
I	ETCBR	0.0067	0.0145	0.0347	0.0595	0.0220	0.8625
	LWCBR	0.0158	0.1145	0.3845	0.0960	0.0179	0.3713
	RWCBR	0.1704	0.1890	0.1488	0.1886	0.1596	0.1436
II	ETCBR	0.0089	0.0311	0.0477	0.0766	0.0314	0.8042
	LWCBR	0.0877	0.0752	0.2550	0.0016	0.3244	0.2561
	RWCBR	0.2190	0.2222	0.0954	0.2203	0.1325	0.1106
III	ETCBR	0.0068	0.0265	0.0391	0.0654	0.0243	0.8377
	LWCBR	0.0175	0.1780	0.2481	0.1188	0.1584	0.2793
	RWCBR	0.1274	0.2603	0.1144	0.2837	0.1092	0.1051
IV	ETCBR	0.0076	0.0259	0.0383	0.0643	0.0247	0.8392
	LWCBR	0.0001	0.3524	0.0682	0.4252	0.1484	0.0056
	RWCBR	0.1627	0.2266	0.1279	0.2206	0.1233	0.1388
V	ETCBR	0.0065	0.0223	0.0345	0.0581	0.0213	0.8573
	LWCBR	0.0250	0.0036	0.1628	0.2751	0.3219	0.2116
	RWCBR	0.2205	0.2186	0.1024	0.2334	0.1076	0.1175

$$\text{Precesion} = \frac{\sum \text{true positive}}{\sum(\text{true positive} + \text{false positive})}$$

$$\text{Recall} = \frac{\sum \text{true positive}}{\sum(\text{true positive} + \text{false negative})}$$

$$\text{F-1 score} = 2 \cdot \frac{\text{precision} \cdot \text{recall}}{(\text{precision} + \text{recall})}$$

$$\text{G-measure} = \sqrt{\text{precision} \cdot \text{recall}}$$

With the retrieved case for each target case, the class label of the target case was predicted according to Eq. (1), and the prediction results were used to compute the information indices at each fold according to the above definitions.

The resulting information indices at each fold are summarized on Table 4, and the comprehensive statistics using the minimum (MIN), average, (AVG), standard deviation (STD) and the maximum (MAX) for each index are summarized on Table 5. Among the models, RWCBR and SVM consistently showed good performances over different sample sets in predicting the class labels with plasma proteomic profiles in comparison with others, but the performance of RWCBR was slightly better. In case of Precision and Recall indices, LWCBR had the biggest range from the minimum of 33% to the maximum of 80% and from the minimum of 29% to the maximum of 100%, respectively while SVM had the smallest range from the minimum of 85.7% to the maximum of 100% in both indices. However, RWCBR showed the highest average value of 91% among the all models in both Precision and Recall, and the performance was maintained at least 71%. ETCBR and RWCBR showed better performance than CLCBR in both Precision and Recall, but LWCBR worked poor in comparison with CLCBR by showing lower mean values in all indices although we generally expected a weighted CBR approach to perform better than CLCBR. Comparing CLCBR to SCUCC, a statistical approach, average precision index of CLCBC was lower, but average recall index was higher. F-1 score and G-measure were similar between the two, so it appears that CBR approaches do not always work well with plasma proteomic profiles. Regarding F1-score and G-measure, SVM also maintained the shortest ranges, but RWCBR showed the best performance at most aspects of summary statistics among the seven models. In particular, it maintained the smallest standard deviations in comparison with the other models.

The retrieved cases for each target case from the test set by RWCBR model at the first fold are displayed on Fig. 2. The black solid lines represent the 14 target cases from the test set, and the red solid lines are the most similar cases retrieved from the case-bases according to the similarity measure of Eq. (4).

Table 4 Information indices by 5-Fold CV

Fold	Measures	K-NN	SVM	SCUCC	CLCBR	ETCBR	LWCBR	RWCBR
I	Precision	0.5000	0.8571	1.0000	0.6667	1.0000	0.8000	1.0000
	Recall	0.7143	0.8571	0.2857	0.5714	0.7143	0.5714	0.7143
	F1-score	0.5882	0.8571	0.4444	0.6154	0.8333	0.6667	0.8333
	G-measure	0.5976	0.8571	0.5345	0.6171	0.8452	0.6761	0.8452
II	Precision	0.8571	0.8571	1.0000	0.8000	0.7500	0.3333	1.0000
	Recall	0.8571	0.8571	0.8571	0.5714	0.8571	0.2857	0.8571
	F1-score	0.8571	0.8571	0.9231	0.6667	0.8000	0.3077	0.9231
	G-measure	0.8571	0.8571	0.9258	0.6761	0.8018	0.3086	0.9258
III	Precision	0.6000	0.8571	0.8333	0.7500	0.8333	0.7778	0.7778
	Recall	0.8571	0.8571	0.7143	0.8571	0.7143	1.0000	1.0000
	F1-score	0.7059	0.8571	0.7692	0.8000	0.7692	0.8750	0.8750
	G-measure	0.7171	0.8571	0.7715	0.8018	0.7715	0.8819	0.8819
IV	Precision	0.7500	1.0000	1.0000	1.0000	0.8750	0.7778	1.0000
	Recall	0.8571	1.0000	0.5714	1.0000	1.0000	1.0000	1.0000
	F1-score	0.8000	1.0000	0.7273	1.0000	0.9333	0.8750	1.0000
	G-measure	0.8018	1.0000	0.7559	1.0000	0.9354	0.8819	1.0000
V	Precision	0.5455	0.8571	0.7000	0.6000	1.0000	0.6000	0.7778
	Recall	0.8571	0.8571	1.0000	0.8571	1.0000	0.8571	1.0000
	F1-score	0.6667	0.8571	0.8235	0.7059	1.0000	0.7059	0.8750
	G-measure	0.6838	0.8571	0.8366	0.7171	1.0000	0.7171	0.8819

Table 5 Comprehensive statistics for information indices

Measures	Statistics	K-NN	SVM	SCUCC	CLCBR	ETCBR	LWCBR	RWCBR
Precision	MIN	0.5000	0.8571	0.7000	0.6000	0.7500	0.3333	0.7778
	AVG	0.6506	0.8857	0.9067	0.7633	0.8917	0.6578	0.9111
	STD	0.1490	0.0639	0.1362	0.1529	0.1087	0.1985	0.1217
	MAX	0.8571	1.0000	1.0000	1.0000	1.0000	0.8000	1.0000
Recall	MIN	0.7143	0.8571	0.2857	0.5714	0.7143	0.2857	0.7143
	AVG	0.8285	0.8857	0.6857	0.7714	0.8571	0.7428	0.9143
	STD	0.0639	0.0639	0.2748	0.1917	0.1429	0.3097	0.1278
	MAX	0.8571	1.0000	1.0000	1.0000	1.0000	1.0000	1.0000
F1-score	MIN	0.5882	0.8571	0.4444	0.6154	0.7692	0.3077	0.8333
	AVG	0.7236	0.8857	0.7375	0.7576	0.8672	0.6861	0.9013
	STD	0.1067	0.0639	0.1795	0.1514	0.0965	0.2320	0.0637
	MAX	0.8571	1.0000	0.9231	1.0000	1.0000	0.8750	1.0000
G-measure	MIN	0.5976	0.8571	0.5345	0.6171	0.7715	0.3086	0.8452
	AVG	0.7221	0.8857	0.7649	0.7624	0.8708	0.6931	0.9070
	STD	0.1088	0.0639	0.1451	0.1488	0.0951	0.2345	0.0593
	MAX	0.8571	1.0000	0.9258	1.0000	1.0000	0.8819	1.0000

Note: *MIN* the minimum, *AVG* average, *STD* standard deviation, *MAX* the maximum

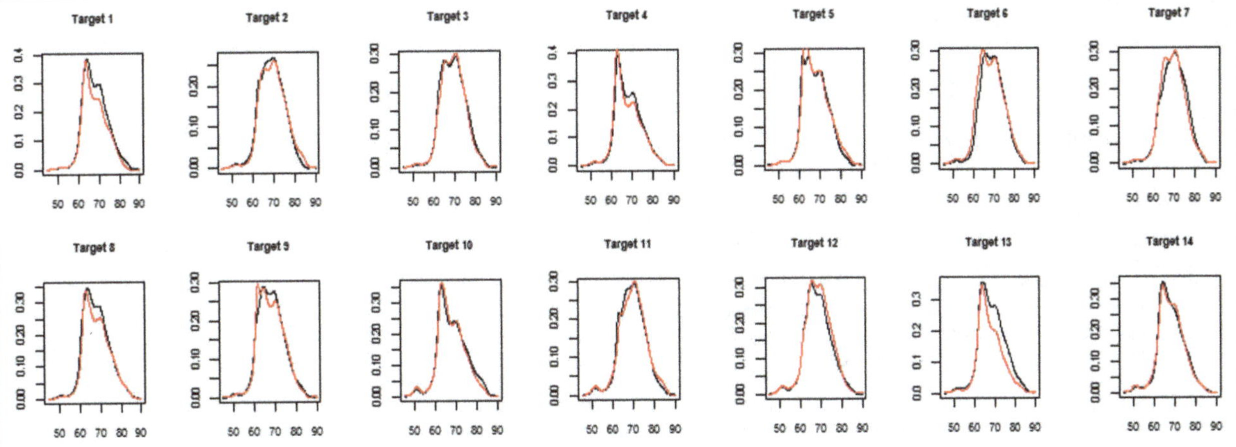

Fig. 2 The retrieved cases by RWCBR at Fold 1. The figure illustrates 14 cases of proteomic profiles at fold 1. Black-solid lines represent target cases, and red-solid lines represent the solutions optimized by RWCBR

Conclusion and Discussion

Plasma proteomic profiles have been regarded as a potential biomarker to diagnose certain diseases according to their specific patterns. It is challenging to precisely predict the clinical status based solely on the patterns of profiles because some profiles do not frequently follow the general patterns, which leads to large within-subject variance. The prediction based on CBR based approaches may be effective in that case. The CBR classifier predicts the clinical status of a target case by retrieving the most similar case from the case-base, so it would be advantageous in prediction because it can avoid the risk to make decision according to deviated overall means due to the outlying pattern. However, CBR classifier often shows low predictability, and some studies made efforts to enhance the predictability using weight optimization for features. There is still no golden standard to optimize or allocate the feature weights, which can be dependent upon the characteristics of the data we encounter.

The present study suggests a rank-based weighted CBR classifier (RWCBR) to predict the clinical status of plasma proteomic profiles. The rank-based weighted CBR classifier uses a weighted similarity based on rank-order information of distance metrics to retrieve the most similar case from the case-base where the feature weights are optimized from Wilcoxon's rank sum statistics. We conducted numerical experiments to validate the performance of RWCBR. As reference methods, two machine learning techniques, *k*-NN and SVM, a statistical method, SCUCC, a classical CBR (CLCBR) and two differently weighted CBR, ETCBR and LWCBR methods were compared in terms of Precision, Recall, F-1 score and G-measure. According to the results, SVM showed the lowest standard deviation and the highest minimum value for Precision, Recall, but RWCBR outperform in average value in all information indices, and it maintained the lowest standard deviation in F-1 score and G-measure. Also, LWCBR showed lower performance than CLCBR in most information indices. A weighted CBR approaches do not always perform well, so the weight allocation or optimization methods should take into accounts the characteristics of the data set to enhance the performance of CBR classifier.

The sample size of the plasma proteomic profiles was small in the present study. However, RWCBR approach showed potential to predict the clinical status based solely on plasma proteomic profiles as a robust classifier over different sample sets in the present study.

Abbreviations

AVG: Average; CBR: Case-based reasoning; CLCBR: Classical CBR; CV: Cross-Validation; ETCBR: Entropy-based CBR; k-NN: k-Nearest neighbor; LWCBR: Logistic regression-based Weighted CBR; MAX: The maximum; MIN: The minimum; RWCBR: Rank-based Weighted CBR; SCUCC: Statistically classified using composite coefficient; STD: Standard deviation; SVM: Support vector machine

Acknowledgements

We thank Assistant Professor NC Garbett at James Graham Brown Cancer Center in the University of Louisville for providing us with the data set and valuable comments. Also, we give thanks to Assistant Professor M. Ouyang at U Mass Boston for thorough scientific reviews and valuable comments.

Funding

This work was supported by the Korea University, Sejong, Korea [K1720701, 2017], and also supported by College of Public Policy, Korea University, Sejong, Korea [K1729001, 2018].

Author's contributions

AMK do the model development, the numerical experiment and manuscript writing. The author read and approved the final manuscript.

Competing interests

The author declares that she has no competing interests.

References

1. Burke EK, MacCarthy B, Petrovic S, MacCarthy B, Petrovic S, Qu R. Structured cases in case-based reasoning-re-using and adapting cases for time-tabling problems. Knowledge Based Syst. 2000;13:159–65.
2. Althoff KD, Auriol E, Barletta R, Manago M. A review of industrial case-based reasoning tools, an AI perspective report. AI intelligence; 1995. p. 3–4.
3. Aamodt A, Plaza E. Case-based reasoning: foundational issues, methodological variations and system approach. AI Commun. 1994;7:39–59.
4. Garbett NC, Miller JJ, Jenson AB, Chaires JB. Calorimetry outside the box a new window into the plasma proteome. Biophys J. 2008;94:1377–83.
5. Chang WL. A CBR-based Delphi model for quality group decisions. Cybern Syst. 2011;42:402–14.
6. Huang YS, Chiang CC, Shieh JW, Grimson E. Prototype optimization for nearest-neighbor classification. Pattern Recogn. 2002;35:1237–45.
7. Zhao K, Yu X. A case-based reasoning approach on supplier selection in petroleum enterprises. Expert Syst Appl. 2011;38:6839–47.
8. Liang C, Gu D, Bichindaritz I, Li X, Zuo C, Cheng W. Integrating gray system theory and logistic regression into case-base reasoning for safety assessment f thermal power plants. Expert Syst Appl. 2012;39:5154–67.
9. Yan A, Shao H, Guo Z. Weight optimization for case-based reasoning using membrane computing. Inf Sci. 2014;287:109–20.
10. Domingos P. Context-sensitive feature selection for lazy learners. Artif Intell Rev. 1997;11:1–5.
11. Skalac DB. Prototype and feature selection by sampling and random mutation hill climbing algorithms. Proceedings of the 11th international conference on machine learning, vol. 2; 1994. p. 293–301.
12. Ahn H, Kim K. Global optimization of case-based reasoning for breast cytology diagnosis. Expert Syst Appl. 2009;36:724–34.
13. Gu DX, Liang CY, Li XG, Yang SL, Zhang P. Intelligent technique for knowledge reuse of dental medical records based on Case-Base reasoning. J Med Syst. 2010;34:213–22.
14. Cardie C, Howe N. Improving minority class prediction using case-specific feature weights. Proceedings of the 14th international conference on machine learning; 1997. p. 57–65.
15. Cha SH. Comprehensive survey on distance/similarity measures between probability density functions. Int J Math Model Methods Appl Sci. 2007;1:300–7.
16. Chen Y, Garcia EK, Gupta MR, Rahimi A, Cazzanti L. Similarity-based classification: concepts and algorithms. J Mach Learn Res. 2009;20:747–76.
17. Jain AK, Murty MN, Flynn PJ. Data clustering: a review ACM computing survey. ACM Comput Surv. 1999;31:264–323.
18. Shirkhorshidi AS, Aghabozorgi S, Wah TY. Comparision study on similarity and dissimilarity measures in clustering continuous data. PLoS One. 2015;10: e0144059.
19. Khalifa A. Al., Haranczyk, M., Holliday, J. Comparison of nonbinary similarity coefficients for similarity searching, clustering and compound selection. J Chem Inf Model. 2009;49:1193–201.
20. Alt H, Godau M. Computing the Fre'chet distance between two polygonal curves. Int J Comput Geom Appl. 1995;5:75–91.
21. Li H, Sun J. Ranking-order case-based reasoning for financial distress prediction. Knowl-Based Syst. 2008;21:868–78.
22. Garbett NC, Merchant ML, Helm CW, Jenson AB, Klein JB, Chaires JB. Detection of cervical Cancer biomarker patterns in blood plasma and urine by differential scanning calorimetry and mass spectrometry. PLoS One. 2014;9:e84710.
23. Fish DJ, Brewood GP, Kim JS, et al. Statistical analysis of plasma thermograms measured by differential scanning calorimetry. Biophys Chem. 2005;152:184–90.
24. Powers DMW. Evaluation: from precision, recall and F-measure to ROC, Informedness, Markedness & Correlation. J Mach Learn Technol. 2011;2:37–63.
25. Nicolas PR. Scala for machine learning. Birmingham: PACKT Publishing Ltd; 2015. p. 37–63.

14

Qcorp: an annotated classification corpus of Chinese health questions

Haihong Guo, Xu Na and Jiao Li*

Abstract

Background: Health question-answering (QA) systems have become a typical application scenario of Artificial Intelligent (AI). An annotated question corpus is prerequisite for training machines to understand health information needs of users. Thus, we aimed to develop an annotated classification corpus of Chinese health questions (Qcorp) and make it openly accessible.

Methods: We developed a two-layered classification schema and corresponding annotation rules on basis of our previous work. Using the schema, we annotated 5000 questions that were randomly selected from 5 Chinese health websites within 6 broad sections. 8 annotators participated in the annotation task, and the inter-annotator agreement was evaluated to ensure the corpus quality. Furthermore, the distribution and relationship of the annotated tags were measured by descriptive statistics and social network map.

Results: The questions were annotated using 7101 tags that covers 29 topic categories in the two-layered schema. In our released corpus, the distribution of questions on the top-layered categories was treatment of 64.22%, diagnosis of 37.14%, epidemiology of 14.96%, healthy lifestyle of 10.38%, and health provider choice of 4.54% respectively. Both the annotated health questions and annotation schema were openly accessible on the Qcorp website. Users can download the annotated Chinese questions in CSV, XML, and HTML format.

Conclusions: We developed a Chinese health question corpus including 5000 manually annotated questions. It is openly accessible and would contribute to the intelligent health QA system development.

Keywords: Health Question, Annotation, Classification, Question Answering, Chinese

Background

Seeking health-related information is one of the top activities of today's online users via both personal computers and mobile devices. 59% of the U.S. adults have looked online for health information in 2012[1]. China has 194.76 million Internet health users in 2016 [2], increased 28.0% compared with that in 2015 [3], and will be further stimulated by the development of the Internet and communication technologies, as well as China's "Internet Plus" and "Health Big Data" policies[4, 5]. Despite the widespread need, the search engines often failed in returning relevant and trustworthy health information [6, 7]. Automatic question answering (QA) systems that can comprehend the questions asked by users in natural language and respond with concise and correct answers using natural language processing techniques shall be a good way to solve this problem [8]. Therefore, several efforts have worked on exploring automatic QA systems in health and medical area in recently years [9–14]. However, it is challenging [15–17], one of the main challenges is the lack of large scale corpus of annotated questions for the machines to learn to extract and understand the main information needs from the questions, known as question processing, which will obviously affect the performance of a QA system [18].

Due to the significant roles of annotated questions for QA system research and development, several studies have focused on this task and collected some useful

* Correspondence: li.jiao@imicams.ac.cn
Institute of Medical Information / Medical Library, Chinese Academy of Medical Sciences & Peking Union Medical College, Beijing, China

corpus. For example, the National Library of Medicine of the United States has collected a total of 4,654 annotated clinical questions [19] via endeavored studies [20–25]. This corpus has been applied for training machines to automatically classify question types [26], distinguishing answerable and unanswerable questions [27], recognizing question entailment [28], extracting keywords of the questions [26], as well as separating consumer questions from clinical questions [29]. Other groups have annotated several small scale corpora of health care-related questions in English, so as to automatically identify questions that can be answered by specific EMR notes [30], analyze the user's demographic, cognitive, affective, situational, social environmental information that are implied in the questions [31], classify the types of consumer health questions [32–35], and extract structured information from EHR-related ICU questions [36] and so on. These previous studies on English question corpora have provided useful references for Chinese health question corpus development.

Several studies on Chinese health questions corpus development have been conducted. Yin JW [37] annotated 1,600 Chinese questions related to maternal and infant health care with 8 topics so as to conduct automatic question classification. Zhang N [38] annotated 4,465 Chinese questions related to skin diseases with a self-developed two-layered classification schema so as to automatically classify question topics and help computing their semantic similarity. Tang GY [39] manually classified 1,688 questions related to hyperlipidemia into 241 categories in order to computing their semantic similarity. Compared with the above studies, our corpus featured as: (1) its annotation schema covers a large range of health topics; (2) the annotated questions covered broad diversity of diseases; moreover, (3) the corpus is openly accessible and easily reusable. Our work would help the intelligent system development related to Chinese health QA.

In this paper, we presented the Qcorp database which collects annotated health care-related questions in Chinese on the basis of our previous works [40, 41]. In current release, Qcorp contains 5000 consumer health questions in Chinese that are annotated with 7101 tags by 8 annotators with a two-layered classification schema consisting of 29 topic categories. An empirical study conducted by us [41] showed that the corpus was useful in training machines to automatically assign the topics of consumer health questions. We have made the current Qcorp publicly available and would enrich it in future work/collaboration, thus, the corpus could be more useful and applicable in various scenarios.

Methods

Data collection

The Qcorp database contains 5000 Chinese consumer health questions in total, and they are divided into two parts: data set 1 is the 2000 hypertension related questions collected by our previous work [40, 41], and data set 2 includes 3000 questions we randomly selected from 5 Chinese health websites under 6 broad sections: internal medicine, surgery, obstetrics & gynecology, pediatrics, infectious diseases, and traditional Chinese medicine (Table 1). These websites were selected because of their disease coverage and data accessibility, and a brief introduction of each of the five websites according to their *about us* section can be found in Additional file 1. The YYNET website lacks traditional Chinese medicine section, and the MYB website lacks either chirurgery or traditional Chinese medicine sections. Thus, no such section questions were collected from these two websites.

Here, the "question" is defined as a request on a certain subject posted by a consumer via the Internet to elicit answers from the physicians or the patient support group, which was identified based on meaning, not form. We manually discarded the uncomplicated data, repeated data and irrelevant data, such as advertisements, health education contents, patients' experiences, and other non-health contents. When one question was excluded we randomly selected another question from the same website within the same section so as to keep the sample balance.

Annotation tasks

Since the various consumer health questions could be represented by limited topics and keywords, the question classification plays an important role in an automatic QA system in identifying the information needs of consumers and further improving the accuracy of returned answers. Here, we performed manual annotation of the

Table 1 Sources of the 3000 questions in data set 2

Website	Internal medicine	Surgery	Obstetrics & Gynecology	Pediatrics	Infectious Diseases	Traditional Chinese Medicine	Total
HAODF	100	125	100	100	100	170	695
XYWY	100	125	100	100	100	165	690
120ASK	100	125	100	100	100	165	690
YYNET	100	125	100	100	100	N/A	525
MYB	100	N/A	100	100	100	N/A	400
Total	500	500	500	500	500	500	3000

general topics of 5000 Chinese questions related to health care posted by consumers via the internet, for the purpose of building a high quality annotated corpus for question classification, and further promoting the research and development of intelligent Chinese health QA systems.

Annotation guidelines

On basis of our previous work [40, 41], we used a two-layered *Classification Schema of Consumer Health Questions* in this study. As shown in Fig. 1, the schema consists of 7 broad categories on the first layer and 28 subcategories on the second layer, where, each category was coded by a unique identifier. The subcategories of other under each broad category were coded as main code plus 99, so as to keep the expandability of the classification schema. To guide the annotation and assure the inter-annotator agreement, we also built a list of annotation rules and question patterns for each category of the classification schema. More details of annotation guidelines can be found at our Qcorp website [42].

Annotators

We recruited eight annotators, one half of them have medical education background and the other half are specialized in medical informatics. For the 2000 hypertension related questions, their annotations were completed by five annotators in our previous work [41]. We translated their tags into two-layered tags according to the annotation guidelines in this study. For the rest 3000 questions (i.e., internal medicine, surgery, obstetrics & gynecology, pediatrics, infectious diseases, and traditional Chinese medicine), the annotation processes were performed in 3 rounds: In round 1, a training set of 300 randomly selected Chinese questions related to health care were annotated by four annotators independently so as to conclude and modify the annotation guidelines, ambiguous questions were settled by specifying the annotation rules and the question patterns. Then the four annotators were divided into two groups. In round 2, a testing set of 600 questions randomly selected from the sample were assigned to the two groups, 300 questions for each, and each annotator annotated independently so as to measure the inter-annotator agreement. In round 3, a development set of the remaining 2100 questions were each annotated independently by two of the four annotators. The disparities were discussed to achieve an agreement.

Inter-annotator agreement analysis

The inter-annotator agreement was evaluated by the percentage agreement statistic (Equation 1), which was one of the commonly used metrics to evaluate interrater reliability, and was directly interpretable. As a health question tend to have multiple topic tags, a match was recorded if two annotators agreed with either main or minor tag assignment based on the assumption that it was acceptable to answer any one of them. Therefore,

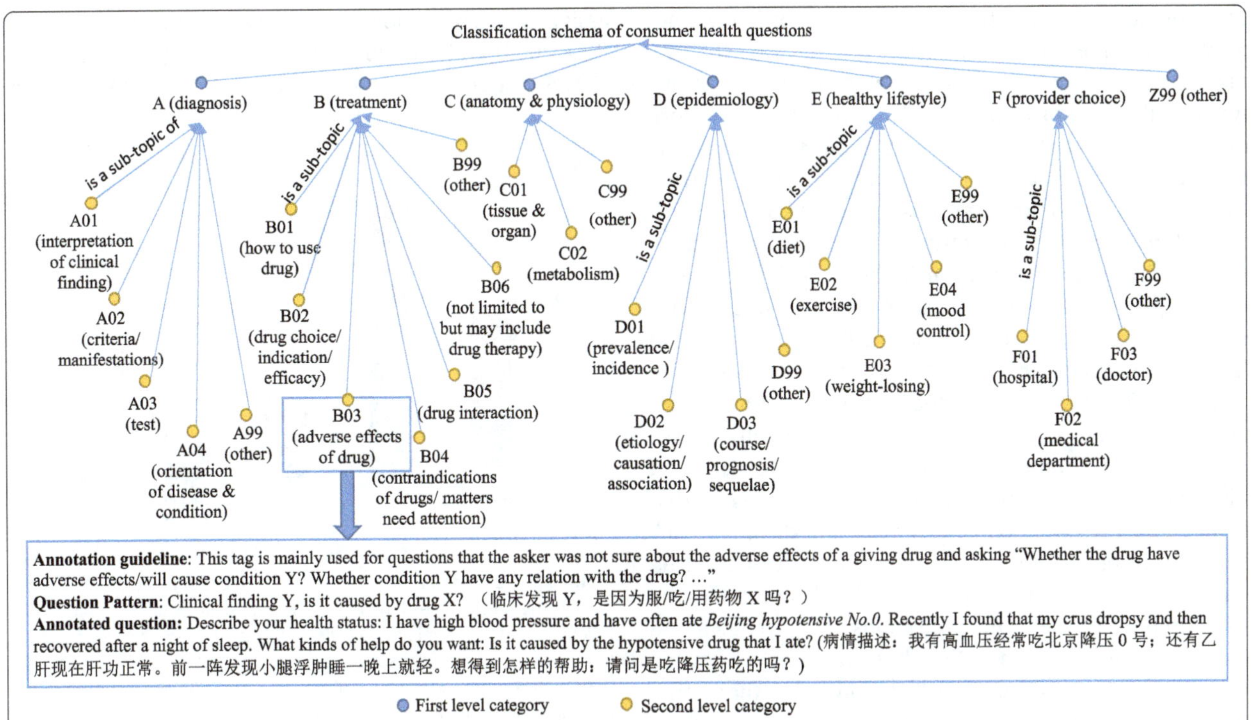

Fig. 1 Classification schema of consumer health questions and an example of the corresponding annotation rules

the kappa statistic that focuses on the inter-annotator agreement on each specific category [43] might not meet the multiple tag assignment measurement. This study used as many as 29 topic categories in annotation, thus, the percentage agreement statistic was more suitable.

$$I = \frac{M}{A} \tag{1}$$

Where M is the number of tag matched questions, and A is the number of all the annotated questions.

Database framework and web interface

Data stored in the Qcorp database were managed by using MySQL. Social network map and descriptive statistics were used to calculate and visualize the distribution and relationship of the annotated tags. The web server of Qcorp was developed based on Java. The Qcorp database is freely available at http://www.phoc.org.cn/healthqa/qcorp/.

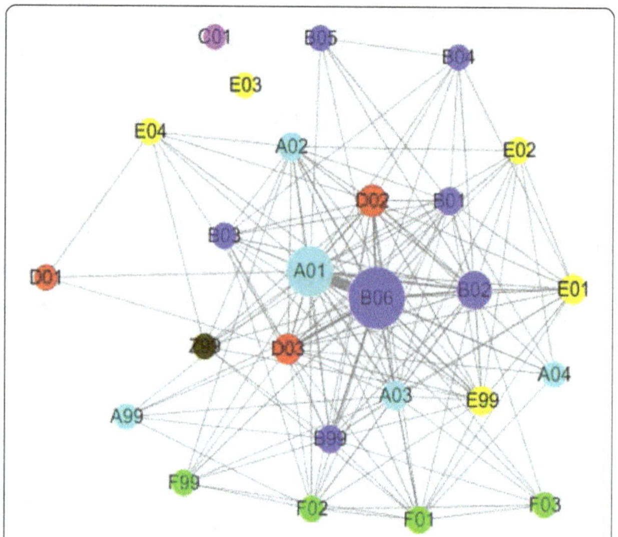

Fig. 2 The network of co-annotated tags on consumer health questions. The bigger the node, the more the corresponding tag is annotated; and the thicker the string, the more the two tags are co-annotated. The meaning of the tags were presented in Fig. 1

Results

Corpus overview

The 5000 Chinese consumer health questions were annotated with 5000 major tags and 2101 minor tags by the two-layered classification schema which consists of 29 topic categories (Fig. 1). One third of the questions (1717, 34.34%) were annotated with multiple tags, demonstrating that consumers tend to ask more than one question at a time, and the sub-questions sometimes belong to multiple topic categories [44], indicating that the task to classify the topics of consumer health questions was a multi-label problem [45]. As shown in the network of the co-annotated tags (Fig. 2), the tag B06 (represents treatments that not limited to but may include drug therapy) was annotated the most (2228, 44.56%), and it was often associated with other tags, mainly A01 (represents interpretation of clinical finding), D03 (represents course, prognosis, and sequelae of disease), B02 (represents drug choice, indications and efficacy of drug) and B99 (represents other issues about treatment) and so on. The tag A01 covered the second amount of the sample questions (1511, 30.22%), besides B06, it was often associated with A02 (represents criteria and manifestation of disease), D02 (represents etiology and causation of disease, and the association of risk facts and disease), D03, and A03 (represents test). The tag B02 (represents drug choice, indications and efficacy of drug) annotated the third amount of the sample questions (784, 15.68%), and it was interesting to see that it sometimes associated with E01 (represents diet), which indicated that some people were seeking for diet to help them recovering from ill condition while looking for drug therapy.

Annotated tag distribution on the first layer

For the seven categories on the first layer of the classification schema (Fig. 3), a total of 3211 (64.22%) questions were assigned to treatment, with 64.44% of the data set 1 (1291/2000) and 64.00% of the data set 2 (1920/3000); 1857 (37.14%) questions were assigned to diagnosis, with 33.65% of the data set 1 (673/2000) and 39.47% of the data set 2 (1184/3000); 748 (14.96%) questions were assigned to epidemiology, with 12.10% of the data set 1 (242/2000) and 16.87% of the data set 2 (506/3000); 519 (10.38%) questions were assigned to healthy lifestyle,

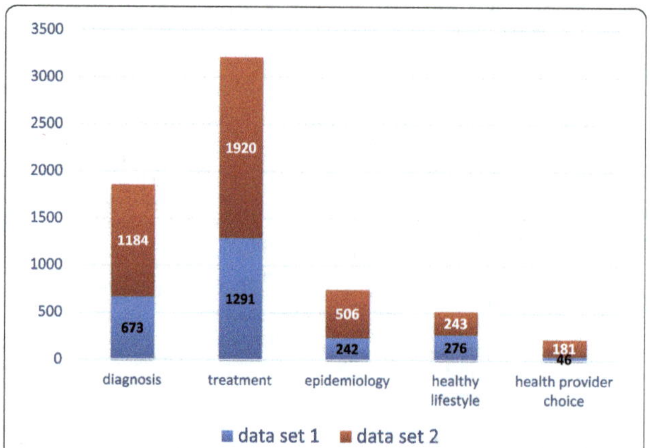

Fig. 3 Annotated tag distribution on the five broad categories of consumer health question classification schema. Data set 1 is the 2000 hypertension related questions collected by our previous work, and data set 2 includes 3000 questions we randomly selected from 5 Chinese health websites under 6 broad sections: internal medicine, surgery, obstetrics & gynecology, pediatrics, infectious diseases, and traditional Chinese medicine

with 13.80% of the data set 1 (276/2000) and 8.10% of the data set 2 (243/3000); 227 (4.54%) questions were assigned to health provider choice, with 2.30% of the data set 1 (46/2000) and 6.03% of data set 2 (181/3000). There was only one question assigned to anatomy & physiology, but we think this category contains many important knowledge about the basic medicine such as tissues and organs, metabolism and so on, so it was kept in the classification schema. 6 (0.12%) questions and 56 sub-questions could not be assigned to any of the above six broad categories.

Annotated tag distribution on the second layer

For questions under the category of diagnosis (Fig. 4), more than 80% of them (1511/1857) were about interpretation of clinical finding, nearly 12% (218/1857) were about test, and almost 10% (182/1857) were about criteria and manifestation of disease. For questions under the category of treatment (Fig. 2.c), almost 70% of them (2228/3211) were seeking treatments that not limited to but may include drug therapy, and nearly one quarter (784/3211) were specified to drug therapy, approximately 6% (173/3211) were about how to use a drug, and lest than 5% (144/3211) were concerned on side effects and contraindications of drugs. Questions under the category of epidemiology were mainly about the course, prognosis, and sequelae of disease (417/748, 55.75%) and etiology and causation of disease, and the association of risk facts and disease (347/748, 46.39%). Half of the Health lifestyle related questions (255/519) were specified to diet, and more than 40% (226/519) were general. For the questions under health provider choice, nearly half (101/227) were asking for a recommendation of hospitals, more than 20% (52/227) were about recommendation of medical departments, about 10% (29/227) were seeking for good doctors, and one quarter (57/227) were asking about the doctor visiting process, doctor appointment and so on.

Inter-annotator agreement

The inter-annotator agreement for the four annotators on the training set (300 questions) of data set 2 was 0.67 in round 1. By discussing on the disparities and further specifying the annotation rules and the question patterns for each category, the inter-annotator agreement for the two groups on the testing set (300 questions for each group) in round 2 increased to 0.88 and 0.92. After further discussion to achieve an agreement on the disparities, the average inter-annotator agreement for the four annotators on the developing set (2100 questions in total, each was annotated by two annotators independently) in round 3 increased to 0.96. And the average inter-annotator agreement for the five annotators on the data set 1 (each question was at least annotated by two annotators) on the second layer of the classification schema was 0.95.

Corpus access and usage

User interface

We provide a user-friendly interface that enable users to access the classification schema, the corresponding annotation rules, as well as the annotated Chinese consumer health questions (Fig. 5). In the "Browse" page, users can browse the classification schema of consumer health questions, and look for the details of each utmost small category with a click, the details of a category include its name in both Chinese and English, category

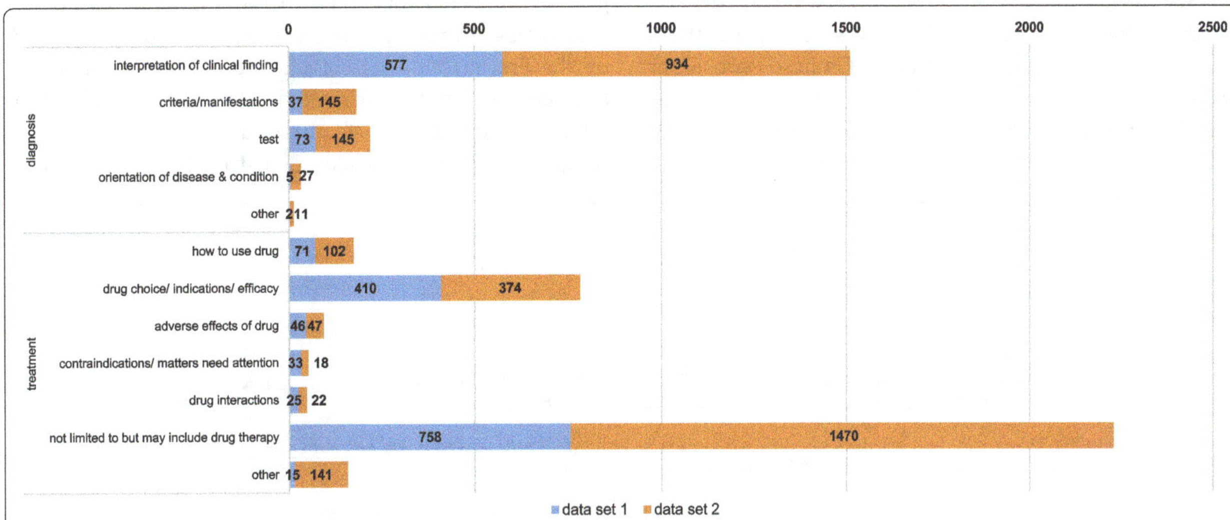

Fig. 4 Annotated tag distribution under the categories of diagnosis and treatment. Data set 1 is the 2000 hypertension related questions collected by our previous work, and data set 2 includes 3000 questions we randomly selected from 5 Chi-nese health websites under 6 broad sections: internal medicine, surgery, obstetrics & gynecology, pediatrics, infectious diseases, and traditional Chinese medicine

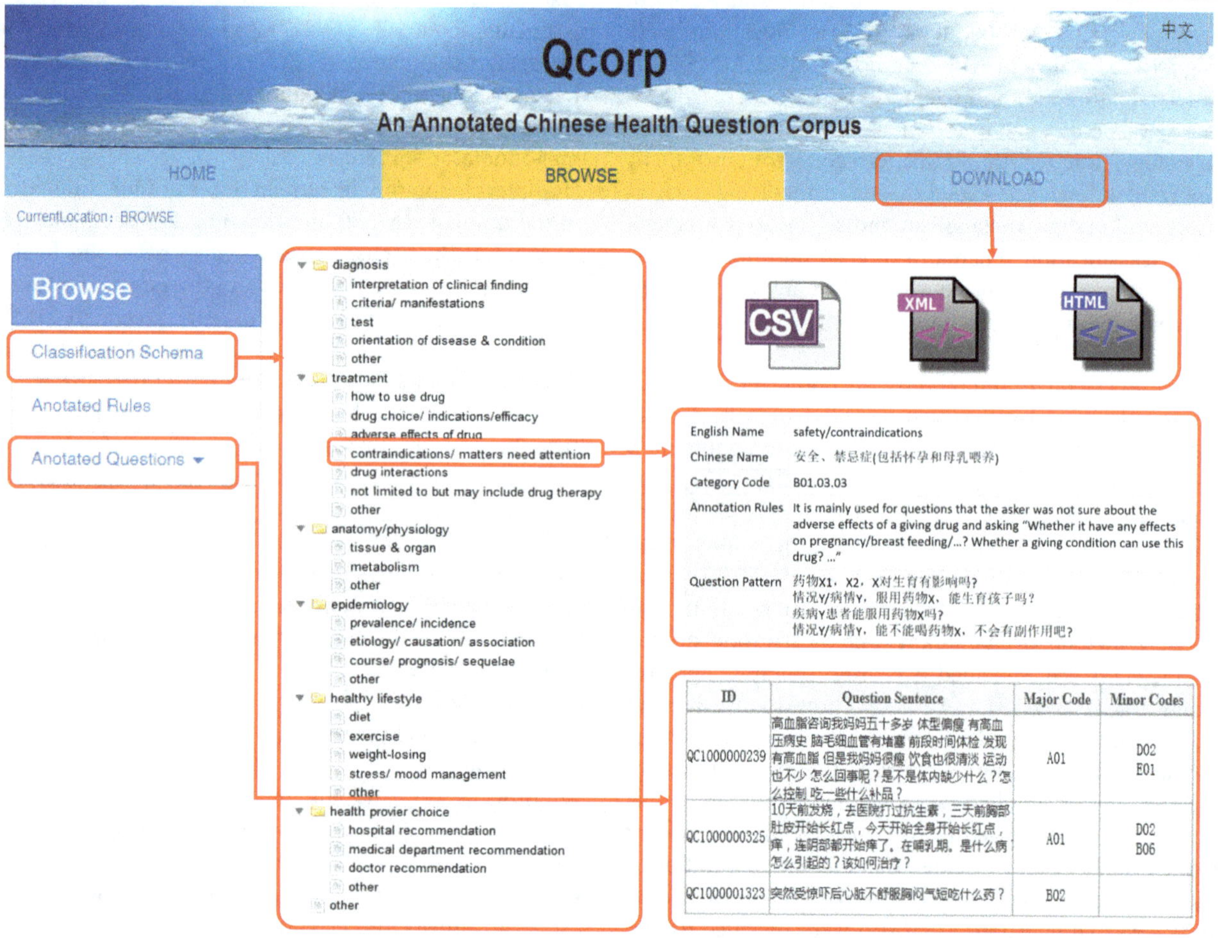

Fig. 5 User interface of Qcorp

code, annotation rules, question patterns and examples. Users can also browse all the annotation rules and browse the annotated questions by the seven broad categories in the first layer. In the "Download" page, users can download all the annotated Chinese consumer health questions in CSV, XML (Fig. 6 shows an example), and HTML format, so as to use them conveniently according to their usage purposes.

Case application of Qcorp corpus

Using the annotated 2000 questions in data set 1 as corpus, we applied a machine-learning method to automatically classify these questions into one of the five topics on the first layer of the classification schema. The Chinese questions were represented as a set of lexical, grammatical, and semantic features, and the features were weighted and selected according to [46]. Among them,

```
<?xml version="1.0" encoding="UTF-8"?>
<!DOCTYPE An_Annotated_Chinese_Health_Question_Corpus SYSTEM "WPRIM_2.dtd">

<Questions URL="http://www.phoc.org.cn/healthqa/qcorp/">
  <Question>
    <Id>QC0000001567</Id>
    <Content>
    最近血压低压高压都有些高，总是胸闷气短，偶尔心慌，头痛以及后脖子和肩膀总是酸酸的，
    浑身没劲，想问是怎么回事？什么病引起的，应吃些什么药？</Content>
    <Code1>A01</Code1>
    <Code1_Name_En>diagnosis--interpretation of clinical finding--symptom</Code1_Name_En>
    <Code1_Name_Cn>诊断--临床发现的解释</Code1_Name_Cn>
    <Code2>B02</Code2>
    <Code2_Name_En>treatment--drug choice/indications/efficacy</Code2_Name_En>
    <Code2_Name_Cn>治疗--药物选择、适应症、效力</Code2_Name_Cn>
  </Question>
```

Fig. 6 An example of annotated questions in XML format

Lexical features include bag-of-words and part-of-speech, grammatical features include interrogative words and corresponding chunks, semantic features include the Chinese Medical Subject Headings concepts and semantic types and so on. The result shows that the question classification achieved the F1-score of 99.13%, 98.55%, 96.35%, 76.02%, and 71.77% for the topics of *Healthy Lifestyle, Diagnosis, Health Provider Choice, Treatment,* and *Epidemiology*, respectively (More details can be found in [41]). This demonstrated that these annotated Chinese questions were applicable for training machines to automatically classify the topics of questions posted by health consumers, facilitating answer generation.

Discussion

Principle findings

Internet is increasingly becoming one of the main resources for consumers to acquire health information. Automatic QA systems that can correctly answer users' questions in natural language shall be a promising way to fulfill this need. A shared corpus of annotated consumer health questions in Chinese is prerequisite for training machines to understand the information needs of Chinese consumers by a health QA system. Thus, we developed the Qcorp database which collects annotated health care-related questions in Chinese. Qcorp currently contains 5000 consumer health questions in Chinese that annotated with 7101 tags by 8 annotators with a two-layered classification schema consisting of 29 topic categories. The corpus was proved to be applicable for training machines to automatically assign the topics of Chinese consumer health questions in an empirical study.

Comparison with other related works

Comparing to other related works on the annotation and corpus building of health and medical questions (Table 2), there are three main specialties in this study. Firstly, the scale of the annotated corpora in our Qcorp database was the biggest. Currently the Qcorp contains 5,000 annotated Chinese health questions, surpass the 4,654 annotated English clinical questions maintained by NLM [19], and the 4,465 annotated Chinese health questions built by Zhang N [38], let alone other small scale corpora. Secondly, the sample questions used in the Qcorp database were randomly selected from multiple sources. Unlike those corpora mainly come from 1 health website [31, 32, 37, 38], our corpus were randomly selected from 5 Chinese health websites so as to improve the representativeness of the corpus. Thirdly, the corpus here covered the relatively more diversity of the diseases. Other similar corpus, especially those Chinese ones, are mainly focused on only one specific kind of diseases, such as genetic and rare diseases [32], cancer [34], maternal and infant diseases [37], and skin diseases [38] and so on. While our corpus were selected from 6 broad sections, including internal medicine, surgery, obstetrics & gynecology, pediatrics, infectious diseases, and traditional Chinese medicine, so as to make it cover as many diseases as possible. To conclude, the Qcorp database is currently the biggest annotated classification corpus of Chinese health questions that from multiple sources and covered relatively more diversity of diseases. Other specialties include that the classification schema modified and applied in this study was quite reliable and with proper layers and number of categories.

Limitations and future studies

The Chinese health question corpus introduced here was only annotated with general topics, and yet was far from precisely representing the health information needs of askers that contained in the questions. There are

Table 2 A comparison of works on the corpus building of health and medical questions

Corpus or Author name	Language	Asker	Corpus scale	Question sources	Disease covering	Annotated categories	Layers
NLM collected clinical questions [19]	En	P	4,654	Clinical settings (5 studies [20–25])	Not limited	64	4
Patrick J [30]	En	P	595	Clinical settings	Not limited	11	4
Zhang Y [31]	En	C	600	1 website	23 subcategories	>50	5
Roberts K [32]	En	C	1,467	1 website	Genetic and rare diseases	13	1
Maroy S [34]	En	C	1,279	6 websites	Cancer	10	2
Yin JW [37]	Cn	C	1,600	1 health APP	Maternal and infant health	8	1
Zhang N [38]	Cn	C	4,465	1 website, books, self-composed	Skin disease	52	2
Tang GY [39]	Cn	C	1,688	4 websites	Hyperlipidemia	241	1
Our Qcorp	Cn	C	5,000	5 websites	6 broad sections	29	2

P refers to physician, and C refers to consumer

much work to do to reveal more detailed information of the Chinese consumer health questions in a structured manner. Our next step is to annotate the named entities and their relationships expressed in the Chinese consumer health questions. We hope that this database mainly developed for Chinese consumer health questions could serve as an important resource for the research and development of intelligent Chinese health QA systems.

Conclusions

We developed a corpus with 5000 Chinese consumer health questions manually annotated using a two-layered classification schema. The corpus, named as Qcorp, was openly accessible with the annotated questions in formats of CSV, XML and HTML, which can be easily used to train machines to understand consumers' health questions in Chinese. To our knowledge, the Qcorp database is currently the annotated classification corpus of Chinese health questions that covered relatively more diversity of diseases and come from multiple sources. Our study would help Chinese health QA system development.

Abbreviations

AI: Artificial Intelligent; CSV: Comma-Separated Values; HTML: Hyper Text Markup Language; MYB: Manyoubang.com; NLM: National Library of Medicine; QA: Question-answering; XML: Extensible Markup Language; YYNET: YYNET.CN

Acknowledgements

This study was supported by the Key Laboratory of Medical Information Intelligent Technology, Chinese Academy of Medical Sciences, the Basal Research Fund from Chinese Academy of Medical Sciences (Grant No. 2016ZX330011), The National Key Research and Development Program of China (Grant No. 2016YFC0901901), the National Population and Health Scientific Data Sharing Program of China, and the Key Laboratory of Knowledge Technology for Medical Integrative Publishing.

Funding

The publishing costs for this manuscript were provided by the Key Laboratory of Medical Information Intelligent Technology, Chinese Academy of Medical Sciences.

Authors' contributions

Jiao Li conducted the Chinese health question classification studies. Haihong Guo and Jiao Li designed the experiment and analyzed the results. Haihong Guo and Xu Na built the classification schema, collected the Chinese consumer health questions, organized the annotation, and did the corpus quality control. Haihong Guo designed the Qcorp website, and Xu Na developed it with the help of an engineer. All the authors wrote and revised the manuscript, all the authors have read and approved the final manuscript.

Competing interests

The authors declare that they have no competing interests.

References

1. Fox S, Duggan M.: Health Online 2013. Pew Research Center Internet & Technology, January 2013, http://www.pewinternet.org/2013/01/15/health-online-2013/, last accessed 21 July 2017.
2. China Internet Network Information Center.: China statistical report on internet development,http://www.cnnic.net.cn/hlwfzyj/hlwxzbg/hlwtjbg/201701/P020170123364672657408.pdf, last accessed 2017/08/20.
3. China Internet Network Information Center.: China statistical report on internet development, http://www.cnnic.net.cn/hlwfzyj/hlwxzbg/201601/P020160122469130059846.pdf, last accessed 2017/08/20.
4. State Council of the People's Republic of China.: Guidance of promoting the "Internet Plus" action, http://www.gov.cn/zhengce/content/2015-07/04/content_10002.htm, last accessed 2017/08/20.
5. Office of State Council of the People's Republic of China.: Guidance of promoting and regulating the application and development of health and medical big data, http://www.gov.cn/zhengce/content/2016-06/24/content_5085091.htm, last accessed 2017/08/20.
6. Pletneva N, Vargas A, Kalogianni K, Boyer C. Online health information search: what struggles and empowers the users? Results of an online survey. Stud Health Technol Inform. 2012;180:843–7.
7. Scantlebury A, Booth A, Hanley B. Experiences, practices and barriers to accessing health information: a qualitative study. International Journal of Medical Informatics. 2017;103:103–8.
8. Wren J D.: Question Answering Systems in biology and medicine – the time is now. Bioinformatics, 27(14): 2025-2026 (2011).
9. Cao Y, Liu F, Simpson P, et al. AskHERMES: An online question answering system for complex clinical questions. Journal of Biomedical Informatics. 2011;44(2):277–88.
10. Cairns BL, Nielsen RD, Masanz JJ, et al. The MiPACQ clinical question answering system. AMIA Annu Symp Proc. 2011:171–80.
11. Ni Y, Zhu H, Cai P, et al. CliniQA: highly reliable clinical question answering system. Stud Health Technol Inform. 2012;180:215–9.
12. Hristovski D, Dinevski D, Kastrin A, Rindflesch TC. Biomedical question answering using semantic relations. BMC Bioinformatics. 2015;16:6.
13. Asiaee AH, Minning T, Doshi P, Tarleton RL. A framework for ontology-based question answering with application to parasite immunology. J Biomed Semantics. 2015;6:31.
14. Liu F, Tur G, Hakkani-Tür D, Yu H. Towards spoken clinical-question answering: evaluating and adapting automatic speech-recognition systems for spoken clinical questions. J Am Med Inform Assoc. 2011;18:625–30.
15. Bauer M, Berleant D. Usability survey of biomedical question answering systems. Human Genomics. 2012;6(1):17–20.
16. Olivera-Lobo MD, Gutiérrez AJ. Evaluation of open- vs. restricted-domain question answering systems in the biomedical field. Journal of Inf Science. 2011;37(2):152–62.
17. Cruchet S, Boyer C, van der Plas L. Trustworthiness and relevance in web-based clinical question answering. Stud Health Technol Inform. 2012;180: 863–7.
18. Zhang N, Zhu L.: A review of Chinese Q & A system questions. Technology Intelligence Engineering, 01-42 (2016).
19. Clinical question collection. https://clinques.nlm.nih.gov/, last accessed 2017/08/23.
20. Gorman P, Ash J, Wykoff L. Can primary care physician's questions be answered using the medical journal literature? Bull Med Libr Assoc. 1994;82: 140–6.
21. Ely JW, Osheroff JA, Ebell MH, Bergus GR, Levy BT, Chambliss ML, et al. Analysis of questions asked by family doctors regarding patient care. Br Med J. 1999;319(7206):358–61.
22. Ely JW, Osheroff JA, Gorman PN, Ebell MH, Chambliss ML, Pifer EA, et al. A taxonomy of generic clinical questions: classification study. British Medical Journal. 2000;321:429–32.
23. Alper B, Stevermer J, White D, Ewigman B. Answering family physicians' clinical questions using electronic medical databases. J Fam Pract. 2001;50: 960–5.
24. Niu Y, Hirst G, Mcarthur G, et al.: Answering clinical questions with role identification. Meeting of the Association for Computational Linguistics, 73-80 (2003). http://www.aclweb.org/anthology/W/W03/W03-1310.pdf, last accessed 23 Aug 2017.
25. Alessandro DM, Kreiter CD, Peterson MW. An evaluation of information seeking behaviors of general pediatricians. Pediatrics. 2004;113:64–9.
26. Cao Y, Cimino JJ, Ely J, Yu H. Automatically extracting information needs from complex clinical questions. J Biomed Inform. 2010;43(6):962–71.

27. Yu H, Sable C, Zhu HR. Classifying medical questions based on an evidence taxonomy. In Workshop of AAAI, (2005). https://www.aaai.org/Papers/Workshops/2005/WS-05-10/WS05-10-005.pdf, last accessed 25 Aug 2017.
28. Abacha AB, Dina DF, Recognizing question entailment for medical question answering. AMIA Annu Symp Proc, 310-318 (2016).
29. Liu F, Antieau LD, Yu H. Toward automated consumer question answering: Automatically separating consumer questions from professional questions in the healthcare domain. Journal of biomedical informatics. 2011;44(6): 1032–8.
30. Patrick J, Li M. An ontology for clinical questions about the contents of patient notes. Journal of Biomedical Informatics. 2012;45:292–306.
31. Zhang Y. Toward a Layered Model of Context for Health Information Searching: An Analysis of Consumer-Generated Questions. Journal of the American Society for Information Science and Technology. 2013;64(6):1158–72.
32. Roberts K, Masterton K, Fiszman M, Kilicoglu H, Demner-Fushman D. Annotating Question Types for Consumer Health Questions. In: In Proceedings of the Fourth LREC Workshop on Building and Evaluating Resources for Health and Biomedical Text Processing; 2014.
33. Roberts K, Kilicoglu H, Fiszman M, Demner-Fushman D. Automatically classifying question types for consumer health questions. AMIA Annu Symp Proc. 2014;2014:1018–27.
34. McRoy S, Jones S, Kurmally A. Toward automated classification of consumers' cancer-related questions with a new taxonomy of expected answer types. Health Informatics Journal. 2015;22(3):523–35.
35. Cronin RM, Fabbri D, Denny JC, et al. A comparison of rule-based and machine learning approaches for classifying patient portal messages. International Journal of Medical Informatics. 2017:110–20.
36. Roberts K, Demner-Fushman D.: Toward a natural language interface for EHR questions. AMIA Jt Summits Transl Sci Proc. 2015 Mar 25:157-161 (2015).
37. Yin JW.: The method of classification and similarity calculation for mobile health questions based on the field dictionary, pp. P42-47. Shenzhen University, Shenzhen (2016).
38. Zhang N. Research on Natural Language Question Analysis Based on Knowledge Organization System. Beijing: Institute of Science and Technology of China; 2016.
39. Tang G, Ni Y, Xie G, et al.: A deep learning based method for similar patient question retrieval in Chinese. In Proceedings of the 16th World Congress on Health and Biomedical Informatics, Hangzhou, China, 23-29 August 2017 (2017).
40. Guo H, Li J, Dai T.: Consumer health information needs and question classification: analysis of hypertension related questions asked by consumers on a Chinese health website, In Proceedings of the 15th World Congress on Health and Biomedical Informatics, São Paulo, Brazil, 19-23 August 2015, Studies in Health Technology and Informatics, IOS Press, 216: 810-814 (2015).
41. Guo H, Na X, Hou L, Li J. Classifying Chinese Questions Related to Health Care Posted by Consumers Via the Internet. J Med Internet Res. 19(6):e220–2017.
42. Qcorp: An Annotated Chinese Health Question Corpus, http://www.phoc.org.cn/healthqa/qcorp/, last accessed 2017/09/29.
43. McHugh ML. Interrater reliability: the kappa statistic. Biochemia Medica. 2012;22(3):276–82.
44. Roberts K, Demner-Fushman D. Interactive use of online health resources: a comparison of consumer and professional questions. J Am Med Inform Assoc. 2016;23(4):802–11.
45. Tsoumakas G, Katakis I.: Multi-label classification: an overview, http://lpis.csd.auth.gr/publications/tsoumakas-ijdwm.pdf, last accessed 26 Aug 2017.
46. Chen YW, Lin CJ. Combining SVMs with various feature selection strategies. In: Studies in Fuzziness and Soft Computing. Berlin, Heidelberg: Springer; 2006. p. 315–24.

15

Design and implementation of an m-health data model for improving health information access for reproductive and child health services in low resource settings using a participatory action research approach

Joseph Thobias[1] and Achilles Kiwanuka[2*]

Abstract

Background: Information and Communication Technologies (ICTs) have been utilised globally for advancing social and economic development. As information becomes key to enlightening development initiatives, the role of mobile technology-based ICT services is becoming more significant. The aim of this study was to design and implement a mHealth data model with an intention of improving mothers' knowledge of Reproductive and Child Health (RCH) services in rural environments and to remind mothers who do not have access to mobile phones to attend antenatal care.

Methods: The methodology adopted in this research was participatory action research. A phased approach was utilised to answer the research question. The phases were: diagnosis of the problem, action planning, action taking, evaluation and reflection. The study was conducted in Chamwino district of Dodoma region, Tanzania. Reproductive and Child Health sections of Buigiri dispensary and Chamwino health centre were purposively selected. Data were collected through key informant interviews, document review, focus group discussion and observation. Content analysis methods were utilised during analysis. Consequently, the data model was designed, implemented and evaluated.

Results: Challenges of information dissemination in low resource settings noted in this study are: mobile phone ownership and access of mothers, vertical coordination of health services and low staffing levels of health workers. Mothers who do not own mobile phones can leverage phone ownership of community leaders, TBAs, CHWs and relatives. This in turn facilitates communication of health messages to mothers.

Conclusions: Although this study was conducted in a low resource setting, mobile network coverage was good and thus SMS technology could be used. Research should be conducted on how to disseminate similar information in remote areas without mobile coverage.

Keywords: Data model, Health information access, Low resource settings, mHealth, Reproductive and child health

* Correspondence: achilles.kiwanuka@mrcuganda.org
[2]Medical Research Council/Uganda Virus Research Institute and London School of Hygiene & Tropical Medicine Uganda Research Unit, P.O. Box 49, Entebbe, Uganda
Full list of author information is available at the end of the article

Background

Information and Communication Technologies (ICTs) have been utilized globally in advancing social and economic development. More so, mobile technology-based ICT services are important in informing development initiatives. In recent years, there has been a tremendous growth in mobile phone usage in developing countries. Many developing countries have skipped fixed-line infrastructure and leapfrogged into mobile technology. Currently, mobile phone usage is the most predominant mode of communication in the developing world. In 2016, over 5.7 billion people (about 78%) of the mobile subscriptions were from developing countries [1]. In Tanzania, by end of June 2016, approximately 39.2 million people (about 78%) had subscribed to mobile phones [2].

Scholars have put forward different definitions of mHealth. According to [3], mHealth is realised as the "medical and public health practice supported through mobile devices for collecting community and clinical health data, delivery of healthcare information to practitioners, researchers, and beneficiaries, real-time monitoring of beneficiary vital signs, and direct provision of care". mHealth is also defined as the use of mobile and wireless technologies to improve health systems [4]. In both definitions, the ultimate goal of using mobile technologies in health is to improve health outcomes. mHealth can be applied in a diversity of contexts including: patient monitoring, health surveys and patient data collection, epidemiological surveillance, health awareness raising, mobile telemedicine, and public health campaigns.

The use of mobile technologies has increased access to healthcare information especially for remote communities [5]. Within the primary health care domain, mobile phones fill the digitization gap at community level. Moreover, mobile phones facilitate health information exchange even during Community Health Workers (CHWs) interaction with beneficiaries. Rapid advances in mobile technologies and applications, rise in new opportunities for integrating mobile health into existing eHealth services, and continued growth in coverage of mobile cellular networks support the achievement of health objectives in developing countries [6].

Mobile based health solutions have been successfully implemented in different parts of the world. In Egypt and Uganda, ICT has reduced the number of preventable maternal deaths [7]. In South Africa, mobile phone technology has been effectively utilised to remind tuberculosis patients to take their medication. Other countries in which such technology has been applied include Cambodia, Rwanda, South Africa, Nicaragua, Bangladesh and India [7].

Information influences social norms and culture by increasing awareness about what other people are doing [8]. The more trusted and credible a source of information is, and the more relevant and resonant it is made to its target audience, the greater is its potential to influence behaviour. Trends in antenatal coverage in Tanzania have risen to 98% while skilled assistance during delivery remains at 64% [9]. As the country aims to reach universal coverage of antenatal services, information communication interventions can encourage mothers to seek antenatal care from skilled health workers, delay pregnancies to healthy ages and ensure healthy intervals between births [8].

Short Messaging Service (SMS) and telephone calls are effective reminders in improving clinic attendance rates [10]. In a randomized control trial that compared various forms of reminders, it was revealed that the attendance rate when adopting SMS reminder was 87.5%, telephone call was 88.3% and un-reminded patient was 80.5% [10]. Although the two systems of reminding patients had almost the same impact, there was a great difference in terms of total cost per attendance with SMS being USD 0.03 and telephone calls being USD 0.06 [10].

Maternal and new born mortalities remain a major public health challenge in Tanzania. The maternal mortality ratio is estimated to be 556 deaths per 100,000 live births while the under-five mortality rate is estimated to be 75 deaths per 1000 live births [9]. To address health related challenges in communities, mobile phone applications have been designed to support outreach services for CHWs in Reproductive and Child Health (RCH) services [11]. In Tanzanian communities, mobile phones have been used to collect birth information of babies delivered outside health facilities through utilising Village Health Workers who are engaged in data collection at household level, data recording in registers, and transferring of the same data to health facilities [12]. Furthermore, through sending reminder messages, RCH services utilisation is increased [13] while at the same time reducing pregnancy related risks.

Mobile phone sharing is common in Sub-Saharan countries [14, 15]. Research has used this opportunity to reach individuals who are disadvantaged to possess mobile phones. Although several mobile based projects have been implemented [14–16], there is no clear data model to guide implementation of mHealth for RCH services particularly reminding mothers to attend clinics in rural areas where women are disadvantaged to own mobile phones. The designed mHealth data model considers women who do not own personal mobile phones. Phone sharing improves mothers' knowledge of RCH services through receiving educative messages using their spouses' or relatives' phones. It is important to note that availability of timely, accessible, accurate and relevant information during perinatal period through mobile technologies plays a key role in shaping knowledge, which in turn is a driver of health-related changes towards seeking delivery in health facilities [16–20].

Methods

Study approach

The methodology adopted in this research was Participatory Action Research. This approach was chosen because there was need for the researcher and the researched to work together throughout the study. Besides, action research empowers individuals and provides practical solutions to community problems [21]. In this study, using mobile phones for spouses and relatives of mothers was seen as a practical solution for mothers who did not possess their own.

This study sought to design and implement a mHealth data model with an intention of improving mothers' knowledge of Reproductive and Child Health (RCH) services in rural environments and to remind mothers who do not have access to mobile phones to attend antenatal care. A phased approach was adopted to answer the research question. The phases adopted in the study were: diagnosis of the problem, action planning, action taking, evaluation and reflection. During diagnosis, authors conducted interviews, observation and document review to find the prevailing challenges in disseminating health information to the community. In action planning, authors analysed hardware and software applications used in the health facilities. Moreover, environments in which software and hardware operate were assessed as well. During action taking, information requirements were elicited and then the data model was designed and implemented. Health workers were trained on how to use the customized prototype in a participatory manner. As part of evaluation, authors conducted focus group discussions and further demonstrated application of the data model to community leaders and health care workers. Through reflection, authors gained knowledge that was used to improve the next phase of the cycle which is further diagnosis and problem formulation.

Study area

This study was conducted in Chamwino district of Dodoma region, Tanzania. Chamwino is among the least developed districts in Tanzania. With the focus of this study being to improve access to RCH information through the use of mHealth, Chamwino was purposively chosen as a representation of poor districts in the country where access to health information is limited. The district economy is almost entirely dependent on agriculture and livestock farming. Agriculture is characterized by low productivity resulting from low and erratic rainfall, high evapo-transpiration and low moisture holding surface soils. The literacy rate in the district has been deteriorating over the years with the current literacy rate being 60%. Peasants constitute about 62% of the general population and the farming seasons take 4–6 months. Seasonal unemployment is well pronounced and becomes higher during the off-farming seasons. Two health facilities were selected for data collection within the district, that is, Buigiri dispensary and Chamwino health centre.

Structure of health services delivery in Tanzania is organised from community level, dispensary, health centre, district, regional to national level. The same applies to RCH services. However, differences exist in services provided and staffing at each level. Community health workers act as links between the community and dispensaries and play a major role in educating communities about prevailing health issues. RCH services in dispensaries are managed by a nurse (certificate or diploma) and a clinical officer whereas as at health centres chances of being attended by a medical doctor or advanced medical officer increase. Specialists and consultants of RCH services are found higher in the hierarchy. All basic RCH services: family planning, antenatal, delivery, postnatal, vaccination, Prevention of Mother to Child Transmission of HIV/AIDS are provided in dispensaries except for caesarean births which are provided in health centres. In case complications arise for any of the services in dispensaries, clients are referred to health centres.

Data collection

Qualitative techniques were employed in data collection. Respondents for the study were mothers attending antenatal and postnatal clinics, health care workers, community health workers, Traditional Birth Attendants (TBAs) and community leaders.

Data were collected through key informant interviews, document review, focus group discussion and observation. The guides used were developed for this particular study. Details of key informant guide and focus group discussion are included as an Additional file 1. Key informants were; 7 health care workers, 6 CHWs, 5 TBAs, 1 RCH coordinator and 4 community leaders. The informants were purposively selected because they were rich of data that was sought. Data sought from the key informants was based on entities and relationships that were used in designing the mHealth model.

The documents reviewed were Information Education Communication (IEC) guidelines of the Ministry of Health. The IEC guidelines contain information that should be provided to RCH clients depending on their gestational age and health status. In addition, Health Management Information System (HMIS) data collection tools were reviewed. The HMIS tools reviewed include antenatal registers and cards. Antenatal cards are kept by the clients and are supposed to be presented at every visit whereas registers contain aggregated data for all clients who visit a particular health facility. Through analysing IEC guidelines, the authors gathered appropriate information which health providers can send to educate the community. In registers, the authors examined adherence to clinical appointments before and after delivery, whereas in antenatal cards, the authors gathered important information requirements useful for developing a prototype.

Six focus group discussions were conducted with women. Group discussions were used to assess ownership and access to mobile phones among women as well as their perceptions in sharing phones. Focus groups constituted five to eight members.

Data were triangulated by using several methods to look for similarities and differences around the main themes under study. Primary and secondary data from health facilities, homes and in village offices were then collated and analysed using content analysis methods. Codes were derived from the data and then grouped into themes in order to get meaning of the wordings.

This study was approved by relevant bodies for graduate studies at the University of Dar es Salaam. Permission to conduct the research was obtained from Chamwino District Medical Office and administrations of Buigiri dispensary and Chamwino health centre. Clients' autonomy to participate in the study was clearly communicated and verbal informed consent was solicited from all participants.

Design data model

Integrating both reminder and educative information to stakeholders of RCH services was fundamental in designing the data model. Entities and proposed relationships are depicted in Fig. 1. The data model gives details of information flow between different entities depending on relationship. Sample attributes to each of the entities have been described in proceeding paragraphs.

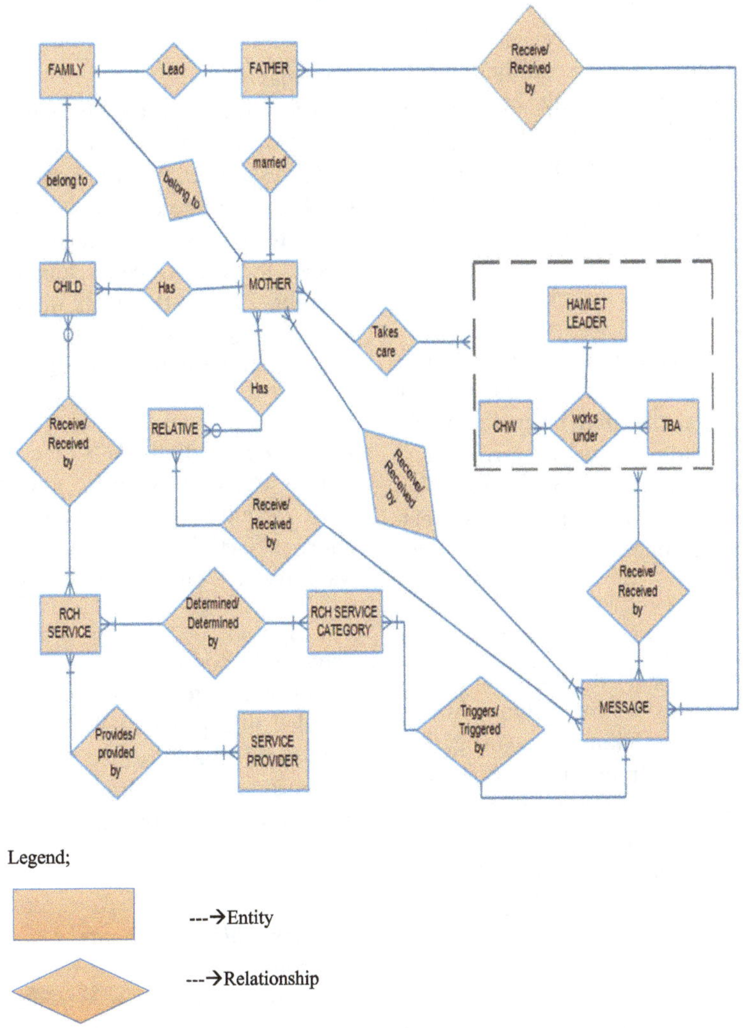

Fig. 1 Data model: Description of relationships between entities and proposed relationships

Mother

The data model accommodates two kinds of index clients, mother and child. Mother is registered as a client for antenatal and/or postnatal services, being allowed to enrol into either category. Examples of mother attributes are: mother ID, mother's first name, mother's last name, date of birth, height, gravidity, parity, blood group, living children, mobile phone number, physical address, gestation age, and expected date of delivery.

Child

Any child eligible for immunisation and other child care services is registered under this category. However, child uses the mother's information identity since she (mother) owns or shares a mobile phone and receives messages. Child attributes include: mothers' identification information, child ID, child's first name, child's last name, date of birth, height, weight, immunisation status, blood group, birth weight, and Apgar score.

Father

This entity is included when a child is registered. When the father is registered as a partner to the mother (client), this will be captured under relative entity. In this case, mother's consent is required for sending information to the father. Nevertheless, father's name and contacts are obtained from mother's entity. A few attributes to include under father are: father's first name, father's last name, age, physical address, and mobile number.

Relative

Relatives of mothers' get registered as part of mother's information. Thus, the relative entity can only exist if there is a related mother. Relative may be male partner (might not be father of child), in-laws or anyone else that mother identifies to be next of kin. Attributes in relative entity may be: first name, last name, type of relationship with mother, mobile phone number and physical address.

RCH services

This includes services provided to clients during antenatal, postnatal and child care visits for instance history taking, physical examination, clinical investigation, immunisation, to mention a few. Information on services is recorded and updated on every visit of the client. Some attributes to include under RCH services are: service ID and service name (blood haemoglobin, blood slide for malaria, sugar in urine, fundal height, blood pressure, and gestation age).

RCH service category

Service provided in RCH are grouped in to four main categories: antenatal care, intra-natal care (delivery) postnatal care and child health services. Each category has a set of services provided to either mother or child. Identifying the service category based on services offered is key in determining kinds of messages and their categories to be disseminated based on the client and type of service. Attributes to be included under this entity are: service category ID, service category name, service category audience (child, mother, relative, community leader or CHW).

Service provider

All health workers that interact with computer application and at the same time interact with clients (mothers and children) fall into this entity. Importance of service providers in this data model is their interaction with the application determining events like updating service records and consequently activating the SMS sending process. Under this entity, attributes can include: service provider ID, service provider first name and service provider last name.

Messages

Categorisation of messages is based on themes to be promoted which may either be reminders or educational. The messages are automatically sent to mothers, their relatives, CHWs, community (hamlet) leaders and TBAs. Some attributes related to messages would include; message ID (code), message category and message group. Messages are sent either to the index mother (as client during pregnancy), child's mother, child's father, mother's relative, TBA, community health worker or community leader.

Community health workers

CHWs are responsible for counselling and following-up clinic defaulters (pregnant mothers and children). Attributes of CHW include: first name, last name, hamlet, ward, district, and phone number.

Community leaders

Responsibility for following-up of mothers and children enrolled in a program lies with community leaders and thus should be informed to remind clients about their appointments. Attributes of community leaders include: first name, last name, hamlet, ward, district and phone number.

Traditional birth attendants

TBAs are included in the data model in order to receive educational messages. Attributes to consider include: first name, last name, date of birth, hamlet, ward, district and phone number.

Implementation of the data model

The model was implemented as a module using District Health Information System (DHIS) Tracker computer application which is a free and open source software [22]. Figure 2 shows information flow architecture used to implement the designed data model.

Health facilities create, update and maintain client information and messages. Health service providers define and enter SMS into content providers. In this case, content provider is the computer database application developed using the model in Fig. 1. Messages are sent in form of Hypertext Transfer Protocol (HTTP) query from the computer application to SMS gateway. The gateway converts HTTP messages into particular Short Message Service Centre (SMSC) format of a particular mobile operator and sends to the SMSC. The SMSC then forwards message to the final destination (mobile phone terminal of a particular community member). Similarly, messages can be sent from mobile terminals to the computer application. Messages are sent to the SMSC using SMSC protocol and then the SMSC forwards the messages to the SMS gateway. The SMS gateway converts the messages into HTTP format and send to the computer application. However, information flow from mobile terminals (mothers, relatives, TBAs, CHWs and community leaders) to health facilities was not explored.

In addition to relatives and spouses, community leaders and CHWs were also registered into the computer application as contact persons of mothers. Reminder messages were then sent to mothers and their contact persons. If the mother owned a phone, an SMS was directly sent to her, otherwise it was sent through another person whom she had decided. It is important to send reminders to both mothers and their community leaders because in some cases, mothers may still not come to clinics regardless of receiving reminders.

Education programs for mothers, male partners, relatives, TBAs and CHWs were customized and implemented. The prototype (DHIS Tracker) was customized to store and disseminate educational messages to TBAs. Traditional birth attendants were registered with their phone numbers and enrolled into DHIS Tracker. Educational messages were sent for a period of 1 year at monthly intervals with altered content.

Testing and evaluating the data model was done after 1000 messages were sent to mothers. 117 (11.7%) of the recipients gave their feedback through phone calls which was used to improve the application. Figure 3 shows the interface which was configured as the SMS gateway.

The study preferred to use BulkSMS gateway for sending SMS from DHIS Tracker to mobile terminals. This gateway was used because once configured there is no need to reconnect every time the computer is started since it just needs an internet connection. Moreover, it can send a bulk of messages at a time and it is simple to configure compared to other gateways.

Results

Results focus on putting forward major challenges related to information dissemination in rural settings. Additionally, the most cost-effective mechanisms in which RCH information can reach community members is described.

Challenges of information dissemination in rural settings

Mobile phone ownership and access

The ownership and access to mobile phones in the study area was not very high as it is among the rural areas having high illiteracy rate and poverty in Tanzania. Many

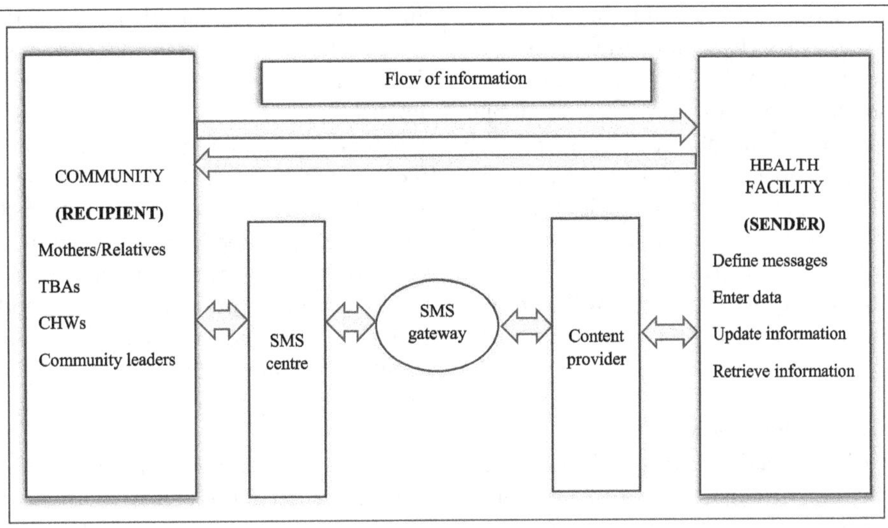

Fig. 2 Information flow architecture: Illustration of information flow architecture used to implement the designed data model

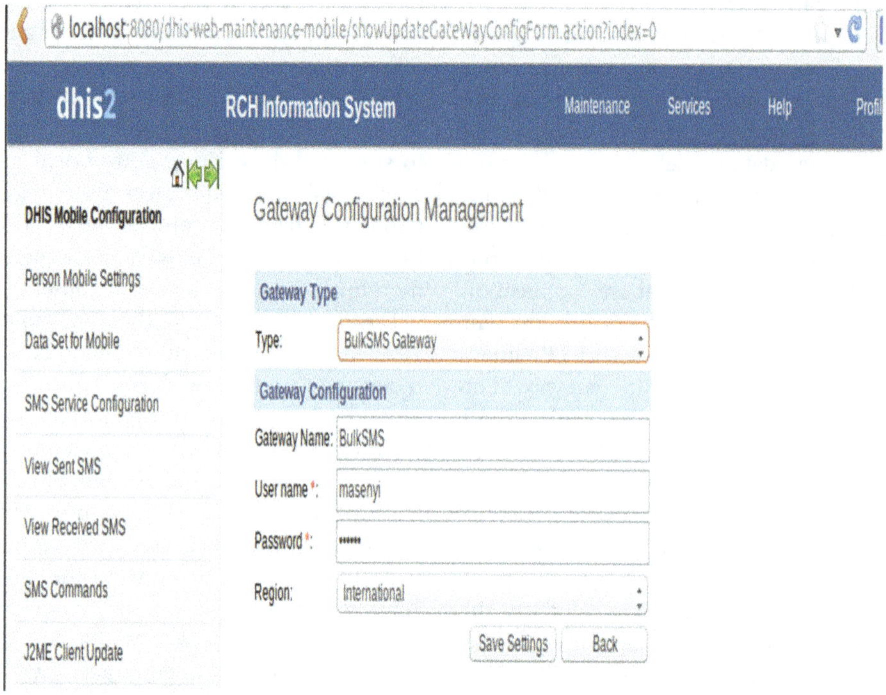

Fig. 3 SMS gateway configuration: Screenshot of the interface which was configured as the SMS gateway

people bought second hand phones which in most cases were not durable. The social construct of men dominance over women and sexual unfaithfulness caused many women not to own mobile phones. The study established that men prevent their spouses from owning mobile phones. This is due to the men's belief that mobile phones facilitate communication of cheating spouses and hence sexual relationships. For example, from the 67 women asked about phone ownership, only 6 (9%) reported to own a mobile phone. However, the study found that most TBAs had mobile phones, as they were old in age and get large support from their children working in towns and cities. The study established that all community leaders (hamlet leaders) and community health workers had mobile phones. Possession of mobile phones by these influential people in villages make it possible to realize the impact of mobile technology in reducing maternal and child mortalities in low income areas despite the low ownership of phones by women. Through using technology, RCH information can be delivered to the community which in turn will improve care provided to mothers and children under-five years in the community.

Vertical coordination of health services

Reproductive and Child Health services in health facilities are part of primary health care, hence integrated within the health care system. Vertical coordination of RCH services also applies to Information Education Communication system where IEC guidelines and relevant materials used are designed and produced by the Ministry of Health Community Development, Gender, Children and the Elderly (MoHCDGEC), to be executed at all health system levels. Nevertheless, health facilities can decide on the kind of information to pass on to clients at a particular time and the best way to pass that information to the community.

Low staffing of health workers

Information opportunities regarding RCH services were limited to the clinic/health facility settings. Due to the low number of health staff, IEC sessions were rarely conducted and normally restricted to mothers who attend antenatal care or postnatal care for the first time. Mothers were required to attend clinics in order to get access to RCH information. This practice benefited parents who usually attended clinics and disregarded those who were not attending clinics for instance male partners and relatives who have influence on reproductive health outcomes of mothers. The study further noted that there was no mechanism of reminding mothers about their appointments before the due date which resulted in many no shows especially for postnatal care.

Improving reproductive and child health information communication in rural areas

The study investigated the most cost-effective mechanism in which information can reach the community by involving different stakeholders that play important roles in delivering RCH information. The sub-sections below present the different actors in the information communication chain of RCH services.

Mothers

These are clients attending RCH clinics. Mothers participate in health education sessions in which various topics are presented by health workers. Through focus group discussions, participants (mothers) revealed that health education sessions did not provide adequate space for them to learn everything they needed. Since health education sessions are conducted in groups, they (mothers) further revealed that health workers assume all clients have the same level of understanding on basic concepts, which is not always the case. The mothers wished that they had more individual focused messages to build their understanding on issues of interest.

Perceptions of mothers regarding mobile phone sharing and secondary delivery of messages were sought. Most mothers thought that it was ideal if a message was directly sent to them, but if that was not possible, then delivering the message through a close relative/friend was a seen as a viable option. The challenge cited though was timely delivery of the messages.

Male partners

Male partners can promote maternal and child health through their effective participation in RCH services. Men are viewed as controllers of family resources in rural settings. Thus, women recommended that men should be involved in birth preparedness planning and couple counselling and testing for Prevention of Mother to Child Transmission of HIV/AIDS. Male participants were more concerned with knowing vaccination schedules for children and danger signs for pregnant mothers so that they could take quick action to save lives of mothers and unborn children once they recognize them. Dissemination of health information through SMS is one of the strategies to engage men to become more supportive to their partners.

Traditional birth attendants

Traditional Birth Attendants play major roles in assisting home deliveries in rural communities. Owing to their impact in the community, improving RCH knowledge of TBAs can minimize home deliveries and hence reduce avoidable maternal deaths. Traditional Birth Attendants can put an end to assisting deliveries and encourage mothers to seek peri-natal care from health facilities. It is important to monitor pregnancy in order to reduce morbidity and mortality risks for mothers and their children during pregnancy, at delivery, and during the post-natal period. Capabilities of mobile technologies facilitate updated educational information delivery to TBAs anywhere and anytime.

Community health workers

Communities choose their own health workers who reside in their localities. Community health workers are lightly trained individuals who act as outreach workers, interfacing between communities and the peripheral of the health system (dispensaries). The strength of CHWs lies in their residence in communities of service and intimacies with health concerns of communities. Responsibilities of CHWs include identifying all pregnant mothers in communities and providing counselling services on health lifestyles, birth planning, complication readiness and need for antenatal care and skilled care at birth. Through reinforcing mobile technologies to send educational messages, CHWs can receive updated health information and hence take on some duties of health service providers in antenatal clinics.

Community (hamlet) leaders

Community leaders are well acquainted with residents in their localities and thus create a link between health facilities and communities. Women who give birth outside health facilities are expected to obtain an introduction letter from their local government leaders before they can receive services at any health facility. The study noted that community leaders followed-up mothers and children who defaulted clinic attendance and also sensitized mothers on child immunisation. During follow-up, a list of defaulters is sent to village chairpersons who then send the list to hamlet leaders. Respect for community leaders compared to CHWs justifies the former's involvement in follow-up. One community health worker mentioned that:

"We are neither respected nor listened to when we approach community members. However, visits with (or by) community leaders are treated with respect and actions are taken accordingly." Community health worker X.

Discussion

Empirical findings show that follow-up of defaulters in RCH clinics involves CHWs and community leaders who are linkages between health facilities and communities. Additionally, during community campaigns, CHWs provide counselling and immunisation services. Through implementation of mobile based systems to disseminate information between health facilities and communities, tracking of defaulters can be improved [16]. Statistics show that only 64% of births are assisted by a skilled health provider [9]. With such a low percentage, community leaders and CHWs can play a big role in tracking the remaining 36% births.

Previous studies have showed benefits of sending educative information to improve health outcomes. Through introduction of mobile software to track antenatal clients, attendance significantly increased compared to the time before the system was introduced [13]. Sending educative messages to females through their male partners has been viewed as the best way to involve males in taking care of pregnancy and children [23]. Phone sharing among individuals exists in Tanzania. Moreover, in order to reduce cost, individuals use mobile phones in creative ways including beeping [15]. This can enable health messages to reach those without phones or even those without credit on their phones. In a study that was carried out in a resource limited setting in Zanzibar, it was established that there is an association between mobile phone intervention and increase in skilled delivery attendance [16].

Since TBAs, CHWs and community leaders own mobile phones, it is important to leverage such resources in improving RCH services. Besides, educating TBAs, CHWs and community leaders with right RCH knowledge can minimize maternal and child mortalities.

The study found out that mothers needed more individualised messages to build their understanding on issues of interest. The mothers revealed that though messages were useful in delivering health messages, sometimes the same messages were not relevant for their situations. The system was designed in such a way that messages are sent depending on recipient, RCH role, and message categorisation. Yet issues like demographic factors were overseen during design of the messages to be delivered. This leaves room for further improvement of the study once such factors are considered. Messages that initiate actions to increase health outcomes basing on various factors yield better RCH results.

Challenges encountered during design included tight schedules of health workers who had to provide services besides participating in customising education content and design of the model. Tight schedules are caused by high patient flows while staffing levels remain low. With user centred design and participatory approaches being at the forefront, the authors assisted health workers in performing some activities like clerical work so that they could spare some to participate in the study. The schedule also affected duration of training on how to use the SMS gateway.

Replicability of the data model is limited to areas in which social cohesion between community leaders, community health workers and community members is strong. In such cases, health information and education to mothers is viewed as part of social responsibility. Besides, structures of CHWs that are well acquainted with community members should be in place for the model to be effective.

Conclusion

Challenges of information dissemination in low resource settings noted in this study are: mobile phone ownership and access of mothers, vertical coordination of health services and low staffing levels of health workers. To address the challenges, the authors present a data model that can leverage phone ownership of community leaders, TBAs, CHWs and relatives to facilitate sending of health education messages to mothers. Entities in this model are: mother, child, father, relative, RCH service, RCH service category, service provider, message, CHW, TBA and community leader. Previous studies of mobile technologies use in RCH stressed providing education messages to mothers, however, this study has shown the viability of sending such messages to mothers who do not mobile phones. Although this study was conducted in a low resource setting, mobile coverage was good and thus SMS technology could be used. Research should be conducted on how to disseminate similar information in remote areas without mobile coverage.

Abbreviations

CHWs: Community Health Workers; DHIS: District Health Information Software; HTTP: Hypertext Transfer Protocol; ICTs: Information Communication Technologies; IEC: Information Education and Communication; MoHCDGEC: Ministry of Health, Community Development, Gender, Elderly and Children; RCH: Reproductive and Child Health; SMS: Short Messaging Service; SMSC: Short Message Service Centre; TBAs: Traditional Birth Attendants

Acknowledgements

Special thanks to Computation and Modeling Research Group (CMRG) at the University of Dodoma for providing technical support for this publication through the secured competitive fund award from the Carnegie - SIG Regional Initiative in Science and Education (RISE).

Funding

This research was funded by the University of Oslo, Norway.

Authors' contributions

JT and AK conceptualized the study design. JT designed the methodology, customized the system and collected the data. JT and AK analyzed and interpreted the findings, prepared the manuscript. Both authors read and approved the final manuscript.

Competing interests

The authors declare that they have no competing interests.

Author details

[1]College of Informatics and Virtual Education, University of Dodoma, P.O. Box 259, Dodoma, Tanzania. [2]Medical Research Council/Uganda Virus Research Institute and London School of Hygiene & Tropical Medicine Uganda Research Unit, P.O. Box 49, Entebbe, Uganda.

References

1. ITU. Mobile cellular subscriptions, by level of development. 2016. http://www.itu.int/ITU-D/ict/statistics/material/excel/2010/Mobile_cellular_00-05-10.xls. Accessed 5 Mar 2017.
2. TCRA. Quartely Communications Statitstics Report April- June 2016. 2016; JUNE:18. https://www.tcra.go.tz/images/documents/telecommunication/CommStatJune16.pdf. Accessed 25 Aug 2016.
3. Germanakos P, Mourlas C, Samaras GA. Mobile agent approach for ubiquitous and personalized eHealth information systems. In: Workshop on "personalization for e-health of the 10th international conference on user modeling (UM"05); 2005. p. 67–70.
4. Boyer E, Ankri R, Zouinar M, Blaisonneau D, Richomme M, Longuet C. mHealth in Senegal : the voices project. In: Cunningham P, Cunningham M, editors. IST-Africa 2012 conference proceedings. IIMC international information management corporation; 2012. p. 1–9. http://www.ist-africa.org/home/outbox/ISTAfrica_Paper_ref_34_4782.pdf.
5. Mechael P, Searle S. Barriers and Gaps Affecting mHealth in Low and Middle Income Countries : Policy White Paper: Columbia University: Center for Global Health and Economic Development Earth Institute; 2010. https://doi.org/10.4103/0019-557X.73274.
6. World Health Organization. mHealth: New Horiz for health through mobile technologies. Geneva: WHO Press; 2011. https://doi.org/10.4258/hir.2012.18.3.231.
7. Chetley A, Trude B, Ramirez R, Shields T, Drury P, Kumekawa J, et al. Improving health, connecting people: the role of ICTs in the health sector of developing countries. A framework paper: information for development program (Infodev) Working paper No. 7. London: Worldlink Worldwide. 2006:1–65.
8. World Health Organization. Analysing Commitments to Advance the Global Strategy for Women's and Children's Health. Geneva: World Heal Organ. 2011; The PMNCH 2011 Report:1–60.
9. Ministry of Health Community Development Gender Elderly and Children (MoHCDGEC) [Tanzania Mainland], Ministry of Health (MoH) [Zanzibar], National Bureau of Statistics [NBS], Office of the Chief Government Statistician [OCGS], ICF. Tanzania Demographic and Health Survey and Malaria Indicator Survey (TDHS-MIS) 2015–16. Dar es Salaam, Tanzania, and Rockville, Maryland: MoHCDGEC, MoH, NBS, OCGS, and ICF; 2016. https://www.dhsprogram.com/pubs/pdf/FR321/FR321.pdf
10. Chen Z, Fang L, Chen L, Dai H. Comparison of an SMS text messaging and phone reminder to improve attendance at a health promotion center: a randomized controlled trial. J Zhejiang Univ Sci B. 2008;9:34–8. https://doi.org/10.1631/jzus.B071464.
11. DeRenzi B, Gaetano B, Jackson J, Kumar VS, Parikh TS, Virk P, et al. Mobile phone tools for field-based health Care Workers in low-Income Countries. Mt Sinai J Med. 2011;78:46–418.
12. Ngoma C, Chawani MS, Herstad J. Adaptation of mobile application to improve flow of birth information from the community to the district level. Lect Notes Inst Comput Sci Soc Telecommun Eng. 2011;64 LNICST:79–92.
13. Kulindwa YK. Development and implementation of software for educating and tracking antenatal care clients using cell phones: the case of Zanzibar. Master of Health Informatics thesis. Dar es Salaam: University of Dar es Salaam; 2010.
14. Kaplan WA. Can the ubiquitous power of mobile phones be used to improve health outcomes in developing countries? Glob Health. 2006;2:9.
15. James J, Versteeg M. Mobile phones in Africa: how much do we really know? Soc Indic Res. 2007;84:117–26.
16. Lund S, Hemed M, Nielsen B, Said A, Said K, Makungu M, Rasch V. Mobile phones as a health communication tool to improve skilled attendance at delivery in Zanzibar: a cluster-randomised controlled trial. BJOG Int J Obstet Gynaecol. 2012;119:1256–64. https://doi.org/10.1111/j.1471-0528.2012.03413.x.
17. Lester RT, Ritvo P, Mills EJ, Kariri A, Karanja S, Chung MH, et al. Effects of a mobile phone short message service on antiretroviral treatment adherence in Kenya (WelTel Kenya1): a randomised trial. Lancet. 2010;376:1838–45.
18. Cole-Lewis H, Kershaw T. Text messaging as a tool for behavior change in disease prevention and management. Epidemiol Rev. 2010;32:56–69.
19. Fjeldsoe BS, Marshall AL, Miller YD. Behavior change interventions delivered by mobile telephone short-message service. Am J Prev Med. 2009;36:165–73.
20. Leong KC, Chen WS, Leong KW, Mastura I, Mimi O, Sheikh MA, et al. The use of text messaging to improve attendance in primary care: a randomized controlled trial. Fam Pract. 2006;23:699–705.
21. Baskerville R, Myers MD. Special issue on action research in information systems: making IS research relevant to practice-foreword. MIS Q. 2004;28(3):329–35.
22. Braa J, Sahay S. Integrated health information architecture: power to the users. New Delhi: matrix Publishers; 2012.
23. Bishanga D, Kimaro H. Mobile phone Technology: a gateway to address gender obstacles in improving access to reproductive and child health services by women and their partners. In: Cunningham P, Cunningham M, editors. IST-Africa 2012 conference proceedings. Dublin: IIMC international information management corporation; 2012. p. 1–7.

16

Metabolic syndrome in hypertensive women in the age of menopause: a case study on data from general practice electronic health records

Šefket Šabanović[1], Majnarić Trtica Ljiljana[1], František Babič[2], Michal Vadovský[2], Ján Paralič[2], Aleksandar Včev[1] and Andreas Holzinger[3*]

Abstract

Background: There is potential for medical research on the basis of routine data used from general practice electronic health records (GP eHRs), even in areas where there is no common GP research platform. We present a case study on menopausal women with hypertension and metabolic syndrome (MS). The aims were to explore the appropriateness of the standard definition of MS to apply to this specific, narrowly defined population group and to improve recognition of women at high CV risk.

Methods: We investigated the possible uses offered by available data from GP eHRs, completed with patients interview, in goal of the study, using a combination of methods. For the sample of 202 hypertensive women, 47–59 years old, a data set was performed, consisted of a total number of 62 parameters, 50 parameters used from GP eHRs. It was analysed by using a mixture of methods: analysis of differences, cutoff values, graphical presentations, logistic regression and decision trees.

Results: The age range found to best match the emergency of MS was 51–55 years. Deviations from the definition of MS were identified: a larger cut-off value of the waist circumference measure (89 vs 80 cm) and parameters BMI and total serum cholesterol perform better as components of MS than the standard parameters waist circumference and HDL-cholesterol. The threshold value of BMI at which it is expected that most of hypertensive menopausal women have MS, was found to be 25.5. The other best means for recognision of women with MS include triglycerides above the threshold of 1.7 mmol/L and information on statins use. Prevention of CVD should focus on women with a new onset diabetes and comorbidities of a long-term hypertension with anxiety/depression.

Conclusions: The added value of this study goes beyond the current paradigm on MS. Results indicate characteristics of MS in a narrowly defined, specific population group. A comprehensive view has been enabled by using heterogeneous data and a smart combination of various methods for data analysis. The paper shows the feasibility of this research approach in routine practice, to make use of data which would otherwise not be used for research.

Keywords: General practice, Research, Routine data, Electronic health records, Computer methods for data anlysis, Menopausal women, Hypertension, Metabolic syndrome

* Correspondence: andreas.holzinger@medunigraz.at
[3]Medical University Graz, Institute for Medical Informatics/Statistic, Auenbruggerplatz 2/V, 8036 Graz, Austria
Full list of author information is available at the end of the article

Background

Strongly founded and evidence-based primary care (PC) is known to significantly improve health of the nations and the efficacy of use of health care (HC) resources [1, 2]. For its position at the interface between population and the HC system, general practice (GP) is the key PC discipline [3]. It is considered that efforts aimed to improve efficiency of GP within the HC system should be taken through strengthening the research capacity of this discipline [4]. This is because GP is a specific discipline, different from specialist medicine, and requires its own knowledge base to improve decision making [4, 5].

Decision making in GP often deals with uncertainty, as many patients present with early symptoms and signs of a disease that do not yet meet criteria for a diagnosis [6]. Older population, that makes the prominent part of GP patients, is usually characterised with multimorbidity (the coexistence of two or more chronic conditions) [7]. These patients are known to have complex HC needs that require solutions that go beyond the disease-based approaches of the traditional medicine, for which also evidence-based medicine (EBM) does not provide adequate answers [8]. This is one of the reasons why EBM, that draws primarily on randomised controlled trials and properly selected populations from tertiary care centres, is difficult to translate to the GP setting [9]. Rather, it is considered that research in GP has to be driven by problems and questions that are derived from its own practice [5].

The first attempt to build the science base of GP at large scale dated back to the end of the past century. To enable a wide access to data in GP, the research elities of this discipline initiated development of practice based research networks across Europe and wider [10]. With the advent of Information and Communication Technology (ICT) and electronic Health Records (eHRs) in PC, this initiative found new opportunities for realisation [11]. In many European countries, individual GP practices have been networked at the national level and episodes of care aggregated in a longitudinal way, to allow the common virtual platform for research [12, 13]. Experience from these countries have helped us learn on how to overcome barriers, while making the best of using the routinelly collected data from GP eHRs for research. It was showed that even from these databases, the number of research questions possible to be investigated is limited, including mostly pharmacoepidemiological and drug-safety issues and health service research [14, 15]. The key barriers, identified to date, include: a limited scope of data recorded in eHRs, non systematically recorded data on socio-economic and lifestyle factors, lack of compatibility in morbidity coding and prescribing guidelines, non uniformity in terminology and content meanings and the lack of links with other HC sectors and databases [16, 17].

In countries where there is no a "gatekeeping "role of GP, but people have the direct access to specialists, the problem is also in non systematically recorded data in GP eHRs [18]. On the contrary, some recent examples, based on integration of GP databases with other national registries, have emphasised the emerging opportunities that the "big data "analytical approaches could have in improving the quality of care and patients outcomes [19, 20]. This would be in a great part possible through using GP eHRS for identification of phenotypes, necessary for predictive modeling [21]. It is considered that opportunities for research that create upon GP databases could be practically endless if data of different types were combined together, including not only structured data (coded and numerical data), that are the easiest for computing, but also text narratives and images, and if different Machine Learning (ML) and other computer methods for complex data analysis were used in the process of problem solving [22].

Motivation for this study

Motivation for this study came from our previous work, where we used multicomponent data sets, composed mostly of data from GP eHRs, and a combination of statistical and data mining methods, for comprehensive analysis of a research question [23–26]. This way, we could answer some important questions associated with uncertainty and complexity in decision making.

Through experience of this work, we came to the conclusion that in GP it is possible to perform a single-site study, without the need of using the common research database, if only structured data (diagnoses, list of medications, numerical data, etc.), known to be consistently recorded, are used for analysis and if the right question is asked of data. To enlarge the scope of data from GP eHRs, some other, but easy-to-obtain data sources have to be added to.

For some of our results we found confirmation in EMB. For some new findings, for which comprehensive analysis has allowed for, we found confirmation later on, in studies of other kind and other authors. Generalisation of these results is still important to achieve, possible through iteration and validation of the same study on other samples, by following the principles of the "bottom-up "research approach. Based on this experience, we believe that reasearch in GP can blow up, in spite of the current situation where the lack of the networked databases and the existence of some unresolved barriers pose limitations to the global use of GP eHRs, for nationwide and cross-country research.

The case study

To illustrate the research approach that we recommend for use in GP, we used the case study on menopausal women with hypertension. This is a complex issue for which, however, the most of data are available in GP eHRs. There were several other reasons to support this choice.

Middle-aged hypertensive women are common attenders in GP. They are at increased risk for developing diabetes and cardiovascular disease (CVD), unless efficient preventive actions are organised [27]. The problem is that the available score systems for CV risk assessment are not sensitive enough to ensure accurate risk stratification of this population group [28]. Thus, research with the potential to provide general practitioners with tools for fast recognition of middle-aged women at high CV risk, would make a substantial contribution to CVD prevention, because in women, as it is in men, CVD are the main cause of death [27].

Hypertension is the main CV risk factors, for its high prevalence in population and great impact on CV morbidity and mortality [29]. There are close, although insufficiently understood relationships between increased body weight (general obesity), abdominal (central) obesity and hypertension [30]. Hypertension is one of the most prominent components of the metabolic syndrome (MS) [31]. It is defined as a cluster of CV risk factors that includes abdominal obesity (indicated with increased waist circumference), glucose intolerance or diabetes type 2 and dyslipidemia characterised with increased triglycerides and decreased HDL-cholesterol. MS, superimposed to hypertension, significantly amplifies CV risk [32].

There are many concerns associated with characteristics of hypertensive women in the age around menopause. In early postmenopausal women, hypertension was found to more oftenly present as a part of MS than as an isolated disease [33]. Transition from pre- to postmenopause, around the age of 50, is the critical period in women's life, when obesity, hypertension and other CV risk factors start to emerge. Also prevention of CVD is then most useful [34, 35]. However, there is a large amount of variation in CV risk factors expression, because of intensive emotional and lifestyle changes taking place during this transition and of possible discordance between the chronological age and the reproductive age at the time of menopause, that may also influence these variations [36, 37]. Several medical conditions and biohumoral alterations, apart from CVD, including e.g. chronic low grade inflammation, renal function decline, anxiety/depression, sleep and cognitive disorders, have been identified to coexist with MS, contributing to variations in phenotypes and CV risk profiles of patients with MS [38–42].

Components of MS and the role they have in development of CVD were found to be gender dependent, indicating the need for different criteria of MS for men and women [43]. There are several working definitions of MS that differ to each other to some extent, both in composition of the components of MS and in their cut-off values [44]. These definitions are clinical constructs, built upon the cut-off for increased CV risk in the referent populations. There is a long lasting debate on whether MS is a syndrome or a mixture of low related phenotypes, the composition of which can vary in different population groups [45].

Objectives

We setted up two main objectives. The first one was to evaluate the appropriateness of the standard definition of MS to apply to this specific, narrowly defined population group. Results are expected to improve our understanding on relationships between hypertension and other components of MS and other CV risk factors, in menopausal women. This knowledge might be useful in improving decision making on this complex issue. The second objective was to improve recognition of women at high CV risk, by identifying relevant markers and phenotypes, including also comorbidities and broader social context, in addition to components of MS. In particular, we wanted to assess the feasibility of data available in GP eHRs, completed with patients interview, to support this phenotype profilling process. Results are expected to inform the composition of the standard data record in GP eHRs and future research. Finally, through this analysis, we wanted to explore the potential of using a combination of methods in getting useful information from the available data.

Methods

Study population and the sample

The study was performed in a GP setting, in an urban-rural area (12.000 inhabitants), eastern Croatia, Central European region. Data were used from six practices located in the same health centre (source population: roughly 9.000 adult patients) (Fig. 1). As evidence says, general practitioners who work in the close vicinity use similar professional vocabulary and content meaning of encoded terminology, that can contribute to data consistency [46]. In addition, physicians who participated in this study were all specialists in GP, with more than 15 years of work experience, that means, skilled in diagnosis and evidence-based prescribing, that could also contribute to the accuracy of data recording.

As the database population, we used women old 47–59 years (650 subjects included) (Fig. 1). We chose this age range as the population selection criterium, being guided with the knowledge on the chronological age that, in women in EU countries, best matches the reproductive periods when MS is most likely to emerge (Fig. 2) [47–49].

As the study population, we used only those women from this age range who were diagnosed with hypertension ($N = 224$) (Fig. 1). Five of them reported surgically

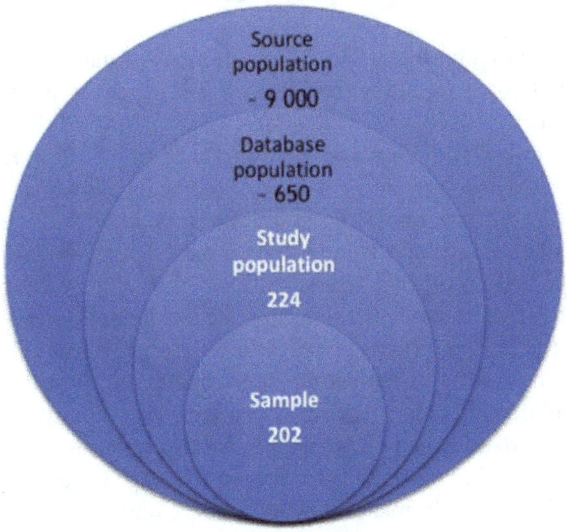

Fig. 1 Study population and the sample

induced menopause and one reported the use of the hormone replacement therapy. They were excluded from the study. Fourteen women did not respond to our call for interview. For two cases, data were incomplete. Thus, the final number of women, included in the study, was 202 (Fig. 1).

Study design

A retrospective and cross-sectional, observational and exploratory study, prepared according to the guidelines for using observational routinely-collected health data (RECORD statement) [50]. On the input data set, composed mostly of data from GP eHRs, we applied a combination of statistical and data mining methods that we supposed appropriate for the objectives. A minor part of data, for which evidence showed their association with MS but that have not been systematically recorded in GP eHRs, we obtained by patients' interview. We also included anthropometric measurements as a part of the interview. Candidate women, we invited by phone, or by using the mobile short message service (sms), or we asked them for the interview when they came to the regular encounter. The team leader physicians had been previously instructed for conducting the interviews.

Croatian PHC ICT system and GP eHRs

In Croatia, PC services have the gatekeeping role. The ICT system and eHRs were firstly developed in PHC and GP settings and boosted several times, primarily to improve connections within the PC services (Fig. 3) [51]. Recently, also e-referrals to specialists have been introduced. In order to improve the quality of care, the panel support tools for chronic disease surveillance and preventive check ups, have been established.

The ICD-10 code (International Statistical Classification of Diseases and Related Health Problems, 10th Revision) is used to support patient encounters. In order to support the prescription procedure, the medication list, together with the prescription rules, are available online to each PC physicians and regulary updated. Reference ranges of blood tests are incorporated in the primary laboratory test report templates.

The main barriers for using data from GP eHRs for research, in Croatia, include a large number of working applications, the lack of eHR data standards and the lack of networking into the common research platform.

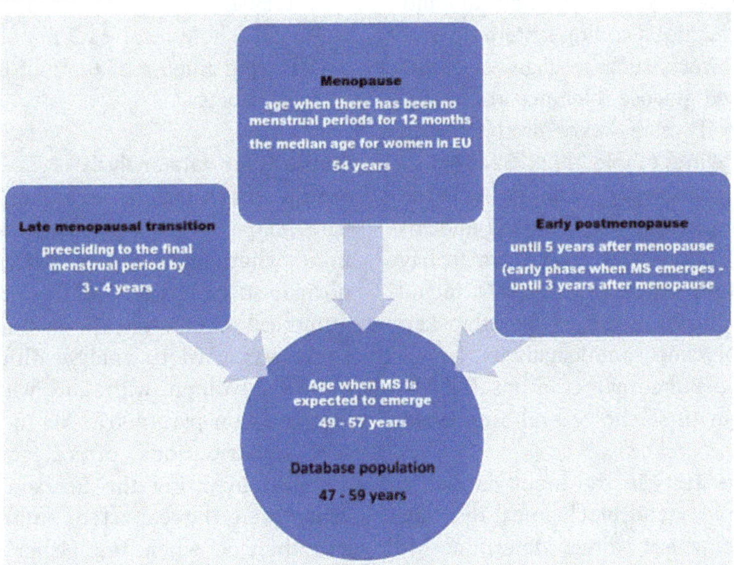

Fig. 2 Evidence that guided the choice of criteria for the database population

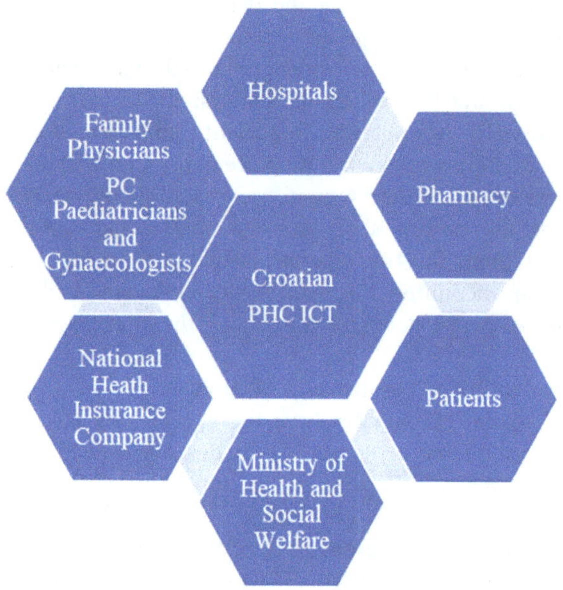

Fig. 3 The Croatian Primary Health Care (PHC) Information Communication Technology (ICT) System

Data set description

The input data set was composed of a total number of 62 parameters, of which 50 parameters were used from GP eHRs (Table 1) and 12 were obtained by patients' interview (Table 2).

From GP eHRs, only structured data were used, including: 1) demographics, 2) diagnoses of chronic diseases, 3) names of medications in a continuous use and 4) results of laboratory tests (Table 1). The high level of data completeness (only two cases of the study populations had incomplete data) was assured according to the fact that this data type are being systematically recorded.

To diagnose some well-defined chronic medical conditions, but for which the diagnosis coding system does not proved the suitable framework, such as stages of chronic renal impairment, impaired glucose tolerance and dyslipidemias, criteria for cut-off values were used from the current international guidelines (Table 3) [28, 52–54].

To improve patients phenotype profiling, we added also medications to the input data set. We used information only on those medications that are known to have the effects on the development of MS or CVD, including: statins (cholesterol lowering drugs), beta-blockers, ace-inhibitors/receptor blockers, anticoagulants, analgesics or non-steroidal anti-inflammatory drugs (NSAD), antibiotics and metformin (first choice oral antidiabetic drug) [55–57].

We included laboratory tests in the input dataset, to identify possible haematology and biochemical disorders that in hypertensive menopausal women determine MS. Of laboratory findings, we used those ones that were old no more than a year and that were performed as a part of the periodic chronic disease surveillance or preventive check ups.

By patients' interview, information were gain on factors known to influence MS, but for which records in GP eHRs were either incomplete or missing (Table 2) [58–60]. Definitions and grading for some of these factors are provided in the Table 3. To diagnose the positive family history on CVD, definition was used from the guidelines [28]. To identify the physical activity level, the scale was used from papers published on frailty syndrome, but modified, to fit the habits of the local elderly population [61]. Description of the socio-economic status relied on the authors' subjective assessment of the living conditions of elderly people in the local community. Self-reported information on impaired sleep patterns, in the last month, was used to diagnose sleep disturbance. Anthropometric measurements, waist circumference and weight and height (for calculation of BMI), were taken from participants during the interview. The WHO classification of categories of BMI, cited elsewhere, was used to differentiate between women with normal weight and those being overweight or obese.

To diagnose MS, we used the definition of the International Diabetes Federation (IDF) (2005), because it fitted well to the objective, to identify women at high risk for CVD [62]. Namely, this definition is sensitive on the abdominal type of obesity and considers also diabetics with MS. In addition, it relies on data available in GP eHRs.

The IDF definition of the metabolic syndrome - the female gender option.

Waist circumference ≥ 80 cm + 2 out of 4 criteria:

1) Diagnosis of hypertension
2) Triglycerides > 1.70 mmol/L
3) HDL-cholesterol < 1.3 mmol/L
4) Fasting glucose ≥5.6 mmol/L or the diagnosis of diabetes

Methods for data analysis

Basic statistics. Differences in distributions

The Shapiro-Wilks normality test was used to determine whether or not numerical parameters take the normal distribution [63]. For normally distributed numerical parameters, the parametric 2-sample Welch's t-test was used to analyse differences in distributions between women with and without MS, otherwise it was the non-parametric Mann-Whitney-Wilcoxon test [64]. Distributions of categorical parameters were assessed by using the Pearson's chi-squared test, except when the expected number of observation was less than 5, when the Fisher's Exact test was more appropriate. For all tests, the level of significance was set up at 0.05.

Table 1 Parameters used from GP eHRs and their abbreviations and descriptions

	Parameter	Description
Age	Age (years)	Numeric < 47, 59>
Hypdu	Hypertension duration (years)	Nominal {< 5, 5–10, > 10}
Hypre	Hypertension regulation	Binary {Normal /No}
DGDM	Dg Diabetes mellitus	Binary {Yes/No}
DMdu	Diabetes duration (years)	Nominal {0, 1–4, 5–10, > 10}
DMtr	Diabetes treatment (oral antidiabetics, oral antidiabetics+insulin, insulin)	Nominal {no, or, or/and, and}
DMco	Diabetes complications: macrovascular (coronary heart disease, cerebrovascular disease, peripheral arterial disease) and microvascular (retinopathy, proteinuric nephropathy, low extremity ulcers)	Nominal {no, mac, mic}
chre	Chronic respiratory diseases (asthma, COPB)	Binary {Yes/No}
allre	Respiratory allergic diseases (rhinitis)	Binary {Yes/No}
CHD	Chronic heart disease (heart failure, cardiomyopathy)	Binary {Yes/No}
CoHD	Coronary heart disease (angina, infarct myocardii, revascularization)	Binary {Yes/No}
CV	Cerebrovascular disease (transitory ischaemic attack, cerebrovascular insult, carotid atherosclerosis)	Binary {Yes/No}
PAS	Peripheral artery disease	Binary {Yes/No}
GI	Upper gastro-intestinal disease (reflux, gastritis, duodenal ulcer)	Binary {Yes/No}
infbo	Inflammatory bowel disease (Crohn disease, ulcerative collitis)	Binary {Yes/No}
hep	Chronic liver disease (chronic virus hepatitis, cirrhosis)	Binary {Yes/No}
mal	Malignant disease (not patients at terminal stage and under therapy)	Binary {Yes/No}
op	osteoporosis	Binary {Yes/No}
OA	Osteo-arthritis	Binary {Yes/No}
Sis	Collagenosis (rheumatoid arthritis, spondylarthritis, systemic lupus, systemic sclerosis, MCTD, dermatomyositis)	Binary {Yes/No}
Uro	Chronic urogenital disease (chr cystitis, pyelonephritis)	Binary {Yes/No}
cogn	Cognitive impairment &dementia	Binary {Yes/No}
thy	Endocrine disease (the thyroid gland disease)	Binary {Yes/No}
depr	Anxiety&depression	Binary {Yes/No}
psy	Psychosis	Binary {Yes/No}
derm	Chronic skin disease (psoriasis, chronic ezcema)	Binary {Yes/No}
chdi	A total number of chronic diseases	Numeric < 1, 10>
sta	statins ≥3 months)	Binary {Yes/No}
BB	beta-blockers (≥ 3 months)	Binary {Yes/No}
anco	anticoagulant drugs (≥ 3 months)	Binary {Yes/No}
anal	Analgesics/Non-steroidal anti-inflammatory drugs (frequent use: ≥3 months in the past year)	Binary {Yes/No}
anbi	Antibiotics (≥2 times per year)	Binary {Yes/No}
met	Metformin (≥ 3 months)	Binary {Yes/No}
Ace	ACE-INH (or AT-receptor antagonist) ≥ 3 months	Binary {Yes/No}
Drug	A total number of oral drugs	Numeric < 1, 9>
FGlu	Fasting glucose (mmol/L)	Numeric < 4.00, 13.00>
TG	Triglycerides (mmol/L)	Numeric < 0.42, 4.49>
cho	Total cholesterol (mmol/L)	Numeric < 3.50, 8.20>
LDL	LDL-cholesterol (mmol/L)	Numeric < 1.02, 5.79>
HDL	HDL-cholesterol (mmol/L)	Numeric < 0.80, 2.60>
cre	Serum creatinine (μmol/l)	Numeric < 43.00, 110.00>
GFR	Glomerular filtration rate (mL/min/1.73 m^2) (MDRD[a] on-line calculator)	Numeric < 40.9, 143.3>
Le	Leukocytes number (10^9/L)	Numeric < 3.90, 11.50>

Table 1 Parameters used from GP eHRs and their abbreviations and descriptions *(Continued)*

	Parameter	Description
CRP	C-reactive protein (mg/L)	Numeric < 0.20, 11.50>
Mo	Monocytes% (in blood differential count)	Numeric < 0.00, 7.00>
Ly	Lymphocytes % (in blood differential count)	Numeric < 5.00, 48.00>
Er	Erythrocytes number (10^{12}/L)	Numeric < 3.66, 5.80>
Hb	Haemoglobin (g/L)	Numeric < 106.00, 155.00>
Htc	Haematocrit (%)	Numeric < 0.29, 0.50>
Fe	Serum iron (μmol/l)	Numeric < 6.30, 26.80>

[a]Modification of Diet in Renal Disease - a formula used for calculation of glomerular filtration rate

Estimation of cut-off values

The Youden method, based on calculation of the Youden's index, $YI(c) = max_c(Se(c) + Sp(c) - 1)$, was used to identify cut-off values of numerical parameters that were showed significant in the analysis of differences [65]. Statistical measures: sensitivity, specificity, positive predictive value (PPV) and negative predictive value (NPV) were used to measure the prediction accuracy for MS of the estimated cut-off values. This method was necessary for the assessment of the appropriateness of criteria provided by the conventional definition of MS to comply with characterististics of MS in the group of hypertensive menopausal women.

Graphical methods for data presentation

Some important numerical parameters, of those found significant in analysis of differences, and their cut-off values, were presented also graphically, as box plot graphs.

Bar graphs were used to make visible frequency distributions of women with and without MS according to the time-dependent categories of the parameters indicating: menopause, hypertension and diabetes duration. These bar graphs added value to information obtained by the LR model, on the effect of these parameters on MS.

Multiple logistic regression

Four models of multiple logistic regression (LR) were developed to determine relationships between particular groups of parameters, indicating different aspects of the patient phenotypes, and the presence of MS, in hypertensive menopausal women. The 95% confidence interval (CI) was used to estimate the precision of odds ratio (OR). The McFadden's R squared test was used to measure the predictive power of the LR models [66].

Four LR models were defined as:

1) metabolic components of MS and associated biohumoral disorders presented as haematological and biochemical tests (parameters: BMI, wei, Fglu, TG, HDL, cho, LDL, cre, GFR, CRP, Le, Mo, Ly, Htc, Er, Hb, Fe)
2) comorbidities, medical histories, socio-economic and lifestyle factors (parameters: CHD, CoHD, infbo, cogn, depr, sle, chdi, drug, OA, op, thy, fhis, chil, abor, soc., phy, smo, alc)

Table 2 Parameters obtained by patients interview and their abbreviations and descriptions

	Parameter	Description
wai	Waist circumference (cm)	Numeric < 78, 120>
BMI	BMI (height, weight) (kg/m^2)	Numeric < 21.11, 38.28>
smo	Cigarette smoking (Yes, stopped, No)	Nominal {Yes, sto, No}
alc	Usual in house alcohol use (for two or more days a week)	Binary {Yes/No}
fhis	Family history of CVD: Yes/No	Binary {Yes/No}
soc	Socio-economic status (good, intermediate, low)	Nominal {g, in, lo}
meno	Menopause duration (age of onset/years after menopause)	Nominal {no, < 1, 1–3, > 3}
chil	Number of children born	Numeric < 1, 5>
abor	Number of abortuses	Numeric < 0, 2>
sle	Sleep quality (good/bad)	Binary {g, b}
phy	Physical activity level (good, intermediate/low)	Nominal {g, in/lo}
HRT	Hormonal replacement therapy: Yes/No	Not applicable (1 case)

Table 3 Definitions and grading of some medical conditions

Parameters	Definitions or grading
Stages of chronic renal impairment	Grading is based on using GFR[a] cut-off values - a measure of renal function decline that is derived from data indicating sex, age, weight and serum creatinine (according to the online available MDRD[b] formula)
Impaired fasting blood glucose	Fasting blood glucose ≥6.1 < 7.0 mmol/L
Diabetes type 2 diagnosis	Fasting blood glucose ≥7.0 mmol/L
Normal blood lipids values	Total cholesterol < 5.0 mmol/L LDL-cholesterol ≤3.0 mmol/L HDL-cholesterol ≥1.2 mmol/L (F) Triglycerides ≤1.7 mmol/L
Categories of BMI	BMI < 19 - malnutrition BMI 19–24.9 - normal weight BMI 25–29.9 - overweight BMI ≥30 - obesity
Physical activity level	Good: sport activities, farming or out of house work (at least twice a week) Intermediate: housekeeping, walking for an hour or more (at least twice a week) Low: sedentary lifestyle and lower-energy in house activities
Socio-economic status	Good: bigger house or flat residency and income at the average or above the average for Croatia Intermediate: smaller house or flat residency and income below the average for Croatia but still sufficient to meet the existential needs Low: [c]poor housing and low income, below the existential needs
Positive family history on CVD	Defined as an early onset of coronary heart disease, at or before 50 years of age, for the father and brothers, and at or before 60 years of age, for the mother and systers

[a]Glomerular filtration rate
[b]Modification of Diet in Renal Disease
[c]Only two subjects registered

3) medications (parameters: sta, BB, met, anal, ace, anbi, anco)
4) age, menopause duration, hypertension duration and regulation, diabetes diagnosis, diabetes duration, treatment and complications (parameters: age, meno, Hypdu, Hypre, DGDM, DMdu, DMco, DMtr)

Decision trees method

The C5.0 algorithm, an advanced binary decision trees (DT) method, was used to define simple, practically useful rules, to help general practitioners recognise hypertensive menopausal women with MS [67]. Characteristics of this method, such as a small number of rules that it produce, made it appropriate for the development of rules that draw upon the full-range of data used in the input.

In order to improve the diagnostic capacity of these rules, to go beyond the framework of the conventional definition of MS, two DT models have been performed: 1) on the full-range of data and 2) on the input data set after the parameters indicating conventional components of MS, including: waist circumference, BMI, triglycerides, HDL-cholesterol and fasting blood glucose, had been removed.

Results

Differences in distributions

Women with MS, compared to those without, showed significant differences in a wide range of numerical (Table 4, bolded) and categorical parameters (Table 5, bolded).

Estimation of cut-off values

Table 6 represents cut-off values of those numerical parameters that in the Table 4 have been presented as significant. Parameters: indicating BMI, waist circumference, total serum cholesterol and triglycerides, showed best statistical performance measures of their cut-off values (bolded).

Graphical presentations of some results

How well cut-off values of the significant numerical parameters: triglycerides, BMI and waist circumference, discriminate between hypertensive menopausal women with and without MS, it is better visible when differences in these parameters are presented graphically, as box plot graphs (Fig. 4, left, middle, right).

Frequency distributions of women with and without MS according to the categories of parameters: menopause duration, diabetes duration and hypertension duration, were presented graphically, as bar graphs (Fig. 5, left, middle, right).

LR models

The overall predictive accuracy of this LR model is 70.1%. Parameters significantly associated with MS indicate: BMI, fasting blood glucose, triglycerides, total serum cholesterol, leukocytes number and monocytes % in blood differential count. The parameter indicating haematocrit, although showed no significant association with MS, is presented with the big OR (Table 7).

Table 4 Differences in distributions of numerical parameters between hypertensive menopausal women with and without metabolic syndrome

Parameter	Mean (±Standard deviation)		Variance		*p*-value**
	MS (yes)	MS (no)	MS (yes)	MS (no)	
BMI (kg/m^2)	29.02 ± 3.670	24.76 ± 2.606	13.467	6.790	**5.27e-16**
TG (mmol/L)	1.939 ± 0.581	1.434 ± 0.304	0.338	0.092	**1.27e-14**
wai (cm)	93.48 ± 8.639	84.74 ± 5.280	74.636	27.872	**5.84e-14**
cho (mmol/L)	6.315 ± 0.885	5.25 ± 0.735	0.783	0.541	**1.52e-13**
LDL (mmol/L)	3.366 ± 1.023	2.552 ± 0.824	1.046	0.680	**3.82e-09**
FGlu (mmol/L)	5.924 ± 1.031	5.333 ± 0.402	1.063	0.161	**7.35e-08**
chdi	5.214 ± 1.445	4.304 ± 1.458	2.092	2.127	**4.07e-05**
CRP (mg/L)	3.295 ± 1.575	2.57 ± 1.275	2.481	1.625	**0.0018**
Drug	4.321 ± 1.618	3.565 ± 1.728	2.619	2.985	**0.0021**
Age	52.79 ± 1.977	52.07 ± 2.024	3.908	4.098	**0.0054**
cre (μmol/l)*	79.75 ± 11.545	75.81 ± 12.534	133.282	157.096	**0.0319**
Er (10^{12}/L)	4.641 ± 0.361	4.521 ± 0.395	0.130	0.156	**0.0292**
Htc (%)	0.3899 ± 0.043	0.3733 ± 0.033	0.002	0.001	**0.0302**
Hb (g/L)	136 ± 9.127	133.7 ± 8.375	83.307	70.137	0.0659
GFR (mL/min/1.73 m^2)	71.44 ± 13.102	74.71 ± 15.537	171.657	241.402	0.0816
Fe (μmol/l)	16.16 ± 3.338	15.38 ± 2.614	11.143	6.832	0.1684
Ly (% in blood differential count)	22.61 ± 7.928	20.54 ± 4.337	62.855	18.811	0.2123
Chil	2.023 ± 0.956	1.884 ± 0.932	0.915	0.869	0.2869
Abor	0.1832 ± 0.443	0.2174 ± 0.481	0.197	0.231	0.6139
Le (10^9/L)	6.676 ± 1.488	6.777 ± 1.349	2.213	1.820	0.9261
HDL (mmol/L)	1.346 ± 0.424	1.306 ± 0.329	0.179	0.108	0.9263
Mo (% in blood differential count)	3.023 ± 1.551	3.043 ± 1.288	2.407	1.660	0.9584

*Welch two sample t-test; ** significant parameters were marked with bolded fonts

The overall predictive accuracy of this LR model is 29.9%. Parameters that showed significant associations with MS or the big ORs indicate: diagnosis of anxiety/depression, alcohol use, intermediate to low socio-economic status, diagnoses of CVD (including both chronic heart disease and coronary heart disease), diagnosis of inflammatory bowl disease and psychotic disease (Table 8).

The overall predictive accuracy of this LR model is 40.9%. All parameters from the input indicating

Table 5 Differences in distributions of categorical parameters between hypertensive menopausal women with and without metabolic syndrome

Parameter	*p*-value**	Parameter	*p*-value	Parameter	*p*-value	Parameter	*p*-value
sta	**3.468e-14**	sle	**0.005866**	soc	0.2193	anco	0.6943*
DMtr	**2.452e-10***	CoHD	**0.005915**	thy	0.2198	Uro	0.8019
DMdu	**2.109e-09***	Hypdu	**0.008909**	smo	0.2241	GI	0.9406
DGDM	**4.043e-07**	Hypre	**0.01481**	mal	0.2317	allre	0.9653
met	**3.789e-07**	DMco	**0.0211***	anbi	0.3154	CV	1*
BB	**1.542e-05**	infbo	**0.03989**	OA	0.4277	Sis	1*
depr	**0.0003668**	fhis	0.07321	op	0.4543	ace	1*
meno	**0.001047***	psy	0.07358*	hep	0.4987	phy	0.9952
CHD	**0.004887***	anal	0.09414	PAS	0.5352	chre	0.6319
cogn	**0.005871**	alc	0.09775	derm	0.207*		

*Fisher exact test; **significant parameters were marked with bolded fonts

Table 6 Cut-off values of numerical parameters found significant in the analysis of differences

Parameter	Cut-off	Sensitivity	Specificity	Positive predictive value	Negative predictive value	False positive results	False negative results
Age	55	0.290	0.899	0.844	0.400	7	93
chdi	5	0.702	0.580	0.760	0.506	29	39
Drug	3	0.870	0.348	0.717	0.585	45	17
cre (μmol/l)	77	0.595	0.623	0.750	0.448	26	53
CRP (mg/L)	2.3	0.733	0.565	0.762	0.527	30	35
Er (10^{12}/L)	4.51	0.656	0.551	0.735	0.458	31	45
BMI (kg/m^2)	25.51	**0.855**[a]	**0.797**	**0.889**	**0.743**	**14**	**19**
cho (mmol/L)	6	**0.740**	**0.754**	**0.851**	**0.605**	**17**	**34**
wai (cm)	89	**0.740**	**0.797**	**0.874**	**0.618**	**14**	**34**
TG (mmol/L)	1.7	**0.718**	**0.942**	**0.959**	**0.637**	**4**	**37**
LDL (mmol/L)	3.1	0.573	0.870	0.893	0.517	9	56
FGlu (mmol/L)	5.7	0.542	0.884	0.899	0.504	8	60
Htc (%)	0.41	0.359	0.855	0.825	0.413	10	84

[a]Bolded parameters show the best cut-off values with respect to statistical performance measures

medications were selected in the model, but with variable contributions (ORs) to the diagnosis of MS. Parameters that showed significant associations with MS indicate: use of statins, metformin and beta-blockers (Table 9).

The overall predictive accuracy of this LR model is 27.9%. The parameter that showed significant association with MS indicates menopause of 1–3 years of duration. Parameters that showed no significant associations with MS but that have the big ORs, indicate diagnosis of diabetes and diabetes duration of less than a year (Table 10).

DT models

The overall predictive accuracy of this model is 91.04%. Two major group of rules (phenotypes) were identified: 1) when triglycerides are increased (TG > 1.68) (confirms the diagnosis of MS with the accuracy of prediction of 96.8%) and 2) a set of rules when triglycerides are not increased (TG ≤ 1.68) (Fig. 6).

When triglycerides are not increased, phenotypes that can be used to identify hypertensive menopausal women with MS, include: diagnosis of diabetes ($N = 6$, accuracy 100%); otherwise, increased BMI (> 25.59) and statins use ($N = 11$, accuracy 100%) or increased BMI (> 25.80) and mild renal impairment (GFR ≤ 70) (N = 6, accuracy 83.3%).

The overall predictive accuracy of this model is 89.55%. Two major group of rules (phenotypes) were identified, based on information of whether or not women use statins (Fig. 7).

By the single statement, on statins use, it is possible to recognise a half of the total number of women with MS (66 out of 133), with the accuracy of recognition of 89.4%.

Women with MS who do not take statins, can be recognised according to the phenotypes: 1) treated diabetes, corresponding with overt diabetes ($N = 12$, accuracy 100%) or 2) not treated diabetes, corresponding with a new onset diabetes, to coexist with anxiety/depression, hypertension of more than 5 years of a duration and increased LDL-cholesterol (> 3.1 mmol/L) ($N = 7$, accuracy 100%).

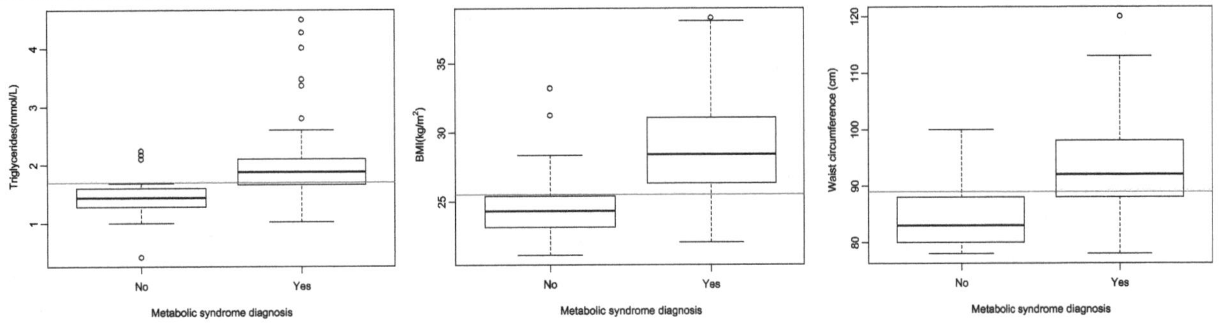

Fig. 4 Graphical presentations of differences in distributions of numerical parameters: triglycerides (left), BMI (middle) and waist circumference (right) with respect to the presence or not of the diagnosis of metabolic syndrome

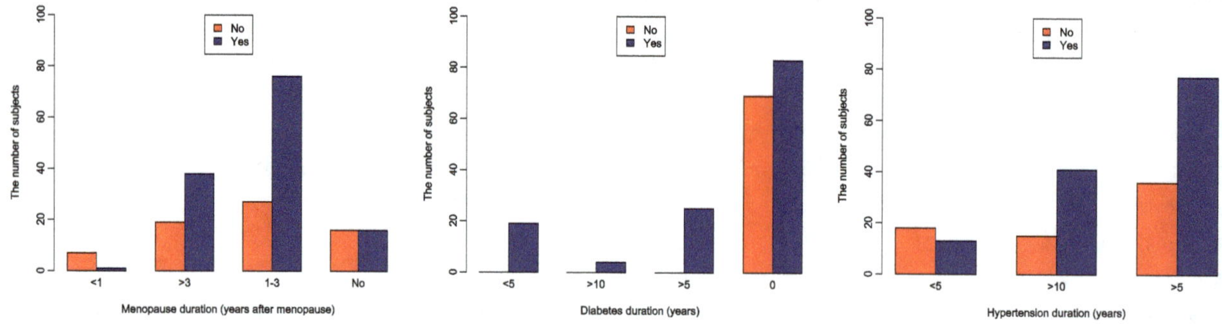

Fig. 5 Graphical presentations of frequency distributions of women with and without MS according to the categories of parameters: menopause duration (left), diabetes duration (middle) and hypertension duration (right)

Discussion

General characteristics of the study population

Chronological age of women in the sample when MS is most likely to emerge was found to be 50–55 years (exactly 50.8–54.8), with the average age of 52–53 years (Table 4). This age range can be used as the screening criterium for women with MS and, in general, for those who are at high CV risk. This is supported with the result of a high percentage (65.8% or 133/202) of women with MS, that is higher than the large-scale studies showed for the general population and even higher than it was found for the selected population of hypertensive patients with uncontrolled blood pressure [68, 69]. In addition, a high percentage of these women with MS also had diabetes (27.2% or 55/202). This percentage is higher than it has been reported e.g. for diabetics in older Croatian population [70]. Taken together, these results implicate the high-grade CV risk of women in the sample. These results are even more remarkable, when taking into account that almost all diabetics had MS

Table 7 Logistic regression model with included parameters indicating conventional components of metabolic syndrome and associated haematology and biochemical disorders

Parameter				CI	
	z value	Pr(>|z|)	OR	5%	95%
BMI	4.24	**0.220e-04*****	2.661	1.821	3.889
wai	−0.39	0.694	0.970	0.856	1.099
FGlu	2.45	**0.014***	5.621	1.762	17.928
TG	2.49	**0.012***	18.455	2.689	126.658
HDL	−1.04	0.299	0.4268	0.110	1.643
cho	3.29	**0.001****	10.897	3.295	36.031
LDL	−0.32	0.749	0.874	0.437	1.746
cre	−0.41	0.684	0.967	0.846	1.105
CRP	0.53	0.594	1.181	0.705	1.981
Ly	1.61	0.107	1.116	0.997	1.249
Er	1.25	0.212	5.788	0.569	58.821
Htc	1.04	0.298	**6.274e04**	0.159e-02	2.473e12
GFR	−1.57	0.116	0.893	0.793	1.005
Le	−2.44	**0.014***	0.444	0.256	0.767
Mo	2.19	**0.028***	1.871	1.168	2.998
Hb	−1.38	0.166	0.932	0.858	1.013
Fe	0.02	0.982	1.003	0.784	1.283

Bolded: parameters with the levels of significance: *** 0.001 ** 0.01 * 0.05 or big ORs

Table 8 Logisitc regression model with included parameters indicating comorbidities, medical histories, socio-economic and lifestyle factors

Parameter				CI	
	z value	Pr(>|z|)	OR	5%	95%
CHD Yes	0.01	0.990	**2.147e07**	0.000	Inf
CoHD Yes	0.01	0.989	**3.103e07**	0.000	Inf
infbo Yes	0.00	0.996	**1.096e-08**	0.000	Inf
cogn Yes	1.35	0.177	3.218	0.772	13.404
depr Yes	2.84	**0.0045****	6.572	2.207	19.573
psy Yes	0.00	0.997	**1.217e07**	0.000	Inf
sle g	0.45	0.652	1.200	0.615	2.343
chdi	1.62	0.105	1.355	0.995	1.847
Drug	1.96	0.050	1.262	1.037	1.536
OA Yes	0.41	0.679	1.195	0.587	2.430
op Yes	−0.80	0.422	0.580	0.190	1.769
thy Yes	0.92	0..357	1.710	0.655	4.464
phy g	0.43	0.666	0.471	0.203	1.666
smo sto	−0.73	0.464	0.672	0.275	1.640
smo Yes	−1.73	0.083	0.466	0.226	0.962
alc Yes	2.67	**0.007****	16.170	2.903	90.047
soc in	2.29	**0.022***	3.956	1.472	10.631
soc lo	0.01	0.995	**5.177e08**	0.000	Inf
fhis Yes	0.53	0.595	1.265	0.610	2.622
chil	1.42	0.155	1.349	0.954	1.910
abor	−0.72	0.473	0.738	0.367	1.480

Bolded: parameters with the levels of significance: ** 0.01 * 0.05 or big ORs

Table 9 Logistic regression model with included parameters indicating medications

Parameter				CI	
	z value	Pr(>|z|)	OR	5%	95%
Sta Yes	5.90	**0.36e-08*** **	15.829	7.329	34.186
BB Yes	2.04	**0.040***	2.685	1.213	5.945
met Yes	3.54	**0.4e-03*** **	44.471	7.622	259.450
anal Yes	1.01	0.311	1.599	0.745	3.433
ace Yes	−1.62	0.106	0.375	0.138	1.017
anbi Yes	−1.70	0.088	0.426	0.187	0.971
anco Yes	− 184	0.066	0.126	0.019	0.805

Bolded: parameters with the levels of significance: *** 0.001 * 0.05

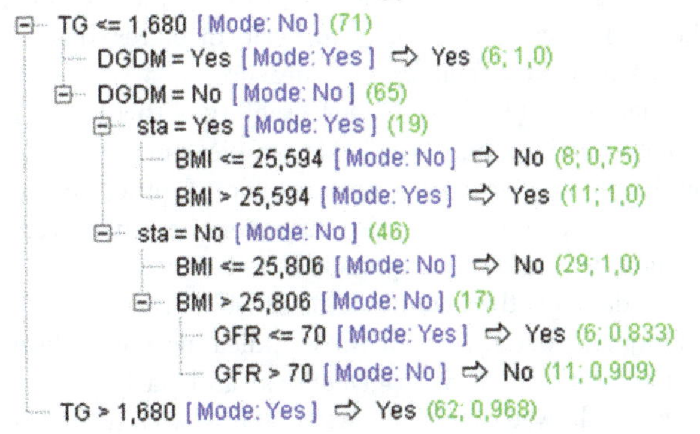

Fig. 6 Decision trees model with all parameters included

(53/55), according to the evidence that diabetics with superimposed MS yield more CV risks [71].

Anthropometric measures and other conventional components of MS

Waist circumference, a measure of the central (abdominal) obesity, is a part of the most of available definitions of MS [44]. On the contrary, a measure of the general obesity, indicated with BMI > 30, makes part of only one definition, in line with evidence that increased body weight may not always be associated with MS [68]. Starting from this background, we proposed that these two anthropometric measures, in the selected women's group, must gain some specific characteristics that are different from criteria provided by the conventional definition, used for analysis. If it is true, these characteristics may be also used for recognition of women at high CV risk.

We found, for women with MS, the waist circumference threshold of 89 cm (Table 6) (Fig. 4, right), that is much above the criterium of 80 cm of the IDF definition, used for analysis, indicating predisposition of these women for abdominal fat accumulation. This predisposition may be due to the effect of both, hypertension and menopause, on abdominal fat accumulation [34, 72]. This observation is supported with the result that also women with isolated hypertension had waist circumference values that are above the standard criterium of 80 cm (84.74 ± 5.28) (Table 4) (Fig. 4, right). When increased body weight is added to these two factors, they all may act synergistically on abdominal fat accumulation, worsening further metabolic and CV status [35, 73]. This pathophysiology chain reaction can be used to explain our results that almost all women with MS had increased body weight (BMI > 25.5 kg/m^2) (Table 6) (Fig. 4, middle). This BMI cut-of value, as based on its good statistical performances to separate women with from those without MS, can be even used as a freestanding rule for recognition of women with MS (Table 5) (Fig. 2, middle). Moreover, because the parameter BMI, but not the parameter waist circumference,

Table 10 Logistic regression model with included parameters indicating: age, menopause duration, hypertension duration and regulation, diabetes diagnosis, duration, treatment and complications

Parameter				CI	
	z value	Pr(>|z|)	OR	5%	95%
Age	0.60	0.548	1.066	0.894	1.242
Meno > 3	1.73	0.084	6.989	1.098	44.453
Meno 1–3	2.18	**0.029***	11.192	1.810	69.181
Meno No	1.28	0.200	4.522	0.652	31.341
Hypdu > 10	1.05	0.296	1.804	0.712	4.570
Hypdu > 5	0.75	0.453	1.438	0.648	3.195
Hypre Normal	−1.90	0.057	0.320	0.119	0.858
DGDM Yes	0.00	0.997	**0.646e-08**	0.000	In0
DMdu > 10	0.00	1.000	1.477	0.000	Inf
DMdu > 5	0.00	1.000	1.094	0.000	Inf
DMdu 0	0.00	0.996	**0.971e-16**	0.000	Inf
DMco mic	0.00	1.000	1.321	0.000	Inf
DMco No	0.00	1.000	1.088	0.000	Inf
DMtr or	0.00	1.000	0.938	0.000	Inf
DMtr or/i	0.00	1.000	2.103	0.000	Inf

Bolded: parameters with the levels of significance: * 0.05 or big ORs

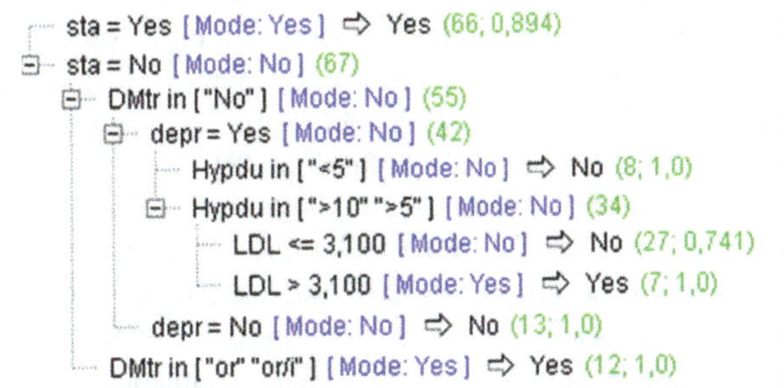

Fig. 7 Decision trees model with excluded parameters closely related to the conventional definition of metabolic syndrome: waist circumference, BMI, triglycerides, HDL-cholesterol and fasting glucose

showed significant association with MS in the LR model, the parameter BMI is likely to perform better, than the standard waist circumference measure, as a part of the MS definition (Table 7). Generalisability of this result, although obtained on a small size sample, can be achieved by its comparison with the results of other studies, where increased BMI, in hypertensive menopausal women, was showed to associate better with subclinical organ damage, than components of MS [74].

Only two parameters of those indicating conventional components of MS, triglycerides and fasting blood glucose, showed significant associations with MS in the LR model (Table 7). Also their cut-off values (of 1.7 and 5.7 mmol/L, respectively) were found congruent with the standard MS criteria, implicating good diagnostic compliance with the examined population group (Table 6). However, when the ability of their cut-off values to discriminate between women with and without MS is considered, then only the parameter triglycerides, but not the parameter fasting blood glucose, can be used as a freestanding MS diagnostic tool for recognition of women with MS (Table 6) (Fig. 4, left). Our results provide even more details, indicating that information on increased serum triglycerides (above the cut-off value for MS) can be used with the high accuracy (of 96.8%) to identify around a half (62/131) of women with MS (DT rules, Fig. 6). Furthermore, based on a high degree of overlap between MS and diabetes, found for women in this sample (53/55), this information can also serve as a screening tool for women at high CV risk. There are pieces of evidence to support this assumption, showing that serum triglycerides are more markedly expressed when MS and diabetes are superimposed to each other, than when either of them stands alone [28, 75]. Distinctly from the parameter triglycerides, the parameter fasting blood glucose does not seem appropriate as a single marker of MS in this selected women's group, because its cut-off value of 5.7 mmol/L failed to accurately classify a large part of women in the sample (Table 6). Explanation for this failure may be found in the fact that a large portion of women with MS have already had a diagnosis of diabetes. Another argument may be a piece of evidence indicating that impaired glucose tolerance, in women, in contrast to men, beter complies with impaired postload than fasting blood glucose, arguing for parameters changes in MS definition [43].

With respect to another conventional component of MS, HDL-cholesterol, our results suggest that the parameter total serum cholesterol and its cut-off value of 6.0 mmol/L perform better as a component of MS, than the parameter HDL-cholesterol. This conclusion is based on the good ability of this cut-off value to recognise women with MS (Tables 4 and 6) and the results of LR modeling, where the parameter total serum cholesterol, but not the parameter HDL-cholesterol, showed significant association with MS (Table 7). Increased total serum cholesterol can be considered the specific characteristic of hypertensive menopausal women, because both factors, hypertension and menopause, were found to increase total serum cholesterol [35]. As our results also suggest, even more favorable marker of MS, than increased total serum cholesterol, might be information on using cholesterol lowering drug statins. High diagnostic accuracy (of 89.4%) of this information to identify a large part of women with MS (66/131) (Fig. 7), is comparative to that on increased triglycerides (62/131) (accuracy 96.8%) (Fig. 6). This information must be, however, used with a caution, because its operative value may depend on how strictly prescription rules for statins are used by family doctors in a local environment. According to the guidelines, statins are prescribed either to diabetics or non diabetics with high serum total cholesterol; in both cases, this information indicates patients at high CV risk [28].

When these results on the diagnostic accuracy of the conventional components of MS, in the selected group of hypertensive menopausal women, are taken together, we can conclude that the best markers of MS, used either separately or as a combination, include: BMI > 25.5 kg/m^2, increased triglycerides > 1.7 mmol/L and increased total serum cholesterol > 6.0 mmol/L, or information on statins use. For a smaller part of hypertensive menopausal women, for which either of these information does not provide the meaningful framework for MS diagnosis, diagnosis of diabetes, or rules based on a mixture of parameters, indicating also comorbidities and socio-behavioural factors, can provide the reasonable means (Figs. 6 and 7).

Comorbidities, socio-demographic and lifestyle factors associated with MS

According to the above discussion and when the overall predictive accuracy of developed LR models is considered (Tables 7, 8, 9 and 10), it allows for a conclusion that the conventional components of MS and related metabolic factors are the best predictable means of MS. However, a full-range of the MS phenotype variability to be achieved, this will require also other factors to be used for predictive modeling. The example is when a range of laboratory parameters showed significant differences between women with and without MS (Table 4) and when many of these parameters were selected in the LR model, contributing to the model's predictive power, along with the conventional components of MS (Table 7). Yet a range of laboratory parameters, taken as a whole, but not any of them, if taken as an alone, allow for pathophysiology disorders to be recognised, for which also other sources of information provide evidence for their associations with MS. Pathophysiology disorders, indicated with these results, include: renal function decline, chronic inflammation and disturbed haemorrheology [38, 39, 76]. We propose that a range of laboratory parameters that are associated with MS can vary in some degrees in different population groups, according to characteristics of patients in the sample and the availability of parameters, although it is not expected to go out of the boundaries of the panel of data that are indicated in this study.

When interpreted in this context, then the parameters monocytes% (Mo) and leukocyte count (Le), that were found significant in the LR model (Table 7), but not in the analysis of differences (Table 4), can be viewed as a part of the common inflammation/disturbed haemorrheology disorder, for which the parameter Htc, indicating increased haematocrit values, yet represents a more general mean [76]. Namely, when a high specificity of the cut-off value of this parameter (Table 4) and its big OR obtained in the LR model (Table 7) are taken into account, that means that only this parameter, of all laboratory parameters examined, is worthy of consideration to be used as a single marker for MS diagnosis. Practical implication is that the haematocrit values above the threshold of 41%, if found in menopausal women with hypertension, could be considered as the MS diagnosis, without the need of having information on conventional components of MS.

As we expected, analysis of comorbidities has provided information that can be used to improve the phenotype profilling of hypertensive menopausal women with MS. As added value, this analysis has enabled some glimpses on mechanisms of MS generation, thus paving the way for future research.

Medical conditions, that had been selected in the first step selection, according to the analysis of differences, were those ones for which also evidence show their associations with MS, including: CVD (parameters CoHD and CHD), sleep disorders, anxiety/depression, cognitive disorders, psychotic disease and inflammatory bowel disease (Table 5) [40–42, 77, 78]. This agreement between the knowledge and our results argues towards the feasibility of the proposed research approach for MS assessment that is based on using data from GP eHRs and a smal size sample. More specific analysis of the second step, based on using LR modeling, showed a more restricted panel of medical conditions as associated with MS, including: CVD, inflammatory bowel disease, psychotic disorders and anxiety/depression (Table 8). Here, a caution must be declared. It is possible that inadequately determined frequencies of the diagnoses of sleep disorders, anxiety/depression and cognitive disorders, for which the ICD-10 coding system shows insufficient, especially when older population is considered, might have influenced their wrong selection into the LR model [79]. For the needs of phenotype profilling, a procedure that relies on a comprehensive analysis of all relevant medical conditions associated with MS, diagnoses of these conditions have to be more accurately determined. This would be routinelly possible, if the available scoring systems for detection of these disorders were included as a part of GP eHRs, ensuring a systematic approach to diagnosis.

Because inflammatory bowel disease and psychotic disease were presented with low frequency in this sample, practical usefulness can be considered for the diagnoses of CVD and anxiety/depression. Of these two, the potential for improving prevention of CVD, in menopausal women, can be considered for the diagnosis of anxiety/depression. This assumption is also supported with the results of the DT model, where this diagnosis was unveiled as a part of the rule for MS recognition, being placed in the same clinical context with the new onset diabetes (indicated with the category "non treated diabetes") and a long-term hypertension (of more than 5 years of duration) (Fig. 7). That anxiety/depression might be a mechanism that in menopausal women drives development of MS and other CV factors, this is indicated, although indirectly, with the results of the LR modeling process, where comorbid disorders were put together with data indicating social factors and lifestyles (Table 8). Based on these results, a social context was identified that in menopausal women can favour MS development, including alcohol use behaviour (a mechanism of how women cut down their intrinsic tensions) and lower socio-economic status (known to produce chronic social stress and unhealthy behaviours, leading to increase in CV risks) [80, 81].

Another comorbid disorder, for which our results also indicate its association with MS, although more indirectly, is impaired renal function, represented with the parameter GFR. It is found as a non significant part of the LR model (Table 7) or as a hidden within the combined DT rules (Fig. 6). Low emphasis that it is put on this parameter, may be due to the low overall level of expression of this disorder in women in the sample, as a progression of this disorder is expected to occur in older age [53].

Although all medications that we used for analysis were also selected in the LR model, indicating that all of them can contribute to MS diagnosis, those ones that showed significant associations with MS were beta-blockers, metformin and statins (Table 9). As we have already stated for statins, information on using these medications can help family doctors recognise the specific women's groups. In this terms, beta-blockers can indicate women diagnosed with CVD and metformin can indicate those diagnosed with a new onset diabetes [82]. Strong emphasis that in our study is put on association between the use of statins and MS, as based on both, results of the LR model and DT rules (Table 9)

(Figs. 6 and 7), can be also reflective of their proposed influence on MS and diabetes development [83]. If proved true, this statement would have implications on changing the prescription rules, from the current "one-fit-all "to a more diversificated approach, that will be able to address, more specifically, narrowly defined patient groups, such as a group of menopausal women with hypertension.

Relationships between menopause, hypertension and diabetes duration and the time when MS does emerge, have become more reliable when presented graphically, than just analysed by the modeling. Namely, results of the LR model showed as the time when MS most intensively emerges the period of 1–3 years after menopause (corresponding with early postmenopause) (Table 10) (Fig. 2). On the bar graph, this period is represented with the big dysproportion in frequency of women with and without MS, indicating intensive transition, placed in the period of 1–3 years of menopause duration (Fig. 5, left). What else was possible to perceive from the graph, but that was not possible otherwise, is an overview of the MS frequency distribution througout the periods of menopause duration. This way, it looks like that the bundles of the MS frequency are devided into the two discrete periods: one less intensive (the option "No"), indicating time close to menopause and corresponding to late menopause transition, and the other more intensive (options 1–3 and > 3), corresponding with early postmenopause (Fig. 2) (Fig. 5, left). These two periods are also emphasised with evidence as critical for the emergency of MS [48]. This gives confidence to our research approach that is based on using a large dataset and a combination of analytical methods, to answer some complex questions.

A new and intruiging finding that arises from these results is related to our impression on the possible coincidence of a new onset diabetes and the emergency of MS. This impression is based on the results of the LR model (Table 10), where parameters "diabetes diagnosis "and "diabetes duration 0", indicating recently developed diabetes, showed significant associations with MS (based on the big ORs). This impression have become even more reliable when results of the LR model were presented graphically (Fig. 5, right). On the bar graph, MS transition is placed into the category of a new onset diabetes (marked with"0"). These results are complementary to the high degree of overlap between MS and diabetes, found for women in the sample (53/55). This idea, on possible simultaneous development of MS and diabetes, as a specific trait of menopausal women with hypertension, is exciting from the preventive aspects and deserves further evaluation, especially because evidence on this issue are also limited. The only report that we found is that on a greater increase in CV risk through the appearance of diabetes, that is a characteristic of women with MS, in contrast to men [84]. Our results provide even more complete information on this issue, by placing the coincidence of MS and a new onset diabetes into a wider clinical context, characterised also with a long-term hypertension (of more than 5 years of duration) and anxiety/depression (Fig. 7) (Fig. 5, middle). This way, pieces of information, provided by different methods for data analysis, converge into a common, complex view.

Practical protocol, for use in GP, for fast recognition and preventive management of menopausal women at high CV risk

The group of women in which CV risk factors are expected to intensivly emerge is in the age of 50–55 years and diagnosed with hypertension. If these women have incresed BMI, this very probably means the diagnosis of MS. Other relatively accurate single-parameter rules, to capture a prevalent part of women with MS, include: increased triglycerides, above 1.7 mmol/L, increased total serum cholesterol, above 6.0 mmol/L, and information on statins use. Frequent follow up of these women on a new onset diabetes is credible, because of the possible simultaneous onset of MS and diabetes. A special attention, in terms of prevention of CVD, should be also put on women with anxiety/depression and mild renal impairment. Women with a new onset diabetes should be provided with intensive treatment of CV risk factors, because of the expected high burden of CV risk factors in this population group.

Conclusions

The added value of this study goes beyond the current paradigm on MS. Results indicate characteristics that can be used to improve the diagnosis of MS according to the narrowly defined specific population group such as menopausal women with hypertension. Although components close to the conventional definition of MS bear the most of the diagnostic capacity for MS, to capture the full-range variability of the phenotypes, a mixture of factors, including also comorbidities and other clinical and socio-behavioural factors, should be used into consideration. Advantages would be in GP, for improving prevention of CVD in women, especially because the current methods for CV risk estimation, for this specific population group, show insufficent.

To enable the routine use of data from GP eHRs for this kind of research, the panel of data that are systematically recorded should include some other parameters, in addition to the usual structured data.

These necessary additional data are information on socio-demographic and lifestyle factors and scoring systems for diagnosing medical conditions for which the standard coded diagnosis system shows limited, such as anxiety/depression and sleep and cognitive disorders. What is also important, is to achieve harmonisation, among family doctors, in diagnosis and prescription rules, mostly related to the diagnoses of diabetes and anxiety/depression and the statins prescription. The challenging issue will be also training of general practitioners in skills for multiple results integration and their harmonisation with knowledge.

Several new findings, specifically associated with the characteristics of the examined population group, have arisen from this study and require further elaboration, for their possible practical implications. These findings include: the existence of the two main lipid disorders represented with increased triglycerides and total serum cholesterol; the possible involvement of statins in the pathophysiology of MS and diabetes development; the possible coincidental development of diabetes and MS; the preventive potential, for the development of MS and diabetes, of recognition of anxiety/depression in menopausal women with a long-lasting hypertension.

Abbreviations

CV: Cardiovascular; DWBC: White blood cell differential; eHRs: Electronic health records; FGlu: Fasting glucose; GFR: Glomerular filtration rate; GP: General practice; HDL: High density lipoprotein; ICD-10: International statistical classification of diseases and related health problems 10th revision; IDF: International diabetes federation; LDL: Low density lipoprotein; MS: Metabolic syndrome; TG: Triglycerides

Acknowledgements

We thank the HCI-KDD expert group for valuable support in discussions and workshops.

Funding

This work is approved by the University of Osijek Common Fund, through cooperative agreements. The views presented here are solely the responsibility of the authors and do not represent the official views of the Faculty of Medicine and the University of Osijek. The work was partially supported by the Slovak Grant Agency of the Ministry of Education and Academy of Science of the Slovak Republic under grant no. 1/0493/16 and The Slovak Research and Development Agency under grant no. APVV-16-0213.

Declarations

The work complies with Ethics Policies of the journal.

Authors' contributions

ŠŠ, LjTM and AV conceptualized and designed the study. ŠŠ acquired the data. FB, MV and JP analysed the data. ŠŠ and LJTM interpreted the results. AH was the coordinating supervisor. ŠŠ, LjTM, FB, MV, JP, AV and AH contributed to the writing of the paper. All authors read and approved the final version of the paper.

Authors' information

ŠŠ is a specialist of Family Medicine and Emergency Medicine and a PhD student under the mentorship of LjTM. LJTM is a specialist of family medicine and Assis. Prof. at the Deparment of Internal Medicine and Family Medicine, Faculty of Medicine, University of Osijek, Croatia. Her main fields of interest are: primary care, clinical medicine, ageing diseases, cardiovascular disease, clinical immunology and knowledge discovery in datasets. She is a member of the Holzinger's HCI-KDD International Network. AV is a Full Prof. in Internal medicine, Head of the Department of Internal medicine and Family medicine and a co-mentor of ŠŠ. FB is Assis. Prof. at the the Department of Cybernetics and Artificial Intelligence, Faculty of Electrical Engineering and Informatics, Technical university of Košice, Slovakia. His research is oriented on data mining and knowledge management. MV is a PhD student supervised by JP at the same department, with the research area in medical data mining. JP is a Full Prof. at the same department and his professional interests are knowledge discovery, knowledge management, scheduling and logistics. AH is head of the Holzinger Group, HCI-KDD, at the Institute of Medical Informatics/Statistics at the Medical University Graz, and Assoc. Prof. of Applied Computer Science at the Institute of Interactive Systems and Data Science at Graz University of Technology. His research interests are in machine learning and knowledge extraction to help to solve problems in health informatics.

Competing interests

ŠŠ declares that he has no competing interests.
LjTM declares that she has no competing interests.
FB declares that he has no competing interests.
MV declares that he has no competing interests.
JP declares that he has no competing interests.
AV declares that he has no competing interests.
AH is member of the editorial board of BMC MIDM but not in this section and he was neither involved in the editorial nor in the review process.

Author details

[1]Department for Internal Medicine, Family Medicine and the History of Medicine, Faculty of Medicine, Josip Juraj Strossmayer University, Osijek, Croatia, Huttlerova 10b, 31 000 Osijek, Croatia. [2]Department of Cybernetics and Artificial Intelligence, Technical University of Košice, Faculty of Electrical Engineering and Informatics, Letná 9/B, 042 00 Košice, Slovakia. [3]Medical University Graz, Institute for Medical Informatics/Statistic, Auenbruggerplatz 2/V, 8036 Graz, Austria.

References

1. Starfield B. Is US health really the best in the world? JAMA. 2000;284:483–5.
2. Wonca Europe. The European definition of general practice/family medicine. 2002; http://www.woncaeurope.org/sites/default/files/documents/Definition%203rd%20ed%202011%20with%20revised%20wonca%20tree.pdf. Accessed 10 Mar 2017.
3. Starfield B. Is primary care essential? Lancet. 1994;344:129–33.
4. De Maeseneer JM, De Sutter A. Why research in family medicine? Ann Fam Med. 2004;2(Suppl 2):17–22.
5. Rosser WW, van Weel C. Research in family/general practice is essential for improving health globally. Ann Fam Med 2004;2 Suppl 2:2–4.
6. Okkes IM, Oskam SK, Lamberts H. The probability of specific diagnoses for patients presenting with common symptoms to Dutch family physicians. J Fam Pract. 2002;51:31–6.
7. Salive ME. Multimorbidity in older adults. Epidemiol Rev. 2013;35:75–83.
8. Van Weel C, Knottnerus JA. Rosser WW. Evidence-based interventions and comprehensive treatment. Lancet 1999;353:916–918.
9. Rosser WW. Aplication of evidence from randomized controlled trials to general practice. Lancet. 1999;353:661–4.
10. Nutting PA, Beasley JW, Werner JJ. Asking and answering questions in practice: practice based research networks build the science base of family practice. JAMA. 1999;281:686–8.
11. Ludwick DA, Doucette J. Adopting electronic medical records in primary care: lessons learned from health information systems implementation experience in seven countries. Int J Med Inform. 2009;78(1):22–31.
12. Carey IM, Cook DG, De Wilde S, Brenner SA, Richards N, Caine S, et al. Implications of the problem oriented medical record (POMR) for research using electronic GP databases: a comparison of the doctors independent network database (DIN) and the general practice research database (GPRD). BMC Fam Pract 2003;4:14.
13. García-Gil Mdel M, Hermosilla E, Prieto-Alhambra D, Fina F, Rosell M, Ramos R, et al. Construction and validation of a scoring system for the selection of high-quality data in a Spanish population primary care database (SIDIAP). Inform Prim Care. 2011;19(3):135–45.

14. De Clercq E, van Casteren V, Jonekheer P, Burggraeve P, Lafontaine M-F, Vandenberghe H, et al. Research networks: can we use data from GPs electronic health records. Stud Health Technol Inform. 2006;124:181–6.
15. Garcia Rodriguez LA, Perez GS. Use of the UK general practice research database for pharmacoepidemiology. Br J Clin Pharmacol. 1998;45(5):419–25.
16. Krish T, Hassey A, Sullivan F. Systematic review of scope and quality of electronic patient record data in primary care. BMJ. 2003;326:1070.
17. Khan NF, Harrison SE, Rose PW. Validity of diagnostic coding within the general practice research database: a systematic review. Br J Gen Pract. 2010;60(572):e128–36.
18. Gijsen R, Poos MJJC. Using registries in general practice to estimate country wide morbidity in the Netherlands. Public Health. 2006;120(1):923–36.
19. Denaxas SC, George J, Herrett E, Shah AD, Kalra D, Hingorani AD, et al. Data resource profile: cardiovascular disease research using linked bespoke studies and electronic health records (CALIBER). Int J Epidemiol. 2012;41:1925–38.
20. Rumsfeld JS, Joynt KE, Maddox TM. Big data analytics to improve cardiovascular care: promise and challenges. Nat Rev Cardiol. 2016;13:350–9.
21. Luke V, Rasmussen BS. The electronic health record for translational research. J Cardiovasc Trans Res. 2014;7(6):607–14.
22. Holzinger A. Introduction to machine learning and knowledge extraction (MAKE). Mach Learn Knowl Extract. 2018;1(1):1.
23. Lj M-T, Vitale B. Systems biology as a conceptual framework for research in family medicine; use in predicting response to influenza vaccination. Prim Health Care Res Develop. 2011;12(4):310–21.
24. Trtica-Majnaric LJ, Zekic-Susac M, Sarlija N, Vitale B. Prediction of influenza vaccination outcome by neural networks and logistic regression. J Biomed Informat. 2010;43:774–81.
25. Yildirim P, Majnarić LJ, Ekmekci OI, Holzinger A. Knowledge discovery of drug data on the example of adverse reaction prediction. BMC Bioinformatics. 2014;15(Suppl 6):7.
26. Babič F, Majnarić LJ, Lukáčová A, Paralič J, Holzinger A. On patient's characteristics extraction for metabolic syndrome diagnosis: predictive modelling based on machine learning. In: Bursa M, Khuri SM, Renda E, editors. Information Technology in Bio-and Medical Informatics. LNSC 20148649. Heidelberg: Springer; 2014. p. 118–132.
27. Mosca L, Barrett-Connor E, Wenger NK. Sex/gender differences in cardiovascular disease prevention. Circulation. 2011;124:2145–54.
28. Reiner Ž, Catapano AL, De Backer G, Graham I, Taskinen M-R, Wiklund O, et al. ESC/EAS guidelines for the management of dyslipidemias. Eur Heart J. 2011;32(14):1769–818.
29. Kearney PM, Whelton M, Reynolds K, Muntner P, Whelton PK, Jiang H. Global burden of hypertension: analysis of worldwide data. Lancet. 2005;365:217–23.
30. Julius S, Valentini M, Palatini P. Overweight and hypertension. A 2-way street? Hypertension. 2000;35:807–13.
31. Eckel RH, Alberti KG, Grundy SM, Zimmet PZ. The metabolic syndrome. Lancet. 2010;375:181–3.
32. Mule G, Cottone S, Nardi E, Andronico G, Cerasola G. Metabolic syndrome in subjects with essential hypertension: relationships with subclinical cardiovascular and renal damage. Minerva Cardioangiol. 2006;54:173–94.
33. Nuzzo A, Rossi R, Modena MG. Hypertension alone or related to the metabolic syndrome in postmenopausal women. Expert Rev Cardiovasc Ther. 2010;8(11):1541–8.
34. Carr MC. The emergency of the metabolic syndrome with menopause. J Clin Endocrinol Metab. 2009;88:2404–11.
35. Chae CU, Derby CA. The menopausal transition and cardiovascular risk. Obstet Gynecol Clin N Am. 2011;38:477–88.
36. Stewart DE, Boydell K. Psychologic distress during menopause: associations across the reproductive life cycle. Int J Psychiatry Med. 1993;23:157–62.
37. Matthews KA, Crawford SL, Chae CU, Everson-Rose SA, Sowers MF, Sternfeld B, et al. Are changes in cardiovascular disease risk factors in midlife women due to chronological aging or to the menopausal transition? J Am Coll Cardiol. 2009;54(25):2366–73.
38. Tracy RP. Inflammation, the metabolic syndrome and cardiovascular risk. Int J Clin Pract Suppl. 2003;134:10–7.
39. Nashar K, Egan BM. Relationship between chronic kidney disease and metabolic syndrome: current perspectives. Diabetes Metab Syndr Obes. 2014;7:421–35.
40. Kahl KG, Schweiger U, Correll C, Müller C, Busch M-L, Bauer M, Schwarz P. Depression, anxiety disorders and metabolic syndrome in a population at risk for type 2 diabetes mellitus. Brain Behav. 2015;5(3):e00306.
41. Hall MH, Okun ML, Sowers MF, Matthews KA, Kravitz HM, Hardin K, et al. Sleep is associated with the metabolic syndrome in a multi-ethnic cohort of midlife women: the SWAN sleep study. Sleep. 2012;35(6):783–90.
42. Panza F, Frisardi V, Capurso C, Imbimbo BP, Vendemiale G, Santamato A, et al. Metabolic syndrome and cognitive impairment: current epidemiology and possible underlying mechanisms. J Alzheimers Dis. 2010;21(3):691–724.
43. Regitz-Zagrosek V, Lehmkuhl E, Weickert MO. Gender differences in the metabolic syndrome and their role for cardiovascular disease. Clin Res Cardiol. 2006;95(3):136–47.
44. Alberti KG, Eckel RH, Grundy SM, Zimmet PZ, Cleeman JI, Donato KA, et al. Harmonizing the metabolic syndrome: a joint interim statement of the international diabetes federation task force on epidemiology and prevention; National Heart, lung and blood institute; American Heart Association; world heart federation; international atherosclerosis society; and International Association for the Study of obesity. Circulation. 2009;120:1640–5.
45. Beaser RS, Levy P. Metabolic syndrome: a work in progress, but a useful construct. Circulation. 2007;115:1812–8.
46. De Lusignan S, van Weel C. The use of routinely collected computer data for research in primary care: opportunities and challenges. Fam Pract. 2006;23(2):253–63.
47. Harlow SD, Gass M, Hall JE, Lobo R, Maki P, Rebar RW, et al. Executive summary of the stages of reproductive aging workshop+10: addressing the unfinished agenda of staging reproductive aging. Climacteric. 2012;15:105–14.
48. Mesch VR, Boero LE, Siseles NO, Royer M, Prada M, Sayegh F, et al. Metabolic syndrome throughout the menopausal transition: influence of age and menopausal status. Climacteric. 2006;9(1):40–8.
49. Dratva J, Gomez Real F, Schindler C, Ackermann-Liebrich U, Gerbase MW, et al. Is age at menopause increasing across Europe? Results on age at menopause and determinants from two population-based studies. Menopause. 2009;16(2):385–94.
50. Benchimol EI, Smeeth L, Guttmann A, Harron K, Moher D, Petersen I, et al. The Reporting of studies Conducted using Observational Routinely-collected health Data (RECORD) Statement. PLOS Med. 2015;doi.org/10.1371/journal.pmed.1001885.
51. E-health Croatia. http://www.ericsson.hr/fgs.axd?id=1747 (2015). Accessed 13 Mar 2017.
52. Levey AS, Coresh J, Greene T, Stevens LA, Zhang YL, Hendriksen S, et al. Chronic kidney disease epidemiology collaboration. Using standardized serum creatinine values in the modification of diet in renal disease study equation for estimating glomerular filtration rate. Ann Intern Med. 2006;145(4):247–54.
53. Inker LA, Astor BC, Fox CH, Isakova T, Lash JP, Peralta CA, et al. KDOQI US commentary on the 2012 KDIGO clinical practice guidelines for the evaluation and management of CKD. Am J Kidney Dis. 2014;63(5):713–35.
54. The Task Force on diabetes, pre-diabetes and cardiovascular diseases of the European Society of Cardiology (ESC) and developed in collaboration with the European Association for the Study of Diabetes (EASD). ESC guidelines on diabetes, pre-diabetes and cardiovascular diseases seveloped in collaboration with the EASD. Eur Heart J. 2013;34:3035–87.
55. Zreikat HH, Harpe SE, Slattum PW, Mays DP, Essah PA, Cheang KI. Effect of renin-angiotensin system inhibition on cardiovascular events in older hypertensive patients with metabolic syndrome. Metabolism. 2014;63:392–9.
56. Devaraj S, Siegel D, Jialal I. Statin therapy in metabolic syndrome and hypertension post-JUPITER: what is the value of CRP? Curr Atheroscl Rep. 2011;13(1):31–42.
57. Rojas LBA, Gomes MB. Metformin: an old but still the best treatment for type 2 diabetes. Diabetol Metab Syndr. 2013;5:6.
58. Montez JK, Bromberger J, Harlow SD, Kravitz HM, Matthews KA. Life-course socioeconomic status and metabolic syndrome among midlife women. J Gerontol B Psychol Sci Soc Sci. 2016;71(6):1097–107.
59. Vryonldon A, Paschou SA, Muscoghuri G, Orlo F, Goulls DG. Metabolic syndrome through the female life cycle. Mechanisms in endocrinology. Eur J Endocrinol. 2015;173:R153–63.
60. Churilla JR, Zoeller RF. Physical activity: physical activity and the metabolic syndrome: a review of the evidence. Am J Lifestyle Med. 2008;2(2):118–25.

61. Fried LP, Ferrucci L, Dover J, Williamson JD, Anderson G. Untagling the concepts of disability, frailty and comorbidity: implications for improved targeting and care. J Gerontol. 2004;59(3):255–63.
62. Alberti KG, Zimmet P, Shaw J. Metabolic syndrome – a new worldwide definition. A consensus statement from the international diabetes federation. Diabet Med. 2006;23:469–80.
63. Shapiro SS, Wilk MB. An analysis of variance test for normality (complete samples). Biometrika. 1965;52(3–4):591–611.
64. Welch BL. On the comparison of several mean values: an alternative approach. Biometrika. 1951;38:330–6.
65. Yin J, Tian L. Optimal linear combinations of multiple diagnostic biomarkers based on Youden index. Stat Med. 2013;33(8):1426–40.
66. McFadden D. Conditional logit analysis of qualitative choice behaviour. In: Zarembka P, editor. Frontiers in econometrics. New York: Academic Press; 1974.
67. Patil N, Lathi R, Chitre V. Comparison of C5.0 & CART classification algorithms using pruning technique. Int J Eng Res Technol. 2012;1(4):1–5.
68. Van Vliet-Ostaptchouk JV, Nuotio M-L, Slagter SN, Doiron D, Fischer K, Foco L, et al. European collaborative study group. The prevalence of metabolic syndrome and metabolically healthy obesity in Europe: a collaborative analysis of ten large cohort studies. BMC Endocr Dis. 2014;14:9.
69. Kjeldsen SE, Naditch-Brule L, Perlini S, Zidek W, Farsang C. Increased prevalence of metabolic syndrome in uncontroled hypertension across Europe: the global Cardiometabolic risk profile in patients with hypertension disease survey. Hypertension. 2008;26:2064–70.
70. Poljicanin T, Pavlić-Renar I, Metelko Z. [CroDiab NET- electronic diabetes registry]. [article in Croatian]. Acta Med Croatica 2005;59(3):185–189.
71. Zadhoush F, Sadeghi M, Pourfarzam M. Biochemical changes in blood of type 2 diabetes with and without metabolic syndrome components. J Res Med Sci. 2015;20(8):763–70.
72. Davy KP, Hall JE. Obesity and hypertension: two epidemics or one? Am J Physiol Regul Integr Comp Physiol. 2004;286:R803–13.
73. Thomas F, Bean K, Pannier B, Oppert J-M, Guize L, Benetos A. Cardiovascular mortality in overweight subjects. The key role of associated risk factors. Hypertension. 2005;46:654–9.
74. Olszanecka A, Dragan A, Kawecka-Jaszcz L, Czarnecka D. Influence of metabolic syndrome and its components on subclinical organ damage in hypertensive perimenopausal women. Adv Med Sci. 2014;59(2):232–9.
75. Ginsberg HN, MacCallum PR. The obesity, metabolic syndrome and type 2 diabetes mellitus pandemic: part I. Increased cardiovascular disease risk and the importance of atherogenic dyslipidemia in persons with the metabolic syndrome and type 2 diabetes mellitus. J Cardiometab Syndr. 2009;4(2):113–9.
76. Toker S, Rogowski O, Melamed S, Shirom A, Shapira I, Berliner S, Zeltser D. Association of components of the metabolic syndrome with the appearance of aggregated red blood cells in the peripheral blood. An unfavorable hemorheological finding. Diabetes Metab Res Rev. 2005;21:197–202.
77. Toalson P, Ahmed S, Hardy T, Kabinoff G. The metabolic syndrome in patients with severe mental illnesses. Prim Care Companion J Clin Psychiatry. 2004;6(4):152–8.
78. Nagahori M, Hyun SB, Totsuka T, Okamoto R, Kuwahara E, Takebayashi T. Prevalence of metabolic syndrome is comparable between inflammatory bowel disease patients and the general population. J Gastroenterol. 2010;45(10):1008–13.
79. Muntingh A DT, van der Feltz-Cornelis CM, van Marwijk HWJ, Spinhoven P, Penninx B WJH, van Balkom A JLM. Is the beck anxiety inventory a good tool to assess the severity of anxiety? A primary care study in the Netherlands study of depression and anxiety (NESDA). BMC Fam Pract 2011;12:66.
80. Tamashiro KL. Metabolic syndrome: links to social stress and socioeconomic status. Ann N Y Acad Sci. 2011;1231:46–55.
81. King AC, Bernardy NC, Hauner K. Stressful events, personality and mood disturbances: gender differences in alcoholics and problem drinkers. Addict Behav. 2003;28(1):171–87.
82. CIBIS-II Investigators and Committees. The cardiac insufficiency Bisoprolol study II (CIBIS-II): a randomised trial. Lancet. 1999;353(9146):9–13.
83. Sattar N, Preiss D, Murray HM, Buckley BM, Welsh P, de Craen AJM, et al. Statins and risk of incident diabetes: a collaborative meta-analysis of randomised statin trials. The Lancet. 2010;375(9716):735–42.
84. Onat A, Hergenc G, Keles T, Doğan Y, Türkmen S, Sansoy V. Sex differences in development of diabetes and cardiovascular disease on the way from obesity and metabolic syndrome. Metabolism. 2005;54(6):800–8.

17

Comprehensive user requirements engineering methodology for secure and interoperable health data exchange

Pantelis Natsiavas[1], Janne Rasmussen[2], Maja Voss-Knude[3], Kostas Votis[4], Luigi Coppolino[5], Paolo Campegiani[6], Isaac Cano[7], David Marí[8], Giuliana Faiella[9], Fabrizio Clemente[9], Marco Nalin[10], Evangelos Grivas[11], Oana Stan[12], Erol Gelenbe[13], Jos Dumortier[14], Jan Petersen[2], Dimitrios Tzovaras[4], Luigi Romano[5], Ioannis Komnios[15] and Vassilis Koutkias[1*]

Abstract

Background: Increased digitalization of healthcare comes along with the cost of cybercrime proliferation. This results to patients' and healthcare providers' skepticism to adopt Health Information Technologies (HIT). In Europe, this shortcoming hampers efficient cross-border health data exchange, which requires a holistic, secure and interoperable framework. This study aimed to provide the foundations for designing a secure and interoperable toolkit for cross-border health data exchange within the European Union (EU), conducted in the scope of the KONFIDO project. Particularly, we present our user requirements engineering methodology and the obtained results, driving the technical design of the KONFIDO toolkit.

Methods: Our methodology relied on four pillars: (a) a gap analysis study, reviewing a range of relevant projects/ initiatives, technologies as well as cybersecurity strategies for HIT interoperability and cybersecurity; (b) the definition of user scenarios with major focus on cross-border health data exchange in the three pilot countries of the project; (c) a user requirements elicitation phase containing a threat analysis of the business processes entailed in the user scenarios, and (d) surveying and discussing with key stakeholders, aiming to validate the obtained outcomes and identify barriers and facilitators for HIT adoption linked with cybersecurity and interoperability.

Results: According to the gap analysis outcomes, full adherence with information security standards is currently not universally met. Sustainability plans shall be defined for adapting existing/evolving frameworks to the state-of-the-art. Overall, lack of integration in a holistic security approach was clearly identified. For each user scenario, we concluded with a comprehensive workflow, highlighting challenges and open issues for their application in our pilot sites. The threat analysis resulted in a set of 30 user goals in total, documented in detail. Finally, indicative barriers of HIT acceptance include lack of awareness regarding HIT risks and legislations, lack of a security-oriented culture and management commitment, as well as usability constraints, while important facilitators concern the adoption of standards and current efforts for a common EU legislation framework.

Conclusions: Our study provides important insights to address secure and interoperable health data exchange, while our methodological framework constitutes a paradigm for investigating diverse cybersecurity-related risks in the health sector.

Keywords: Cybersecurity, Interoperability, Health information technologies (HIT), Digital health, Cross-border health data exchange, User requirements engineering, Gap analysis, Barriers and facilitators for HIT acceptance

* Correspondence: vkoutkias@certh.gr
[1]Institute of Applied Biosciences, Centre for Research & Technology Hellas, Thermi, Thessaloniki, Greece
Full list of author information is available at the end of the article

Background

Advances in Health Information Technologies (HIT) and digital health are transforming healthcare delivery. However, the constantly increasing digitalization and the inherent use of sensitive health data come along with the cost of cybercrime proliferation. Lack of adequate security measures result in patients' and healthcare providers' (HCPs) unwillingness to adopt HIT, as well as investors' skepticism to fund such activities. In the European context, as the number of citizens who travel across Europe for education, training, work and tourism constantly increases, the need for cross-border health data exchange becomes imperative. Especially, people suffering from chronic diseases are facing obstacles in travelling either within or outside their country of residence, due to the lack of an established, systematic and secure framework for data exchange among healthcare organizations across Europe.

KONFIDO is a European Union (EU) funded project [1], which aims to leverage novel approaches and cutting-edge technologies, such as homomorphic encryption [2], photonic Physical Unclonable Functions (p-PUF) [3], a Security Information and Event Management (SIEM) system [4], and blockchain-based auditing [5], in order to develop a holistic paradigm for secure, cross-border exchange, storage and overall handling of health data. It builds its solution upon existing/evolving European frameworks, such as OpenNCP (Open-source and reference version of the NCP software) [6], which is the open-source National Contact Point (NCP) software implementation of its predecessor project named epSOS (European Partners – Smart Open Services) [7], and eIDAS (electronic IDentification, Authentication and trust Services) [8], which stands for the EU regulation on electronic identification and trust services for electronic transactions in the internal market. An overview of the KONFIDO technical solution and its links with the abovementioned frameworks is presented in [9]. Overall, KONFIDO aims to advance the state-of-the-art of HIT along the four key dimensions of digital security, i.e. data preservation, data access and modification, data exchange, and interoperability and compliance. To this end, KONFIDO is organized in four complementary phases, namely, 'User requirements analysis; 'Design'; 'Technology development'; and 'Integration, testing and validation'. The current study focuses on the former phase.

As part of the "User requirements analysis" phase, we first reviewed and mapped applicable technical and legal frameworks as well as ethical and social norms at the European level with a major focus on the KONFIDO pilot-site countries (i.e. Denmark, Italy and Spain). This entailed a gap analysis study for interoperable and secure solutions at the systemic level. We then defined and analyzed user scenarios with major emphasis on cross-border health data exchange and, based on these, we conducted a user requirements elicitation phase starting from the definition of the underlying business processes and proceeding to the identification of respective assets, threats and, ultimately, high-level user goals. Equally important, we pursued intense interaction with the wider healthcare community, in order to validate the methods and the outcomes of our approach, aiming also to identify key barriers and facilitators for HIT solutions acceptance linked with cybersecurity. Overall, HIT acceptance in the clinical environment has been identified as a challenge and has been investigated (mostly focusing on Electronic Health Record (EHR) systems [10, 11]), using models based on psychology, sociology, and consumer behavior. To this end, we conducted a survey targeting all possible relevant stakeholders (i.e. HCPs, hospital staff at IT departments, industrial HIT stakeholders, and patients/citizens), as well as an end-user Workshop.

In this paper, we present the overall methodology concerning the user requirements engineering phase of KONFIDO as well as the obtained outcomes. We conclude by consolidating these outcomes in terms of recommendations for the KONFIDO technical design and we argue about the usefulness of the proposed methodological framework for developing secure and interoperable health data exchange IT solutions.

Methods

The overall methodological framework adopted for user requirements engineering focuses on four pillars (Fig. 1). The methodological pillars are provided in the left-side of Fig. 1, along with the targeted outcomes in the right-side, while the arrows linking pillars illustrate their interrelations. A description of each methodological pillar is provided in the respective subsections below.

Pillar 1: Gap analysis study

Generally, a gap analysis aims to identify "gaps", i.e. the qualitative or quantitative differences, between the *current* and the *target* state of the analyzed subject (e.g. product, process, organization, market, etc.). *Current state* corresponds to the analysis subject's present status (i.e. "where we are") and *target state* defines the desired condition where the analysis subject would satisfy some specific criteria or goals (i.e. "where we want to be"). Such an analysis typically requires the comparison of *current* and *target* state across a range of criteria. For the current study, the conducted gap analysis aimed to identify how well our analysis subjects satisfy a set of requirements regarding HIT cybersecurity and interoperability.

The gap analysis subjects included several relevant European initiatives, projects and their outcomes,

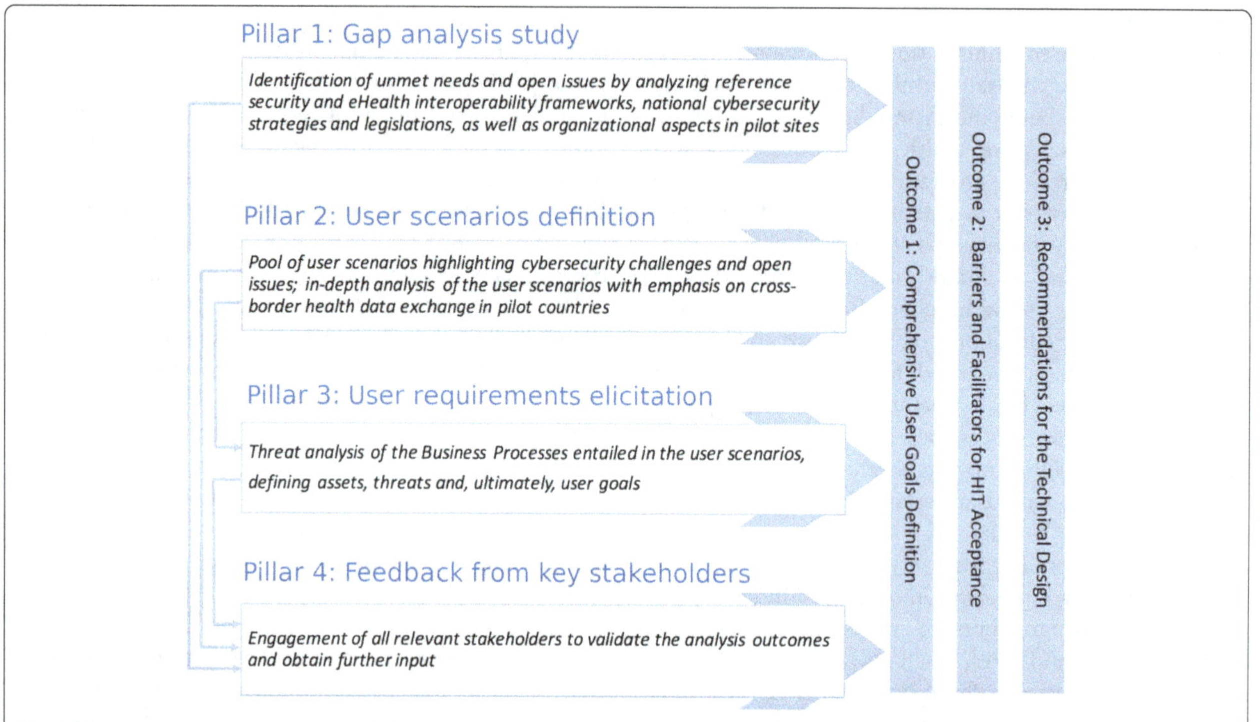

Fig. 1 The user requirements engineering framework: methodological pillars and main outcomes

technological artifacts as well as end-user perspectives and policy strategies across four thematic areas, i.e.:

- *HIT Interoperability Frameworks*: epSOS [7], Antilope [12], the Joint Action to Support the eHealth Network (JASeHN) [13] and SemanticHealthNet [14].
- *HIT Security Software Frameworks*: DECIPHER [15], OpenNCP and STORK 2.0 [16].
- *End-user perspectives across diverse settings in KONFIDO pilot countries*: Santobono Pausilipon Hospital (Italy), Odense University Hospital & Svendborg Hospital (Denmark), and Hospital Clínic Barcelona (Spain).
- *National cybersecurity strategies and reference reports*: Documents regarding the currently applied cybersecurity strategies in the pilot countries and relevant reports (e.g. regarding guidelines or best practices) primarily provided by the European Union Agency for Network and Information Security (ENISA) [17, 18].

The analysis was assigned to Working Groups (WG) per thematic area within the KONFIDO Consortium. The analysis subjects were examined by topic experts in each WG against a gap analysis template (provided in Additional file 1). This gap analysis template defined an explicit set of analysis criteria (a.k.a. *controls*), mostly based on the ISO/IEC 27k information security standards family [19]. In the scope of the presented study, the following ISO standards were employed: (a) ISO/IEC 27002 [20]; (b) ISO/IEC 27010 [21]; (c) ISO/IEC 27040 [22]; (d) ISO 27799 [23]; (e) ISO 22857 [24], and (f) ISO/IEC 25010 [25].

The template was organized on 11 clauses, defining the template's upper–level structure: *Security policy; Organizing information security; Asset management; Human resources security; Physical and environmental security; Communications and operations management; Access Control; Information systems acquisition, development and maintenance; Information security incident management; Business continuity management; Compliance,* and *Usability.* Instructions and relevant examples on how to use the template were given to the WGs. In addition, the respondents became aware that some questions contained in the template might not be relevant for their analysis, due to the specific scope and/or the varying information granularity of the considered analysis subjects. Finally, iterative teleconferences were conducted among WG members to discuss the plan, their progress, and finalize the results.

The gap analysis was mainly conducted via: (a) *Desk research,* by reviewing material regarding the analysis subject, e.g. project reports or deliverables, as well as papers published in scientific journals or conferences. (b) *Interviews / discussions with experts* related with the analysis subject (either directly involved in KONFIDO or not). The overall gap analysis methodology along with some preliminary results were presented in [26].

Pillar 2: User scenarios definition

Given the European dimension of KONFIDO, its user scenarios focus on cross-border health data exchange. In particular, two reference scenarios have been defined, the first focusing on cross-border services for a chronic patient, and the second elaborating on cross-border and cross-regional health data exchange, considering triage services in emergency situations. Several stakeholders have been taken into account in the scenarios' definition, e.g. public and private hospitals, HCPs with different roles and patients with diverse healthcare needs, as well as various technological artifacts (mHealth apps, telemonitoring services, EHRs, etc.). The aim was to address the heterogeneity of the domain, considering the three pilot countries of the project. The second scenario is described in Table 1 [27].

Besides the textual description of each user scenario, a workflow was defined (for its realization) and analyzed in detail.

Pillar 3: User requirements elicitation

The term "user requirements elicitation" can be ambiguous in the varying contexts of user requirements engineering. In the scope of this work, we defined it as the process of exploiting diverse information sources, in order to "*... discover the current project needs and agree upon its vision and goals*" [28]. Our overall approach aimed at specifying high-level *user goals* by first defining the related *business processes* (BPs), based on the methodology described in Park et al. [29]. User goals in turn are defined as *"abstract user requirements, not directly referring to specific technical solutions or components"*. They typically refer to specific user actors, while their definition facilitates early identification of possible conflicts between actors and, consequently, their timely resolution.

The identification of BPs was based on the actions contained in the textual description of each scenario, which is a well-established approach [30]. Typically, "*verbs correlate to operations which can be invoked by components or actors*" [31], in order to facilitate the specification of the system functionality. The user scenario presented in Table 1 is annotated based on the above rationale by highlighting in bold the key-phrases implying BPs. The identified BPs were then analyzed by conducting a *threat analysis*. Typically, this refers to the systematic process of identifying and evaluating spots of vulnerability for a facility, operation, or system, which is also applicable in the context of HIT [32, 33]. Our threat analysis process involved the following steps:

1. *Asset identification*; assets include anything worth to be protected and can be organized in the following indicative categories: *information*, *infrastructure* (physical infrastructure, software, etc.), *persons*, *business functions*.
2. *Threats identification*; threats are uncontrolled circumstances or actions, typically related with malicious people or factors out of control (e.g. weather, physical failures, etc.), which can obtain control of, damage or destroy an asset.

Table 1 The second reference scenario considered in KONFIDO

Phase 1: Milan
Anna is a 45-year-old university professor living in Milan (Lombardy Region), Italy. For the summer holidays, Anna and her daughter are planning a cruise to Barcelona, Spain. Anna suffers from Diabetes type 2, while her 6-year-old daughter Cristina has heart disease since she was born. Being a chronic patient, Anna has learnt how to live with her disease and to manage her daughter's health too, undertaking routine tasks such as **measuring** periodically Cristina's vital signs (e.g., blood pressure), **taking** medicines, or **performing** tasks like glucose measurements and insulin injections. Cristina was enrolled in the Regional Program called CReG (Chronic Related Groups) and together with her mother they use a tele-monitoring service. CReG is a program which delegates the care management of chronic patients to General Practitioners, supporting them in the prescription, monitoring and renewal of care plans. The hospital of Milan has equipped both Anna and Cristina with a tele-monitoring kit for **remote monitoring** of their health condition. The kit includes medical devices and a gateway which sends the measured vital signs to the respective Service Center in Milan.
Phase 2: Naples
Travelling by car for a conference in Naples (Campania Region) with her husband and their daughter, Anna experiences a quite serious car accident and Cristina has serious wounds. The healthcare authorities in Naples, where the accident takes place, offer an innovative telemedicine application empowered by KONFIDO. Particularly, using the national eID technology that KONFIDO recognizes and handles properly, the retrieval of all the information needed to intervene while in the ambulance (patient identification, clinical details, immunization details, and usual therapy) is made possible. Specifically, Cristina's data are retrieved from the EHR system of the healthcare authorities in the Lombardy Region.
Using the telemedicine application and a tablet, Cristina's personal data (including pictures of her wounds) are **transmitted** through the mobile network to the emergency department by paramedics. Using KONFIDO technologies, paramedics can safely **authenticate** her and the encrypted transmission of her medical data is conducted. The application **monitors** the child, **suggests** actions, possibly re-routes the ambulance, and makes sure that everything is ready upon arrival at the hospital with the aim to speed-up the triage process and reinforce the preparedness levels.
Phase 3: Barcelona
After a few weeks, Cristina is discharged from the hospital in Naples and, given her risky heart condition, the doctor in Milan **is immediately informed** by the hospital in Naples that anti-coagulant therapy had to be interrupted. Consequently, the doctor decides to adjust the therapy and **review the monitoring plan**. Cristina and Anna can realize their vacation plans in Spain using the tele-monitoring service.
Anna and Cristina know that in case of problems, any hospital they might have to visit in Barcelona will **have access** to their patient summaries in Italy. During the journey, Anna faints and she is transferred to the nearest hospital in Barcelona to check her health condition. While the Spanish doctor is accessing Anna's patient summary, a cyberattack tries to compromise the data exchange. Specifically, an international hacker group, using a system vulnerability, attacks and takes control of the NCP in the Spanish OpenNCP deployment. Thanks to KONFIDO security mechanisms, Anna's data integrity and confidentiality is protected against the cyberattack and the doctor can make a diagnosis and provide the medical treatment.

Terms highlighted in bold indicate verbs or phrases that have been used to identify the respective BPs in the scenario

Threats may refer to technical, functional, legal, personal and political aspects. We focused on technical threats, which were classified based on the STRIDE model [34]:

(a) ***Spoofing***: refers to gaining access to a system by using a false identity.
(b) ***Tampering***: refers to the unauthorized modification of data.
(c) ***Repudiation***: refers to the denial of specific actions or transactions on the user's behalf (legitimate or not).
(d) ***Information disclosure***: refers to exposure of private or sensitive data.
(e) ***Denial of service (DoS)***: refers to the process of making a system/application unavailable.
(f) ***Elevation of privilege***: refers to gaining access to resources by self-assigning more privileges.

The threat analysis results were combined with best practices and outcomes produced by relevant projects/initiatives, in order to define the user goals per actor. In particular, we took into account: (a) the ISO/IEC 27k family of standards; (b) outcomes of the gap analysis, the end-user survey and Workshop conducted in the scope of the project, as described below; (c) reports from relevant EU projects and initiatives, as well as (d) the recently enforced into practice General Data Protection Regulation (GDPR) [35], which aims to align data privacy laws among EU Member States.

We defined two types of user goals, i.e. *functional* and *non-functional*, corresponding to functional and non-functional requirements, respectively. Functional goals were based on the user scenarios, while the identified threats per BP were combined with other sources of information to pinpoint non-functional goals.

Aiming to consolidate and interpret the identified user goals, a meta-analysis was conducted based on a visual analytics approach. The aim was to illustrate the dependencies among the identified user goals and the respective information sources, BPs, assets and threats, as well as the strongest links among them.

Pillar 4: Feedback from key stakeholders

An end-user engagement strategy was employed to validate the prior methodological pillars and their outcomes, and identify key barriers and facilitators for HIT adoption linked with security and interoperability. In particular, an online, anonymous and confidential survey as well as a Workshop with the participation of key stakeholders were conducted. The goal of the survey was two-fold: (a) to identify the currently applied practices regarding security and interoperability on existing HIT infrastructures for healthcare organizations of varying size and nature (e.g. private and public), and (b) to obtain insights regarding patient/citizen awareness on cybersecurity risks entailed in cross-border health data exchange and document opinions about exchanging health data with HCPs or HIT service providers. Thus, we discriminated two groups of participants in the survey: (a) *HCPs and HIT stakeholders across Europe*, and (b) *patients/citizens*.

The overall survey design was built upon key principles of human psychology [36], while it contained different content per group. Several sources were used for designing the respective questionnaires, such as relevant standards, surveys conducted by other organizations, reports, scientific papers, etc. The questionnaire structures for both participant groups are provided in Additional files 2 and 3, respectively.

For the first group, personal invitations were sent, in order to obtain high-quality, expert feedback. The survey questions for this group were structured as follows:

1. *Organization profile*: referred to the organization's size and structure (e.g. number of employees, activities in the domain, etc.).
2. *Security facts*: focused on security incidents occurred in the organization, targeting IT stuff and managers.
3. *Security policy*: referred to policies applied in the organization (e.g. existence of security and risk management policies, use of encryption, etc.).
4. *Security incident management*: concerned handling security breaches in a technical level, targeting technical stuff and managers.
5. *Barriers and facilitators*: aimed to identify key issues that facilitate or discourage the adoption of cybersecurity best practices.
6. *Personal view*: focused on awareness (e.g. use of publicly available cloud storage services, importance of security in everyday work, etc.) and satisfaction regarding the current cybersecurity state.

Contrary to the survey targeting the first group, the survey for the second group was circulated publicly by using patient forums, mailing lists, and social media. It contained the following sections:

1. *Awareness regarding Information Technology risks*: Focused on identifying the level of the participants' awareness regarding the risks entailed in using HIT.
2. *Legislation*: Aimed to identify the patients'/citizens' familiarity with relevant legislation artifacts.
3. *Cross-border medical treatment*: Aimed to provide insights on whether the participant was medically treated or hospitalized abroad.

4. *Cross-border medical data exchange*: Focused on the participants' opinion regarding the need for cross-border health data exchange.
5. *Barriers and facilitators*: Aimed to identify issues that facilitate or discourage cross-border health data exchange from a patient's/citizen's viewpoint.
6. *Demographics*: Contained key information about the participant, in order to facilitate the statistical analysis of the obtained data.

The end-user Workshop attracted more than 30 stakeholders from the HIT and healthcare sectors across Europe; it was organized to encourage open discussion, exploring the diverse issues concerning cross-border health data exchange. Personal invitations were sent to candidate participants from diverse organizations (healthcare, standards developing organizations, HIT associations, regional healthcare authorities, privacy authorities, research/academia, etc.), aiming to obtain input from the widest possible spectrum of stakeholders composing the European HIT ecosystem. The methodological overview along with preliminary outcomes as regards barriers and facilitators for HIT acceptance were presented in [37].

Results

In this section, we present the main outcomes of the employed methodology (Fig. 1). Given the wide range of the activities carried-out in the scope of this work, we concentrate on the key parts of the findings.

Outcome 1: Comprehensive user requirements definition

The detailed analysis of the user scenarios highlighted the challenges and the open issues of applying them in real-world settings, taking into account the context of the project's pilot sites. Figure 2 depicts a part of the workflow corresponding to the user scenario presented in Table 1, highlighting actions considered in the senario, the entailed challenges and open issues, as well as scenario background information.

The user scenarios analysis resulted in a set of BPs (listed in Table 2). In order to illustrate the user goals definition process, we present the analysis of BP2: "Access

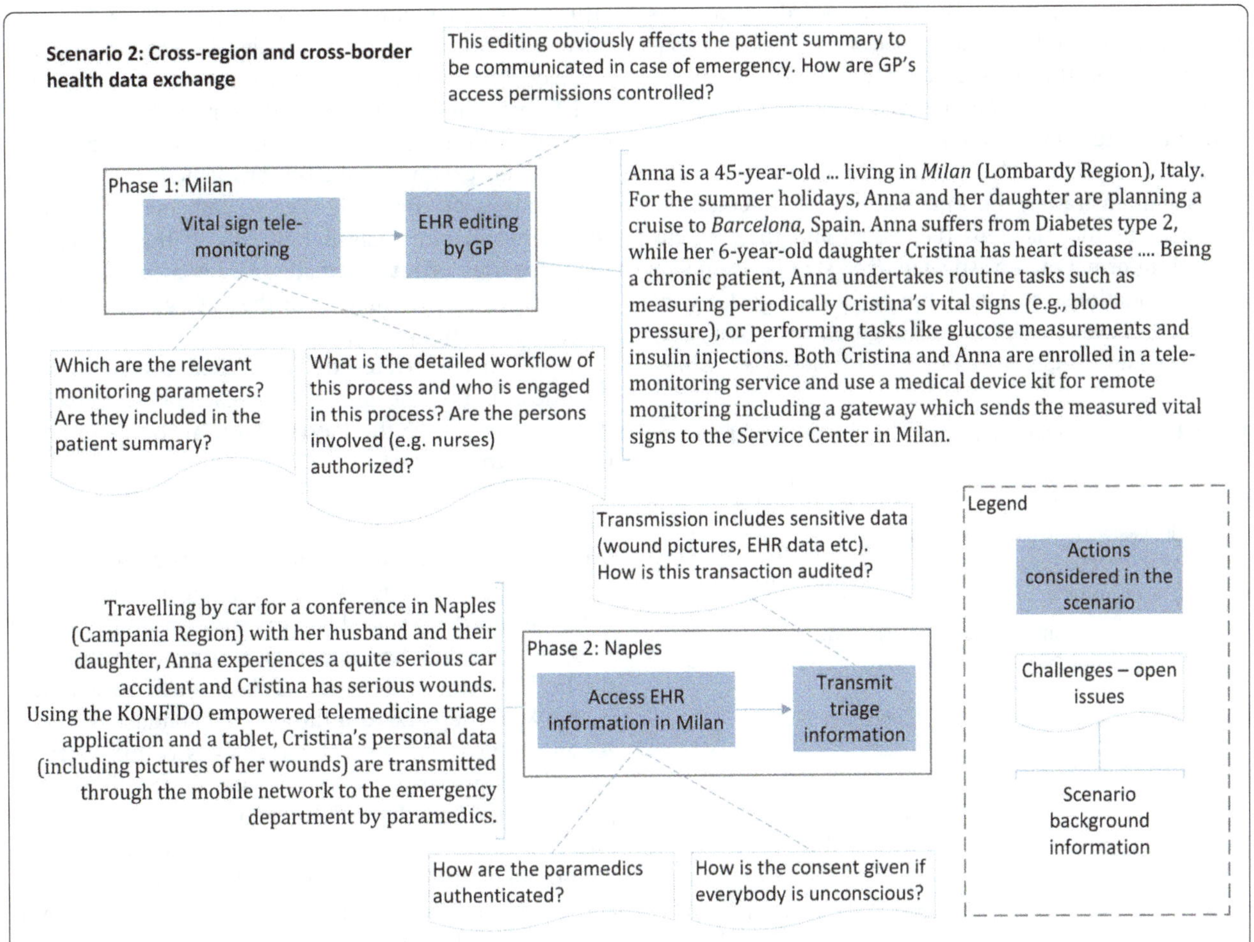

Fig. 2 Partial view of the workflow corresponding to the user scenario described in Table 1

Table 2 Business processes identified from the user scenarios

ID	Business process	Description
BP1	Grant access to own Medical Record	A patient in the visiting country grants the foreign HCP access to his/her medical record to facilitate treatment.
BP2	Access the medical record of a foreign patient	The HCP accesses a foreign patient's medical record, e.g. his/her medical history summary, medication treatment plan, diagnosis and relevant lab examination results.
BP3	User authentication using the national eID infrastructure	The user is being authenticated via his/her nationally-issued eID.
BP4	Transmitting data for remote monitoring	The user transmits data using a telemonitoring service.
BP5	Accessing the patient's medical record while transferred via an ambulance	Paramedics retrieve data from the patient's medical record.
BP6	Exchanging triage information, while the patient is transferred to the hospital via an ambulance	Paramedics transmit triage data to the respective hospital, e.g. wound pictures. The application transmits patient data in the ambulance and may provide guidance to the paramedics.
BP7	Exchange of medical information between HCPs	HCPs exchange medical information directly, e.g. in the case of a medication safety issue, and notify the treating physician accordingly. This BP refers to an active way of communication and not to keeping notes in the patient's medical record.

the medical record of a foreign patient", demonstrating this way indicative results in each step of the analysis (Table 3 depicts the assets and Table 4 the identified threats for BP2, respectively).

These threats were analyzed, taking also into account further information sources, e.g. ISO standards, guidelines produced by other European projects, etc. Based on our analysis, a set of 30 user goals were defined in total (Tables 5 and 6 demonstrate two example goals associated with BP2).

Aiming to further analyze the identified user goals, we conducted a meta-analysis using visual analytics. Diagrams demonstrating the link among the outcomes of intermediate analysis steps (i.e. assets and threats), the original information investigated (i.e. standards, policy recommendations, etc.) and the final user goals, were produced. This visualization highlighted the complexity of these links for specific intermediate outcomes, information sources and user goals, and gave a broader overview concerning the overall contribution in the user goals' definition by grouping the intermediate analysis steps and the original information investigated according to their category. Figure 3 provides an indicative example visualization, depicting a subset of the links among information sources (e.g. standards, BPs, reports on the left side of the figure), intermediate outcomes (assets and threats, in the middle) and user goals G7, G8 and G12 (on the right side of the figure). Respectively, Fig. 4 provides an example visualization depicting the overall contribution of the categories of information sources considered in our analysis (left side of the figure) and the categories of intermediate analysis steps (i.e. assets and threats, in the middle) in the user goals definition (right side of the figure).

Table 3 Assets identified for BP2: "Access the medical record of a foreign patient"

ID	Description	Category	Comments
A1	Medical record information	Information	The main asset to be protected.
A2	HCP credentials	Information	e.g. usernames, passwords etc.
A3	HCP authentication means	Infrastructure	e.g. eID card
A4	Intention of accessing medical record	Information	The intention of accessing a patient's medical record is crucial. On the one hand, it could imply an attack attempt and, in this case, the medical record owner should be notified. On the other hand, it should be protected as it clearly implies that the doctor intends to conduct a medical transaction, and this could contain sensitive information.

Table 7 demonstrates the quantified contribution of the most important information categories. Evidently, ISO standards were the most influential source of information in this respect.

Outcome 2: Barriers and facilitators for HIT acceptance

The gap analysis study provided the initial input for this outcome, since it revealed barriers and constraints as well as open issues and challenges for information security in the health sector. This input has been further elaborated in the Workshop and also through the conducted survey. As an example, we present the analysis of the everyday operational processes applied in one of the KONFIDO pilot sites, the Santobono Pausilipon Hospital (PAUSIL) in Naples, Italy. PAUSIL is a specialized pediatric hospital with more than 1000 employees and it demonstrated high adherence to the controls contained in the gap analysis template and the respective underlying standards. Nevertheless, some indicative gaps were identified (Table 8).

Table 4 Threats identified for BP2: "Access the medical record of a foreign patient"

ID	Type	Assets	Malicious actors	Description/Example scenario
T1	Spoofing	All information assets	Other actors without a clear role in the BP	An external actor could pretend to be legitimate, in order to get the HCP credentials and use them to access information (e.g. patient's medical record), on behalf of the HCP.
T2	Tampering	All information assets	Other actors without a clear role in the BP	A malicious user could (perhaps combined with a spoofing attack) modify the information assets (e.g. the patient's medical record or the HCP's credentials) in a malicious way for social, financial or for personal reasons.
T3	Repudiation	All information assets	HCPs	Deny accessing medical information to avoid legal consequences upon an HCP (e.g. in a case of a medical error).
T4	Information disclosure	All information assets	HCPs and other actors without a clear role in the BP	An HCP could provide access to a patient's medical record, aiming at patient's financial or personal harm or for personal financial benefit.
T5	Denial of Service	Medical record information	Other actors without a clear role in the BP	Hinders access to the respective services, aiming to cause damage to the patient or the healthcare organization providing the medical services.
T6	Privilege Elevation	Medical record information	Other actors without a clear role in the BP	Assign privileges to one or multiple medical records aiming at exploiting or damaging data, or alternatively aiming at patients' financial or personal harm.
T7	Physical stealing	Physical authentication means	Other actors without a clear role in the BP	Stealing the eID card of the HCP could facilitate spoofing, information disclosure and privilege elevation.

Overall, the main issues identified through the gap analysis for the considered analysis subjects can be summarized as follows:

1. Full adherence to the targets set by international standards for information security is currently not universally met. For example, the processes applied in the considered hospitals demonstrated high adherence with the controls proposed by information security standards. However, compliance with standards was not evident in the review of the considered interoperability and software security frameworks.
2. The analysis of national cybersecurity strategies and reference reports highlighted the difficulty in balancing between a high-level document and actionable information. As a consequence, this material can be ambiguous for users and, therefore, the adherence is partly incentivised and arbitrarily localized.
3. As technology evolves at rapid pace, cybersecurity artifacts can quickly become outdated. A sustainability plan for the employed technologies should be undertaken, in order to enhance user trust. In some cases, legacy or vulnerable technologies were identified in the investigated technology frameworks.
4. Lack of integration towards a holistic security approach was clearly identified. While, various interesting technologies are being developed in parallel, it seems that each project focuses on a specific technological aspect and integration is not taken into account to leverage cybersecurity of HIT as a whole.

The survey focusing on selected stakeholders, i.e. HIT experts, managers, HCPs and health IT stuff working in hospitals, resulted in 35 submissions. The open survey targeting patients/citizens attracted 437 submissions. The analysis of the submitted responses led to the identification of barriers and facilitators regarding HIT acceptance. For example, barrier B1: *"Lack of awareness regarding information technology risks"* was identified due to the analysis of the responses to the questions *"Have you ever thought about your privacy regarding your health data?"*

Table 5 Goal 11: "Prevent tampering attacks"

G11	Prevent tampering attacks
Goal Type	Non-functional
Actor(s)	Other actors without a clear role in the BP
Reference(s)	BP2
Description	As someone could (perhaps combined with a spoofing attack) modify the information assets (e.g. the patient's medical record or the HCP's credentials) in a malicious way for social, financial or personal reasons, KONFIDO should be able to prevent such kind of malicious actions.

Table 6 Goal 12: "Prevent ambiguity issues"

G12	Prevent ambiguity issues
Goal Type	Functional
Actor(s)	HCP, Patient
Reference(s)	BP1, BP2, JASeHN deliverable D5.3 (section IV)
Description	Semantic ambiguity can be a burden in cross-border health data exchange. Referencing to diseases and medication might be confusing in clinical practice due to different drug brand names, clinical protocols/procedures, etc. KONFIDO should promote semantic interoperability in order to minimize these risks.

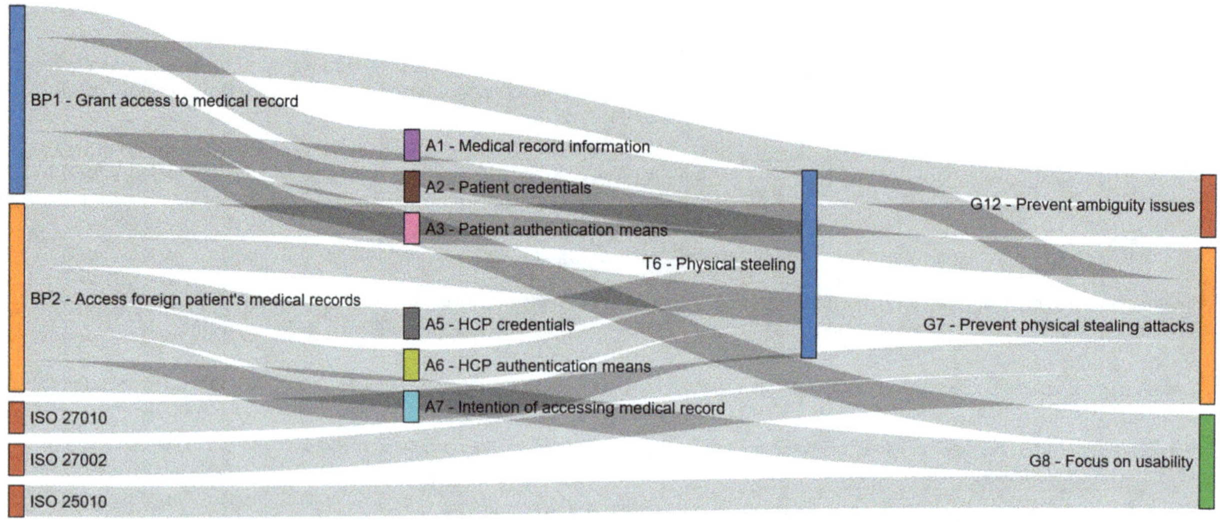

Fig. 3 Sankey diagram illustrating an indicative view of links among specific information sources considered in the analysis

(depicted in Fig. 5) and *"Do you feel well-informed regarding possible health data security risks?"* (depicted in Fig. 6), provided by the patients/citizens group.

As another example, facilitator F6: *"Wide recognition of the need for a security policy based on standards"* was partly identified due to the responses to the question *"Please rank the importance of the issues that you think might facilitate the adoption of security-oriented best practices"* provided by the selected stakeholders group (Fig. 7). Similarly, answers to question *"Please rank the following barriers, hindering acceptance of cross-border health data exchange"* provided by the patients/citizens group (Fig. 8) were linked with barrier B2: *"Lack of end-user confidence on their overall electronic health data handling"*.

Overall, the analysis of the survey responses and the outcomes of the Workshop led to the identification of a comprehensive set of barriers and facilitators regarding HIT acceptance (shown in Tables 9 and 10, respectively). The barriers identified in Table 9 are grouped with respect to awareness, interoperability, legislation, trust, and usability.

Outcome 3: Recommendations for the technical design

Based on the outcomes from all methodological pillars (Fig. 1), we concluded with a list of recommendations for the design phase of the KONFIDO toolkit. Notably, not all the produced recommendations concern technical aspects that can be overcome in the context of KONFIDO. Some of them are quite generic, exceeding the KONFIDO scope.

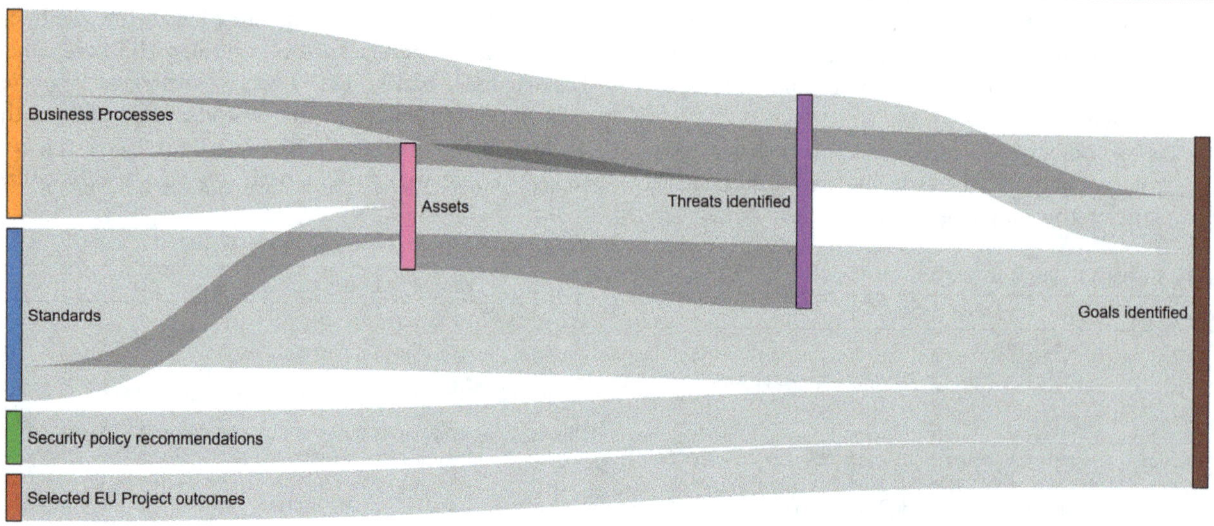

Fig. 4 Sankey diagram illustrating the overall contribution of the categories of information sources considered in the analysis for goal definition

Table 7 Origin of user goals with respect to the information asset categories considered in our meta-analysis

Original source category	Percentage of goals referring to the category
Standards	29%
Business Processes	24%
Threats	13%

Nevertheless, since these can be useful for the designers of cybersecurity tools in the health domain, we cite below the full list of recommendations:

R1. Strive for high adherence to standards as this reinforces end-users' trust in HIT.
R2. Leverage existing technical frameworks of the domain (in the European context, e.g. OpenNCP and eIDAS), but also follow a flexible design to address technical dependencies to the extent possible.
R3. Implement state-of-the-art cybersecurity technologies and measures, while ensuring sustainability of the technical solutions.
R4. Consider how and where consent is registered as well as accessed by patients and HCPs.
R5. Adopt a clear and comprehensive data handling scheme, in order to facilitate its understanding (for both patients and HCPs).
R6. Usability should be a first-class priority in cybersecurity technical developments, given that this constitutes a key acceptance factor for the end-users.
R7. Implementation details should target the three pilot countries as there are too many open issues to plan and conclude in the development of an EU-wide robust technical solution. A prototype toolkit targeting the three pilot countries can be used as an example for the future development of an EU-wide solution.
R8. Carefully take into account the diversity of organizational and information workflows applied in healthcare organizations, and adapt the technical design accordingly.
R9. Comply with all applicable laws and regulations in the involved regions and countries, but also with EU regulations related to HIT. At the same time, be adaptable to prominent changes regarding legal issues and take into account that legislation is not aligned among EU Member States.
R10. The lack of budget to address security aspects by healthcare organizations dictates that new cybersecurity technologies shall be cost-effective, contributing to practical solutions.

Discussion

Principal results

The current study provided a comprehensive set of user requirements and a set of barriers and facilitators for HIT acceptance associated with the design of secure and interoperable HIT, concluding with recommendations for the technical design phase of cybersecurity solutions focusing on health data exchange and the KONFIDO toolkit in particular.

According to the gap analysis, full adherence with information security standards is currently not universally met. In view of the rapid pace of cybersecurity technologies, sustainability plans shall be defined for adapting existing/evolving frameworks to the state-of-the-art. Overall, lack of integration in a holistic security approach was clearly identified. For each user scenario, a comprehensive workflow has been defined, highlighting challenges and open issues for their application in our pilot sites. The threat analysis resulted in a set of 30, high-level user goals in total, which were documented in detail, while links among our information sources and assets, threats and goals were identified as part of a meta-analysis. The survey and the Workshop with key stakeholders validated the above-

Table 8 Indicative gaps identified in the PAUSIL hospital

Gap analysis template clause	Gap analysis objective	Question/security control	Current status and gap mitigation
Security Policy	Information security policy	Does the analysis subject facilitate or promote the idea of information security policy document?	A formal information security policy document does not yet exist; however, PAUSIL is planning to introduce operational procedures and policies regarding security.
Physical and environmental security	Secure areas	Does the analysis subject facilitate or promote protecting against external and environmental threats?	Protection against external and environmental threats is not centrally documented/planned.
Usability	Effectiveness	Does the analysis subject facilitate or promote the operability regarding the respective security aspects?	The process of changing user passwords could be improved in terms of usability.
Communications and operations management	Media handling	Does the analysis subject facilitate or promote management of removable media?	No formal procedures are enforced for the management of removable media

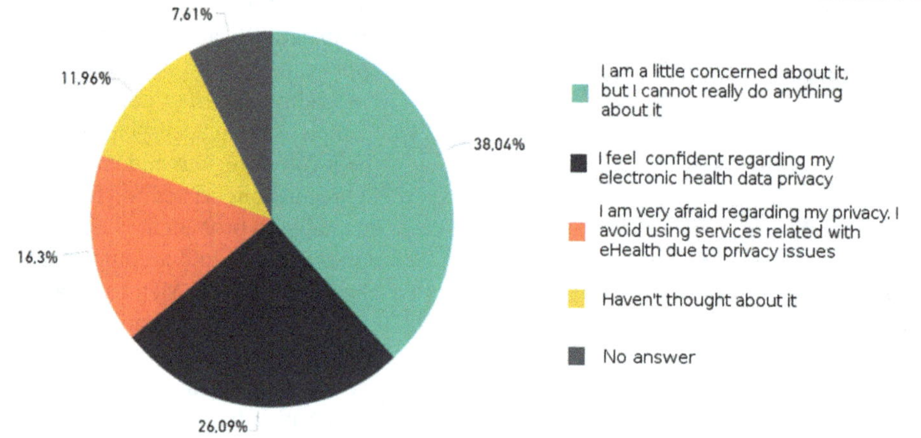

Fig. 5 Answers to question "Have you ever thought about your privacy regarding your health data?"

mentioned outcomes. Indicative barriers of HIT acceptance include lack of awareness regarding HIT risks and legislations, lack of a security-oriented culture as well as usability constraints, while important facilitators concern the adoption of standards and the efforts to establish a common legislation framework across EU. To this end, GDPR is a significant step forward which will certainly affect the management of patient data and the design of HIT systems. However, its detailed analysis exceeds the scope of our user requirements engineering methodology and, therefore, GDPR is not further elaborated in this paper.

The overall outcomes obtained from the presented user requirements engineering methodology were consolidated as recommendations for the design of cybersecurity solutions. Despite the fact that some of these recommendations do not concern technical aspects that can be overcome in the context of KONFIDO, we stress their importance, as they can provide significant insights for the design and development of cybersecurity solutions in the healthcare domain at large.

Limitations

As our study relies on multiple methodological steps, various limitations per step can be identified. In particular, the gap analysis study entails the subjectivity in both the obtained responses and the interpretation of the analysis subjects. As a mitigation action, we extensively discussed and tried to clarify cases of vague/unclear input across the respective WGs. When necessary, we contacted the producers of the analysis subjects (e.g. consortia of the considered projects) for clarifications. The employed gap analysis framework (template) did not specifically address cross-border data exchange, storage and management, which is the main objective of our project. In addition, while relying on ISO standards and having an adequate level of detail concerning information security, the employed gap analysis template might not cover all possible conditions. Nevertheless, we believe that potential missing aspects will be identified and addressed as the technical development evolves.

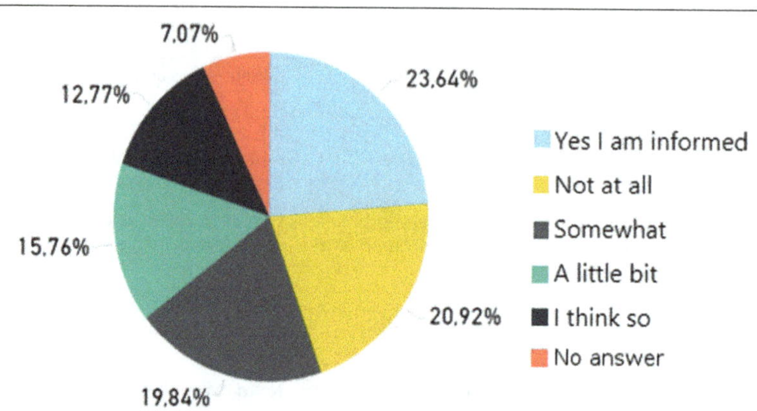

Fig. 6 Answers to question "Do you feel well-informed regarding possible health data security risks?"

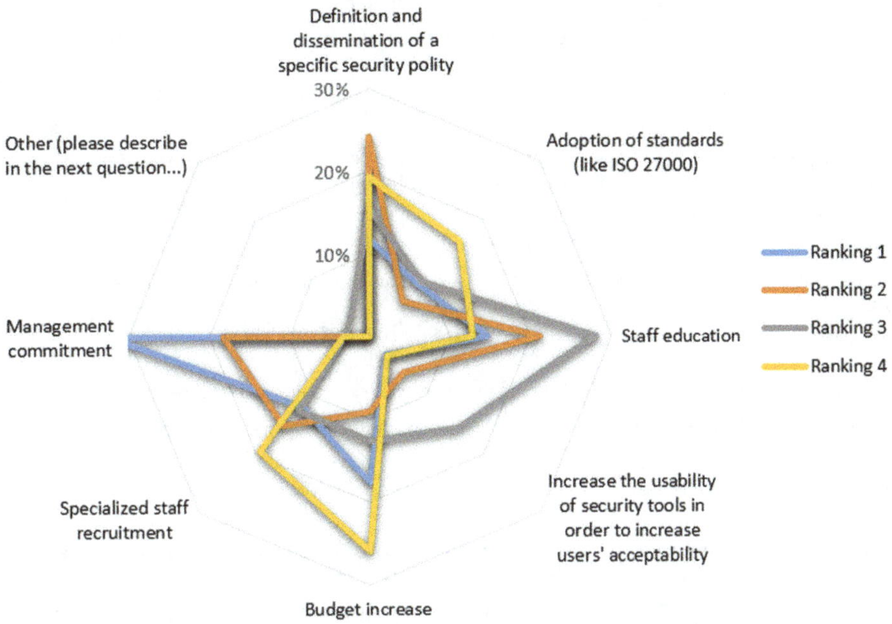

Fig. 7 Answers to question "Please rank the importance of the issues that you think might facilitate the adoption of security-oriented best practices" (for readability, only the most popular responses are presented)

The user scenarios were driven by the current setting of the KONFIDO pilot sites. Given the project setup, the pilot studies for assessing the KONFIDO toolkit will be conducted in three European countries. Thus, it is possible that our analysis missed cybersecurity-related aspects that are applicable in other European countries. In order to overcome this limitation, the conducted end-user survey targeted a broad audience, aiming to obtain input from the widest possible spectrum of stakeholders composing the European eHealth ecosystem.

Overall, as the study of other HIT ecosystems (e.g. the case of exchanging health data among different hospitals in US) is out of the current work's scope, the European focus of the study can be considered as a limitation per se. Nevertheless, the heterogeneity which is met across the different national healthcare systems in Europe constitutes

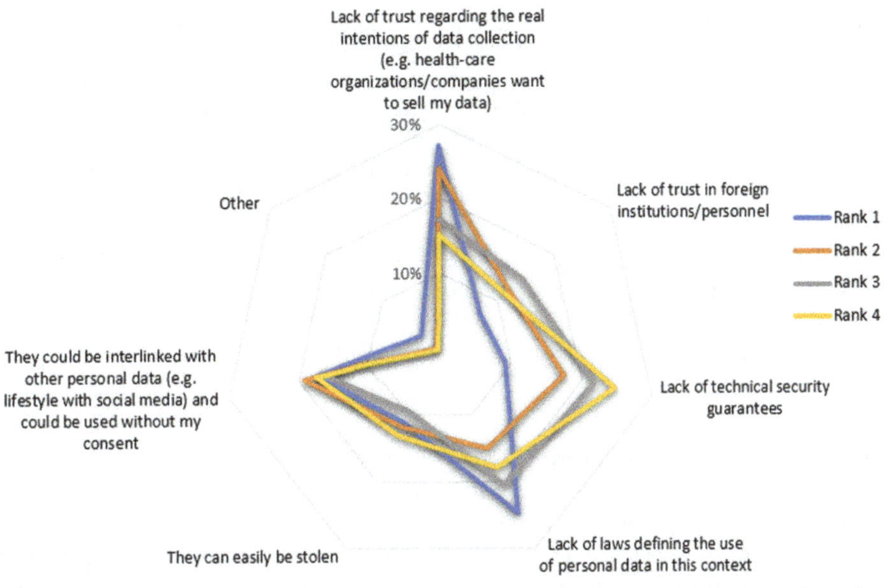

Fig. 8 Answers to question "Please rank the following barriers, hindering acceptance of cross-border health data exchange"

Table 9 Barriers for HIT acceptance linked with cybersecurity and interoperability

ID	Description	Expected impact on technical design and/or the overall KONFIDO project activities	Category
B1	Lack of awareness regarding information technology risks	Need to reinforce awareness on cybersecurity risks associated with healthcare delivery.	Awareness
B2	Lack of end-user confidence on their overall electronic health data handling	The technical design shall account for a comprehensive and transparent data handling scheme.	Trust
B3	Lack of trust to private companies providing HIT services	The solution should focus on using infrastructure in the most transparent way possible.	Trust
B4	Lack of interest regarding the "Terms and Conditions" for using HIT services	▪ Need to make "Terms and Conditions" more comprehensive for all users. ▪ Need to support the implementation of a comprehensive and transparent data handling scheme.	Trust
B5	Inadequate level of legislation awareness	Need to promote awareness on legislation aspects.	Awareness
B6	Lack of perceived effectiveness of legislation by end-users	Need to explain and illustrate the effectiveness of legislation to end-users.	Trust
B7	Lack of clear and transparent consent processes currently applied	Need to design a comprehensive consent mechanism.	Trust
B8	Legislation not aligned among EU Member States	Need to track ongoing legislation initiatives and adapt the technical design accordingly.	Legislation
B9	Immaturity of existing frameworks	Need to reduce strong dependencies with such frameworks to the extent possible.	Usability
B10	Partial lack of management commitment	Need to raise awareness on cybersecurity risks associated with healthcare delivery.	Awareness
B11	Lack of a cybersecurity-oriented culture in everyday operations	Need to raise awareness on the cybersecurity risks associated with healthcare delivery.	Awareness
B12	Lack of budget	Need to raise awareness on the impact of cybersecurity incidents and the economic burden that these may entail.	Awareness
B13	Usability reduced due to IT security measures	Need to prioritize usability in the technical design process.	Usability
B14	Inadequate use of established cybersecurity mechanisms (e.g. active directory, intrusion detection systems, etc.)	Need to promote the use and added value of novel/standard cybersecurity mechanisms.	Awareness
B15	Diversity of information workflows among organizations	Need to contextualize the technical design, in order to accommodate the requirements of local healthcare delivery processes and therefore increase end-user acceptance through enhanced usability.	Usability
B16	Free-text content in different languages	Need to employ reference medical terminologies/encodings to address interoperability.	Interoperability
B17	Legislation not aligned among EU Member States	Need to follow ongoing legislation initiatives and adapt the design according to EU directives.	Legislation
B18	Legal issues not clarified (e.g. data ownership, liability etc.)	Focus on provenance and auditing mechanisms, in order to clarify details if/when needed and, therefore, increase trust on the overall data exchange process.	Legislation
B19	Lack of inter-organizational trust	Need to promote robust and transparent cybersecurity measures while illustrating the added value of health data sharing (e.g. considering patient safety, quality of care, etc.).	Trust
B20	Complexity of consent process	Need to design a comprehensive consent mechanism for patients.	Usability
B21	Lack of available IT expertise in organizations	Need to raise awareness about the required personnel to address cybersecurity risks in organizations delivering healthcare services.	Awareness
B22	Data exchange agreement's complexity	Need to establish data exchange agreements compliant with legal norms.	Usability

a unique characteristic that is worth investigating. Our study outcomes could also be generalized and exploited in the context of exchanging data in other contexts, e.g. with other countries outside EU. For example, the Trillium-II project [38], which focuses on EU-US cooperation and particularly on exchanging patient summary data, could find our outcomes useful both regarding barriers, facilitators and end-user goals, as well as our technical advances. Raising awareness about cybersecurity for health data exchange requires intensive synergies, in order to build the necessary cybersecurity-oriented culture and address the respective barriers that were identified in our study.

Table 10 Facilitators for HIT acceptance linked with cybersecurity and interoperability

ID	Description	Expected impact on technical design and/or the overall KONFIDO project activities
F1	The need for HIT services and applications tends to overcome the insecurity regarding personal data misuse	It confirms the need for solutions that provide added value in real-world healthcare settings, while still promoting a holistic security approach.
F2	End-users support cross-border data exchange (even for research)	It confirms the value of the KONFIDO key concepts. Does not affect design decisions.
F3	Common legislation activities between EU Member States	GDPR and other initiatives will form the legal base for the solution and guide the respective design decisions (e.g. on the consent process).
F4	Technical EU initiatives are currently ongoing	The design will create a liaison with and build upon existing/evolving frameworks in Europe (epSOS, OpenNCP, eIDAS).
F5	Standards already established and widely accepted	The design and implementation will follow security standards, such as those from ISO/IEC 27k.
F6	Wide recognition of the need for a security policy based on standards	The technical solution should be based on widely-accepted standards and therefore implicitly increasing compatibility with standard based security policies.
F7	Exchange of data between organizations is based on agreements following GDPR	The design shall take GDPR into account wherever applicable (e.g. in the design of the consent process).
F8	Common mechanism of eID currently built (eIDAS)	The design of the solution shall be based on eIDAS, which is expected to be the de-facto standard among EU Member States.
F9	Cloud services, compatible with medical data exchange legislation	KONFIDO will be able to use cloud infrastructure being compatible with the respective legislation.
F10	Credible network services available	Facilitate the engagement in high mobility scenarios.

Comparison with prior work

To the best of our knowledge, this is the first systematic study presenting and applying a comprehensive, user requirements engineering methodology for the design of secure and interoperable HIT. Our methodology included a broad range of activities, starting from a gap analysis study which reviewed a wide range of relevant projects/initiatives, technological artifacts as well as end-user organizations' policies and national cybersecurity strategies. User scenarios have been defined and analyzed in detail, focusing on three pilot sites and cross-border health data exchange. The respective user requirements elicitation phase containing a threat analysis of the business processes entailed in the user scenarios, defined assets, threats and, ultimately, high-level user goals. Finally, an end-user survey and a Workshop with the participation of diverse stakeholders validated the obtained outcomes of the previous steps and identified key barriers and facilitators for HIT adoption linked with cybersecurity. Overall, the presented methodology is aligned with best practices [39] and established methods in the domain of requirements engineering for digital health, with respect to requirements elicitation and validation [40], as well as security requirements identification [41].

Conclusion

This study enabled us to define a comprehensive set of user requirements, a set of barriers and facilitators for HIT acceptance and, ultimately, a set of recommendations for designing a toolkit for secure and interoperable health data exchange in Europe. We argue that our results provide important insights to the domain, while our methodological framework constitutes a paradigm that can be reused for investigating other kinds of cybersecurity-related risks in the health sector. Equally important, the identified barriers and facilitators for HIT acceptance may constitute a useful guide for HIT stakeholders in reinforcing the adoption of their solutions by the targeted end-users (i.e. HCPs and patients/citizens).

Abbreviations

BP: Business Process; EHR: Electronic Health Record; eID: electronic IDentification; eIDAS: electronic IDentification, Authentication and trust Services; ENISA: European Union Agency for Network and Information Security; epSOS: European Partners – Smart Open Services; EU: European Union; GDPR: General Data Protection Regulation; HIT: Health Information Technologies; HCP: Healthcare Provider; IEC: International Electrotechnical Commission; ISO: International Organization for Standardization; ISO/IEC 27k: The ISO/IEC 27000 suite of standards; IT: Information Technology; JASeHN: Joint Action to Support the eHealth Network; mHealth: Mobile Health; NCP: National Contact Point; OpenNCP: Open-source and reference version of the NCP software; p-PUF: photonic Physical Unclonable Functions; SIEM: Security Information and Event Management; SQuaRE: Systems and software Quality Requirements and Evaluation; STORK: Secure idenTity acrOss boRders linked; STRIDE: Spoofing – Tampering – Repudiation – Information disclosure - Denial of service – Elevation of privilege; WG: Working Group

Acknowledgements

The authors would like to thank the Advisory Board members of the KONFIDO project for their feedback on the presented user requirements engineering methodology.

Funding

The research leading to these results has received funding from the European Union's Horizon 2020 research and innovation programme under grant agreement No 727528 (KONFIDO - Secure and Trusted Paradigm for Interoperable eHealth Services).
This paper reflects only the authors' views and the Commission is not liable for any use that may be made of the information contained therein.

Authors' contributions

PN, JR, MV-K, KV, LC, PC, IC, DM, GF, FC, MN, EvangelosG, OS, ErolG, JD, JP, DT, LR, IK and VK contributed in the gap analysis study (supervised by JR, JP and VK), validated the questionnaires of the end-user survey, and contributed in the realization of the end-user Workshop. MV-K, GF, MN, IC and DM conducted the user scenarios analysis. PN and VK defined the overall user requirements engineering approach and conducted the user requirements elicitation phase as well as the end-user survey. VK supervised the entire study. All the authors read, reviewed and approved the content of the paper.

Competing interests

One of the authors (namely, VK) is an Associate Editor with BMC Medical Informatics and Decision Making in a different section (i.e., "Decision Support") compared to the section that the current paper has been submitted to (i.e., "Healthcare Information Systems"). The authors declare that they have no competing interests.

Author details

[1]Institute of Applied Biosciences, Centre for Research & Technology Hellas, Thermi, Thessaloniki, Greece. [2]MedCom, Odense, Denmark. [3]Sundhed.dk, Copenhagen, Denmark. [4]Information Technologies Institute, Centre for Research & Technology Hellas, Thermi, Thessaloniki, Greece. [5]Department of Engineering, University of Naples "Parthenope", Naples, Italy. [6]Bit4id S.r.l, Naples, Italy. [7]IDIBAPS, Hospital Clinic de Barcelona, Universitat de Barcelona, Barcelona, Spain. [8]eHealth R&D Unit, EURECAT, Barcelona, Spain. [9]Fondazione Santobono Pausilipon, Naples, Italy. [10]Telbios S.r.l, Milan, Italy. [11]Eulambia Advanced Technologies Ltd, Athens, Greece. [12]CEA, LIST, Point Courrier 172, 91191 Gif-sur-Yvette Cedex, France. [13]Department of Electrical and Electronic Engineering, Imperial College of Science, Technology and Medicine, London, UK. [14]Time.lex, Brussels, Belgium. [15]Exus Software Ltd, London, UK.

References

1. KONFIDO project website. http://www.konfido-project.eu/konfido/. Accessed 18 May 2018.
2. Yi X, Paulet R, Bertino E. Homomorphic Encryption. Homomorphic Encryption Appl. Cham: Springer; 2014. p. 27–46. https://doi.org/10.1007/978-3-319-12229-8_2.
3. Mesaritakis C, Akriotou M, Kapsalis A, Grivas E, Chaintoutis C, Nikas T, Syvridis D. Physical Unclonable function based on a multi-mode optical waveguide. Sci Rep. 2018;8:9653. https://doi.org/10.1038/s41598-018-28008-6.
4. Bhatt S, Manadhata PK, Zomlot L. The operational role of security information and event management systems. IEEE Secur Priv. 2014;12(5):35–41. https://doi.org/10.1109/MSP.2014.103.
5. Angraal S, Krumholz HM, Schulz WL. Blockchain technology: applications in health care. Circ Cardiovasc Qual Outcomes. 2017;10(9):e003800 PMID:28912202.
6. Fonseca M, Karkaletsis K, Cruz I, Berler A, Oliveira I. OpenNCP: a novel framework to foster cross-border e-health services. Stud Health Technol Inform. 2015;210:617–21. https://doi.org/10.3233/978-1-61499-512-8-617.
7. epSOS project website. https://ec.europa.eu/digital-single-market/en/news/cross-border-healthproject-epsos-what-has-it-achieved. Accessed 18 May 2018.
8. eIDAS website. https://www.eid.as/home/. Accessed 18 May 2018.
9. Staffa M, Sgaglione S, Mazzeo G, Coppolino L, D'Antonio S, Romano L, Gelenbe E, Stan O, Carpov S, Grivas E, Campegiani P, Castaldo L, Votis K, Koutkias V, Komnios I. An OpenNCP-based solution for secure eHealth data exchange. J Netw Comput Appl. 2018;116(15):65–85. https://doi.org/10.1016/j.jnca.2018.05.012.
10. Tubaishat A. Perceived usefulness and perceived ease of use of electronic health records among nurses: application of technology acceptance model. Inform Health Soc Care. 2017;18:1–11. https://doi.org/10.1080/17538157.2017.1363761.
11. Tavares J, Oliveira T. Electronic health record portal adoption: a cross country analysis. BMC Med Inform Decis Mak. 2017;17(1):97. https://doi.org/10.1186/s12911-017-0482-9.
12. Antilope project website. https://www.antilope-project.eu/front/index.html. Accessed 18 May 2018.
13. JAseHN project website. http://jasehn.eu/. Accessed 18 May 2018.
14. SemanticHealthNet project website. http://www.semantichealthnet.eu/. Accessed 18 May 2018.
15. DECIPHER project website. http://www.decipherpcp.eu/. Accessed 18 May 2018.
16. STORK 2.0 project website. https://ec.europa.eu/digital-single-market/en/content/stork-take-your-eidentity-you-everywhere-eu. Accessed 18 May 2018.
17. Liveri D, Sarri A, Skouloudi C. Security and resilience in eHealth infrastructures and services, Security Challenges and Risks; 2015. https://doi.org/10.2824/217830.
18. European Union Agency for Network and Information Security. Cyber security and resilience for Smart Hospitals; 2016. https://doi.org/10.2824/28801.
19. ISO/IEC 27000 standards family - Information security management systems. Geneva; 2016. https://www.iso.org/isoiec-27001-information-security.html. Accessed 18 May 2018.
20. ISO/IEC 27002:2013 - Information technology -- Security techniques -- Code of practice for information security controls. 2013. https://www.iso.org/standard/54533.html. Accessed 18 May 2018.
21. ISO/IEC 27010:2015 - Information technology -- Security techniques -- Information security management for inter-sector and inter-organizational communications. 2015. https://www.iso.org/standard/68427.html. Accessed 18 May 2018.
22. ISO/IEC 27040:2015 - Information technology -- Security techniques -- Storage security. 2015. https://www.iso.org/standard/44404.html. Accessed 18 May 2018.
23. ISO 27799:2016 - Health informatics -- Information security management in health using ISO/IEC 27002. 2016. https://www.iso.org/standard/62777.html. Accessed 18 May 2018.
24. ISO 22857:2013 - Health informatics -- Guidelines on data protection to facilitate trans-border flows of personal health data. 2013. https://www.iso.org/standard/52955.html. Accessed 18 May 2018.
25. ISO/IEC 25010:2011 - Systems and software engineering -- Systems and software Quality Requirements and Evaluation (SQuaRE) -- System and software quality models. 2011. https://www.iso.org/standard/35733.html. Accessed 18 May 2018.
26. Rasmussen J, Natsiavas P, Votis K, et al. Gap analysis for information security in interoperable solutions at a systemic level: the KONFIDO approach. Precision Medicine Powered by pHealth and Connected Health, vol. 66. Singapore: Springer; 2017, IFMBE Proceedings. p. 75–9. https://doi.org/10.1007/978-981-10-7419-6_13.
27. Coppolino L, D'Antonio S, Romano L, Staffa M. KONFIDO project: a secure infrastructure increasing interoperability on a systemic level among eHealth services across Europe. Proc. IEEE Int Conf Internet of Things (iThings) and Green Computing and Communications (GreenCom) and Cyber, Physical and Social Computing (CPSCom) and Smart Data (SmartData). 2017;342–7. https://doi.org/10.1109/iThings-GreenCom-CPSCom-SmartData.2017.57.
28. Wong LR, Mauricio DS, Rodriguez GD. A systematic literature review about software requirements elicitation. J Eng Sci Technol. 2017;12(2):296–317.
29. Park G, Fellir F, Hong J-E, Garrido JL, Noguera M, Chung L. Deriving use cases from business processes: a goal-oriented transformational approach. Proc Symp Appl Comput - SAC '17. New York: ACM Press; 2017. p. 1288–95. https://doi.org/10.1145/3019612.3019789.
30. Kof L. Requirements analysis: concept extraction and translation of textual specifications to executable models. Natural Language Processing and Information Systems (NLDB 2009). Lecture Notes in Computer Science, vol. 5723. Berlin: Springer; 2010. p. 79–90. https://doi.org/10.1007/978-3-642-12550-8_7.

31. Drechsler R, Soeken M, Wille R. Automated and quality-driven requirements engineering. IEEE/ACM Int Conf Comput Des IEEE. 2014;2014:586–90. https://doi.org/10.1109/ICCAD.2014.7001410.
32. Nematzadeh A, Camp LJ. Threat analysis of online health information system. Proc 3rd Int Conf PErvasive Technol Relat to Assist Environ - PETRA '10. New York: ACM Press; 2010. Article No. 31. https://doi.org/10.1145/1839294.1839331.
33. Schneider RM. A comparison of information security risk analysis in the context of e-government to criminological threat assessment techniques. Proc 2010 Inf Secur Curric dev Annu Conf (InfoSecCD'10). 2010;107–16. https://doi.org/10.1145/1940941.1940966.
34. Meier JD, Mackman A, Dunner M, Vasireddy S, Escamilla R, Murukan A. Threats and countermeasures. 2003. https://msdn.microsoft.com/en-us/library/ff648641.aspx. Accessed 18 May 2018.
35. The EU General Data Protection Regulation (GDPR). https://www.eugdpr.org/. Accessed 18 May 2018.
36. Shaughnessy JJ, Zechmeister EB, Zechmeister JS. Research methods in psychology. 10th ed. New York: McGraw-Hill Education; 2015. ISBN:978-0-07-782536-2.
37. Natsiavas P, Kakalou C, Votis K, et al. Identification of barriers and facilitators for eHealth acceptance: the KONFIDO study. Precision Medicine Powered by pHealth and Connected Health, vol. 66. Singapore: Springer; 2017, IFMBE Proceedings. p. 81–5. https://doi.org/10.1007/978-981-10-7419-6_14.
38. Trilium II project website. https://trillium2.eu/. Accessed 20 July 2018.
39. Fricker SA, Grau R, Zwingli A. Requirements engineering: best practice. Requir Eng Digit Heal. Cham: Springer International Publishing; 2015. p. 25–46. https://doi.org/10.1007/978-3-319-09798-5_2.
40. Volk M, Falk-Andersson N, Sedlar U. How to elicit, analyse and validate requirements for a digital health solution. Requir Eng Digit Heal. Cham: Springer International Publishing; 2015. p. 155–88. https://doi.org/10.1007/978-3-319-09798-5_8.
41. Brost GS, Hoffmann M. Identifying security requirements and privacy concerns in digital health applications. Requir Eng Digit Heal. Cham: Springer International Publishing; 2015. p. 133–54. https://doi.org/10.1007/978-3-319-09798-5_7.

18

The effect of model selection on cost-effectiveness research: a comparison of kidney function-based microsimulation and disease grade-based microsimulation in chronic kidney disease modeling

Shusuke Hiragi[1,2*], Hiroshi Tamura[1], Rei Goto[3,4] and Tomohiro Kuroda[1]

Abstract

Background: Cost effectiveness research is emerging in the chronic kidney disease (CKD) research field. Especially, an individual-level state transition model (microsimulation) is widely used for these researches. Some researchers set CKD grades as discrete health states, and the transition probabilities between these states were dependent on the CKD grades (disease grade-based microsimulation, MSM-dg), while others set estimated glomerular filtration rate value which determines the severity of CKD as a main variable describing patients' continuous status (kidney function-based microsimulation, MSM-kf). MSM-kf seems to reflect the real world more precisely but is more difficult to implement. We compared the calculation results of these two microsimulation models to evaluate the effect of model selection on CKD cost-effectiveness analysis.

Methods: We implemented simplified MSM-dg and MSM-kf emulating natural course of CKD in general, and compared models using parameters derived from an IgA nephropathy cohort. After checking these models' overall behavior, life-years, utilities, and thresholds regarding intervention costs below which the intervention is thought as dominant (V0) or cost-effective (V1) were calculated. In addition, one-way and probabilistic sensitivity analyses were performed.

Results: With base-case parameters, the calculated life-years was shorter in MSM-dg (73.89 vs. 75.80 years) while the thresholds were almost equal (86.87 vs. 90.43 (V0), 132.29 vs. 146.25 [V1 in 1000 USD]) compared to MSM-kf. Sensitivity analyses showed a tendency of the MSM-dg to show shorter results in life-years. V0 and V1 were distributed by approximately ±100,000 USD (V0) and ± 150,000 USD (V1) between models.

Conclusions: Estimated cost-effectiveness thresholds by both models were not the same and its difference distributed too wide to be ignored. This result indicated that model selection in CKD cost-effectiveness research has large effect on their conclusions.

Keywords: Chronic kidney disease, Health economics, Cost effectiveness analysis, Disease modeling

* Correspondence: hiragi.shusuke.4x@kyoto-u.ac.jp
[1]Division of Medical Information Technology and Administration Planning, Kyoto University Hospital, 54 Kawaharacho, Shogoin, Sakyo-ku, Kyoto 606-8507, Japan
[2]Department of Nephrology, Kyoto University Hospital, 54 Kawaharacho, Shogoin, Sakyo-ku, Kyoto 606-8507, Japan
Full list of author information is available at the end of the article

Introduction

Chronic kidney disease (CKD), defined as impaired kidney function, is a very common disease that causes a high mortality rate and lowers quality of life (QOL) [1]. Progression of CKD to end-stage renal disease (ESRD) necessitates the renal replacement therapy (RRT, e.g. hemodialysis, peritoneal dialysis, or kidney transplantation), a costly [2] and lifelong treatment. As it is impossible to reverse renal impairment in CKD, in general, the effectiveness of management is judged by the extent to which disease progression is delayed.

CKD is said to progress gradually in a certain rate, depending on the underlying disease [3]. Various treatments developed to slow CKD progression have been investigated [4–6], and some researchers have evaluated the cost-effectiveness of these treatments [7–9]. One of the most utilized statistics for the measurement of cost-effectiveness is the incremental cost-effectiveness ratio (ICER), which is defined as the additional cost of a given treatment divided by the additional units of effects produced by the treatment. However, when we intend to analyze in a longer time horizon like CKD, which is lifelong disease, it is difficult to observe health utilities derived from treatments directly, because following patients for such a long time is typically not feasible.

Currently, computer simulations based on mathematical modeling are utilized to emulate patients' prognoses in longer time horizon [10], and in particular, the decision analytic models are widely used. When evaluating a target intervention (e.g. drug, treatment), researchers first develop a disease prognosis model using parameters such as mortality rate, disease progression speed, cost, and QOL derived from epidemiological and in vitro data [11, 12]. Once the model is validated, the next step is to calculate the time courses of virtual patients using computer software and extract cost-effectiveness results.

In the decision analytic model, there are several ways to emulate the prognosis of a disease including decision tree analysis, and state transition modeling (STM). Decision tree analysis becomes unwieldy when many possible outcomes exist or when the follow-up period is very long [13] as with CKD. Comparably, STM is suitable for modeling lifelong diseases because these models are relatively simple and simulations can be carried out recursively. In STM, researchers define possible discrete health states that the patient can develop and input transition probabilities between them [14–16]. There are two types of STM: cohort-level STM and individual-level STM (microsimulation). Cohort-level STM simulates the average experience of the patients in a cohort, while individual-level STM, also called as microsimulation (MSM), simulates individual patient histories over time. Both STM models assume state transition occurs at once per predetermined time cycle [17].

CKD is defined by abnormalities of kidney structure or function, present for more than 3 months, with implications for health [18]. Structural abnormality is detected using urine sediment or imaging and so on, while functional abnormalities are defined by a glomerular filtration rate (eGFR) less than 60 mL/min/1.73 m^2. The disease is classified into six grades according to eGFR (Table 1) [18], and sometimes the severity of kidney function impairment advances from grade 5 CKD to the condition named ESRD, in which patients are dependent on RRT for survival. eGFR is considered to reflect the total capacity of body waste filtration by tiny renal components known as nephrons. Two million nephrons are thought to exist in normal kidneys, which individually lose function for various reasons such as nephritis or diabetes. Therefore, eGFR is thought to decline steadily over time, which is supported by epidemiological study [19].

STM basically assumes discrete health statuses which patients can become. Therefore, researchers have used CKD grades as discrete health states between which transition probabilities are dependent on these grades (hereinafter referred to as disease grade-based microsimulation, MSM-dg). A research group also tried to find out these transition probabilities between these states in general population [20]. MSM-dg is easy to implement with commercially available software, but from the clinical viewpoint, the assumption that CKD stages are discrete states and transition probabilities are constant within a certain

Table 1 Glomerular filtration rate (GFR) categories in chronic kidney disease (CKD). Patients with CKD G1 and G2 have normal eGFR value and have other evidence of kidney damages (e.g. proteinuria)

GFR category	GFR (mL/min/1.73 m^2)	Terms
G1	≥90	Normal or high, with evidence of kidney damage
G2	60–89	Mildly decreased, with evidence of kidney damage
G3a	45–59	Mildly to moderately decreased
G3b	30–44	Moderately to severely decreased
G4	15–29	Severely decreased
G5	< 15	Kidney failure

CKD Chronic kidney disease, *G* Grade, *GFR* Glomerular filtration rate, *eGFR* Estimated glomerular filtration rate

grade is unrealistic because severity of the disease is defined by eGFR, which is continuous variable declining constantly. In contrast, STM using eGFR as a constantly changing variable (hereinafter referred to as kidney function-based microsimulation, MSM-kf) has also been implemented [21], in spite of its difficulty in implementation, and it seems to emulate real world more precisely. Aforementioned models are based on different assumptions; health states are discrete or continuous, and thus it is possible that they show different results for the same research topic. So far, there is no research examining the difference in calculation results between these models, which can affect the conclusion of cost-effectiveness research. Hence, we aimed to compare the calculation results of these modeling methods and evaluate the effect of model selection on research conclusion to provide information for future CKD health economics investigators.

Methods

We implemented simplified MSM-dg and MSM-kf models that were not intended to describe a specific kidney disease but instead to simulate the natural course of CKD in general, for use in comparing results derived from them. The details of development and the comparisons are described below.

Implementing disease grade-based microsimulation (MSM-dg)

We implemented individual-level STM (microsimulation, MSM) in which we set CKD grades as health states and assumed transition probabilities between states were dependent on these grades only (Fig. 1), adhering to conventional STM assumption. Once the kidney is damaged, the damage generally cannot be fully cured. Thus, the target population in cost-effectiveness research for treating kidney disease can be assumed to have grade 1 or more advanced CKD stages, or ESRD. With this model, the virtual cohort's time course was computed as shown in the flowchart on Additional file 1: Figure S1. Mortality rates were set as a function of age, sex, and CKD grade and that of patients in the predialysis and dialysis periods were set separately. Time cycle was set as 1/4 years based on the Japanese CKD guideline which recommends every CKD patient should be followed-up with eGFR measurement every 3 months [22]. In general, visiting an internal medicine clinic once every 3 months is common practice [23]. We repeated the process for each individual in the virtual cohort and acquired historical data including each individual's health state, accumulated cost, and utility.

Implementing kidney function-based microsimulation (MSM-kf)

Next, we implemented MSM-kf in which we set only two health states (alive and dead), but the alive state has

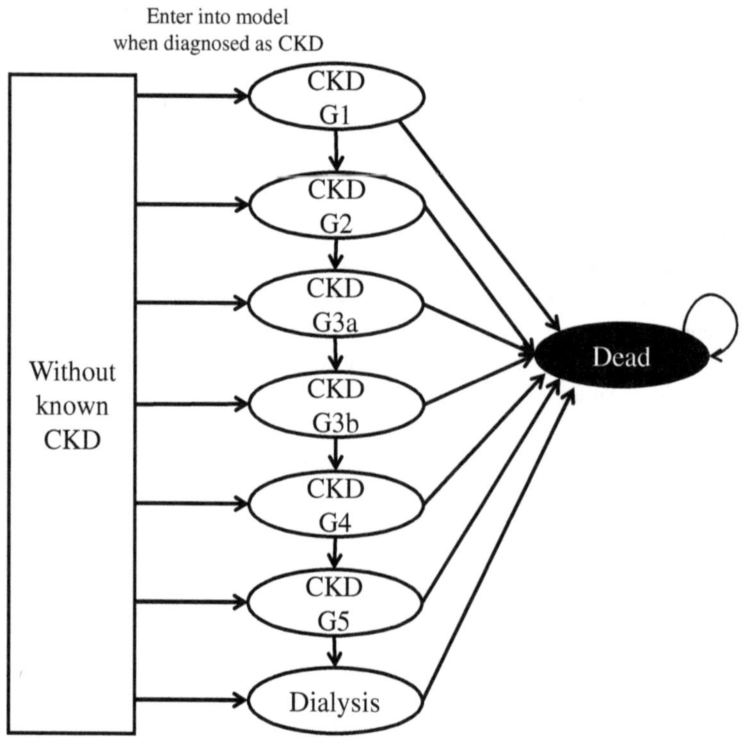

Fig. 1 State transition diagram of disease grade-based microsimulation (MSM-dg). The transition probabilities between states depend on CKD grades

eGFR value as constantly declining variable (Fig. 2). The decline rates were sometimes said to be non-linear [24], but we assumed widely-believed constant decline rate for simplicity. The transition probability between alive and dead states is dependent on CKD grades, which is determined only by the eGFR value. We assumed the decline rates are different by person to person. The mean and standard deviations of the rate are already well examined [25–27], and we utilized these data when developing our model. We assumed a log-normal distribution for the rates of eGFR decline [28], with assumption that no patient had continuously increasing eGFR value.

The simulation flowchart is shown in Additional file 2: Figure S2. Mortality rates, accumulated costs, and utilities were analyzed as described for the MSM-dg implementation. The conversion from eGFR to CKD grade was based on the aforementioned KDIGO definition, and we assumed that patients with an eGFR < 7 mL/min/1.73 m^2 were ESRD who required RRT according to the IDEAL study [29]. We also set time cycle as 1/4 years with the same reason explained in MSM-dg implementation section. The historical data of each patient was obtained using methods similar to those described for MSM-dg, and we calculated several parameters discussed below.

Parameter translation for model comparison

When comparing MSM-dg and MSM-kf, it is essential to translate parameters. In particular, transition probabilities in MSM-dg and eGFR decline rates in MSM-kf. Generally, previous researchers obtained the transition probabilities for MSM-dg from medical records [20, 30]. That is, they compared the eGFR of patients at two visits and calculated the fraction of those who proceeded to the next grade among all patients with a particular CKD grade. On the contrary, investigators applying MSM-kf used eGFR decline rates obtained from previous cohort studies [21, 31]. Therefore, we at first performed our MSM-kf with parameters obtained from existing epidemiological data. Next, from the historical eGFR data acquired with the MSM-kf, we randomly sampled the grade transition between two consecutive visits and estimated the transition probabilities to emulate the method described above to acquire transition probabilities. Finally, we inputted the calculated transition probabilities for MSM-dg (Fig. 3). By implementing the aforementioned translation, we could calculate transition probabilities from eGFR decline slope, resulting in comparison between MSM-dg and MSM-kf with same conditions.

Comparison of estimation results with MSM-dg and MSM-kf

We compared MSM-dg and MSM-kf to evaluate the differences in the calculation results. In this study, we set MSM-kf as reference model, considering its potential to reflect the reality more than MSM-dg. As base case analysis parameters, we used data from prior epidemiological study on IgA nephropathy, a major cause of CKD [32]. Clinically, utility changes from the disease and natural course represent those of typical CKD and cost structure may be the same, suggesting the data was suitable for our purpose. The study, named VALIGA [33], consisted of patients from 13 European countries. Adhering the data, we made our virtual cohort include equal numbers of 37-year old men and women with an eGFR of 76 mL/min/1.73 m^2. Mortality rates were acquired from general population of Ontario [34–36], Canada and dialysis patients from Japan [37] due to limited available data (Detail is described in supplementary material provided as Additional file 3). The study showed immunosuppressant therapy for IgAN can slow the rate of eGFR decline from − 2.2 ± 6.5 to − 1.3 ± 8.5 mL/min/1.73 m^2/year. We set the initial parameters as shown in Table 2. At first, we checked these models' behavior by means of Kaplan-Meier plot of renal survival rates. Renal survival rate is a ratio of patients not requiring RRT at a point of certain time, which is common indicator in nephrology research. Afterwards, we calculated and compared unadjusted life years, discounted quality-adjusted life-years (QALYs), costs, and new parameters defined below with both MSM-dg and MSM-kf.

Here, we introduced two new parameters indicating cost thresholds below which an interventions of interest are dominant strategy, and cost-effective (Fig. 4). In particular: the maximum present value of the cost of an

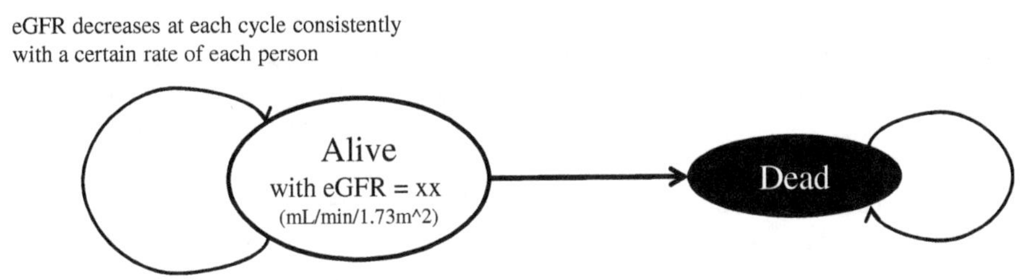

Fig. 2 State transition diagram of kidney function-based microsimulation (MSM-kf). The transition probabilities between states depend on eGFR value which constantly decreases at each time cycle with a certain rate

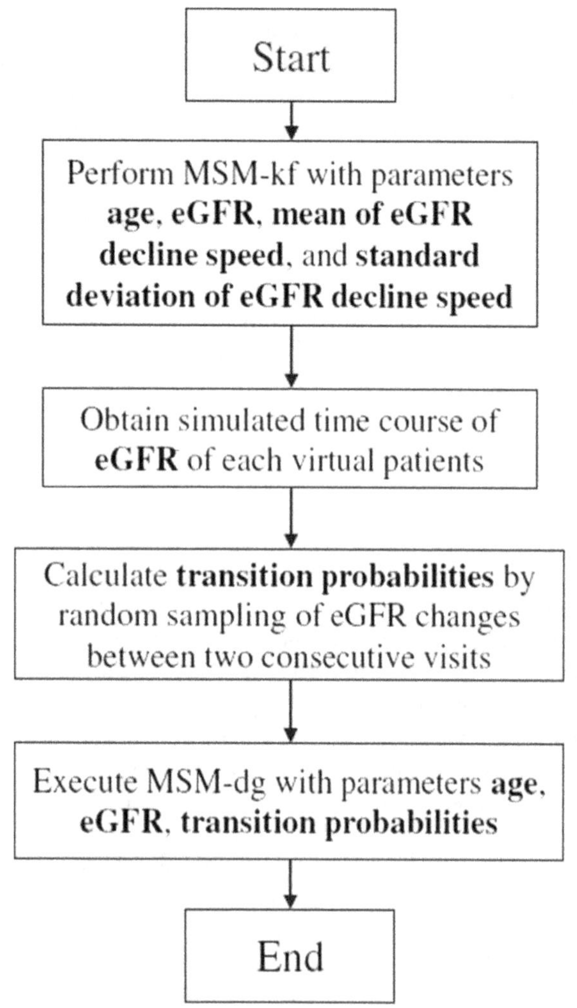

Fig. 3 Parameter adjustment and comparison of MSM-dg and MSM-kf flowchart

intervention below which the intervention can be dominant over the control (named V0 in this study) under the assumption that utility increases by the intervention, and the maximum present value of the cost of an intervention below which the intervention can be thought as cost-effective (V1). For this study, we assumed the threshold of cost-effectiveness was 50,000 USD / QALY adhering to prior literature [38]. The formulas used to calculate V0 and V1 are:

$$V0 = Ca\text{–}Cb \text{ (under the assumptions of } Ub > Ua\text{) and } V1 = 50,000 \times (Ub\text{–}Ua) + (Ca\text{–}Cb)$$

Where Ca = total cost of disease without intervention, Cb = total cost of disease with intervention (excluding intervention costs), Ua = total utility without intervention, and Ub = total utility with intervention. When Ca > Cb + cost of intervention, the intervention is dominant over the control. Hence, V0 = Ca – Cb. When (Cb + cost of intervention – Ca) / (Ub – Ua) < 50,000, the intervention will be seen as cost-effective. Hence, V1 = 50,000 × (Ub – Ua) + (Ca – Cb).

These variables represent the value we can pay for the intervention (detail is shown in Fig. 4). By calculating them with MSM-dg and MSM-kf, we can evaluate the effect of modelling methods on researchers' conclusion whether a new expensive intervention is cost effective or not.

Sensitivity analysis

There was unavoidable uncertainty in the parameters extracted from the VALIGA cohort, which provided only cohort-level information. Therefore, we performed one-way sensitivity analysis to overcome this limitation. We altered eGFR (30–90 mL/min/1.73 m^2), initial age (30–60 years old), mean eGFR decline rate (0.5–10.0 mL/min/1.73 m^2/year), standard deviation of the eGFR decline rate (0.5–10.0 mL/min/1.73 m^2/year), and other variables listed in Table 2 and calculated difference between estimated life years, utilities, costs, V0 and V1.

Researchers may be interested in not only IgAN, but also other diseases causing CKD, in other cohorts. Thus, we also performed probabilistic sensitivity analysis of these parameters and plotted the estimated life years, utilities, costs, and V0 and V1, from both models.

We used the Numpy and Math libraries. (Source codes are provided as Additional files 4 and 5). For visualization, we used R 3.4.2 software [39] and "survminer" package [40] to draw the Kaplan-Meier curve.

Results

Comparison of models

Figure 5 shows the Kaplan-Meier plot of the renal survival rates in both models. That of 5-years follow up in VALIGA cohort was also shown in zoomed area in lower left for comparison. Renal survival rates at 5 years were 99.8% in MSM-dg, 97.8% in MSM-kf, and 97.8% in VALIGA cohort.

The estimated life-years determined using MSM-dg were 73.89 ± 12.14 years (control) and 75.80 ± 12.82 years (immunosuppressant therapy). The estimated life-years using MSM-kf were 76.35 ± 12.44 years (control) and 78.80 ± 12.62 years (immunosuppressant therapy). The expected utilities (discounted) from the starting point calculated by MSM-dg were 19.43 ± 4.06 QALYs (control) and 20.00 ± 4.33 QALYs (immunosuppressant therapy). The expected utilities calculated by MSM-kf were 20.34 ± 4.08 QALYs (control) and 21.12 ± 4.08 QALYs (immunosuppressant therapy). The present values of expected lifetime costs calculated by MSM-dg were 286.85 ± 350.27 thousand dollars (control) and 213.42 ± 365.60 thousand dollars (immunosuppressant therapy, excluding intervention costs).

Table 2 Parameters of base case and sensitivity analyses. There were no CKD 1 patients as the initial eGFR was below 90 mL/min/1.73 m^2. Hence, we did not perform sensitivity analyses of mortality rate, utility, and cost for CKD 1 patients

Parameters	Baseline values	Sensitivity analyses		Ref.
		Lower limit	Upper limit	
Mean of eGFR decline speed (mL/min/1.73 m^2/year)	2.2	0.1	10	[33]
Standard Deviation of eGFR delcline speed (mL/min/1.73 m^2/year)	6.5	0.1	10	[33]
Initial age (years)	37	30	60	[33]
Initial eGFR (mL/min/1.73 m^2)	73	30	75	[33]
Baseline mortality rate of predialysis patients	$3.338 \times 10^{-5} \times e^{0.091 \times age}$(male) $1.615 \times 10^{-5} \times e^{0.098 \times age}$(female)	× 0.8	× 1.2	[34, 35]
Mortality rate of CKD 1 patients	Baseline × 1	× 0.9	× 1.1	[36]
Mortality rate of CKD 2 patients	Baseline × 1	× 0.9	× 1.1	[36]
Mortality rate of CKD 3a patients	Baseline × 1.2	× 1.1	× 1.3	[36]
Mortality rate of CKD 3b patients	Baseline × 1.8	× 1.7	× 1.9	[36]
Mortality rate of CKD 4 patients	Baseline × 3.2	× 3.0	× 3.4	[36]
Mortality rate of CKD 5 patients	Baseline × 5.9	× 5.6	× 6.2	[36]
Mortality rate of dialysis patients	$1.32 \times 10^{-3} \times e^{0.060 \times age}$	× 0.8	× 1.2	[36]
Utility of CKD 1 patients	1	0.9	1	[12]
Utility of CKD 2 patients	0.9	0.8	1	[12]
Utility of CKD 3a patients	0.87	0.77	0.97	[12]
Utility of CKD 3b patients	0.85	0.75	0.95	[12]
Utility of CKD 4 patients	0.85	0.75	0.95	[12]
Utility of CKD 5 patients	0.85	0.75	0.95	[12]
Utility of dialysis patients	0.72	0.62	0.82	[12]
Cost of CKD 1 (1000 USD / year)	1.6	0.8	3.2	[46]
Cost of CKD 2 (1000 USD / year)	1.7	0.9	3.4	[46]
Cost of CKD 3a (1000 USD / year)	3.5	1.8	7.0	[46]
Cost of CKD 3b (1000 USD / year)	3.5	1.8	7.0	[46]
Cost of CKD 4 (1000 USD / year)	12.7	6.4	25.4	[46]
Cost of CKD 5 (1000 USD / year)	12.7	6.4	25.4	[46]
Cost of dialysis patients (1000 USD / year)	84.6	42.3	169.1	[2]
Improve rate of eGFR decline slope	0.59	0.1	0.9	[33]
Annual discount rate for costs	0.03	0	0.1	
Annual discount rate for utilities	0.03	0	0.1	

CKD Chronic kidney disease, *eGFR* Estimated glomerular filtration rate, *Ref* Reference

The present values of expected lifetime costs calculated by MSM-kf were 199.98 ± 298.13 thousand dollars (control) and 122.99 ± 265.59 thousand dollars (immunosuppressant therapy, excluding intervention costs). The V0 values calculated from acquired data were 86,870 USD (MSM-dg) and 90,430 USD (MSM-kf). The V1 values calculated from the same data were 132,290 USD (MSM-dg) and 146,250 USD (MSM-kf) (Table 3). In base cases, the MSM-dg results showed shorter life-years, lower utilities, and greater costs than MSM-kf did. As a result, MSM-dg showed smaller result in both V0 and V1 compared to MSM-kf in this circumstance.

Sensitivity analysis

The results of the one-way sensitivity analysis revealed that MSM-dg showed shorter and lower life-years and utilities than MSM-kf in most cases, respectively. Also similar to the base case analyses, the calculated costs determined using MSM-dg were greater by approximately 50,000–100,000 USD in most cases. The difference in V0 and V1 values did not show specific tendencies, and the differences distributed within approximately − 50,000 to 100,000 USD (V0) and − 100,000 to 150,000 USD (V1). The detailed result of one-way sensitivity analyses are shown in Additional file 6: Figure S3.

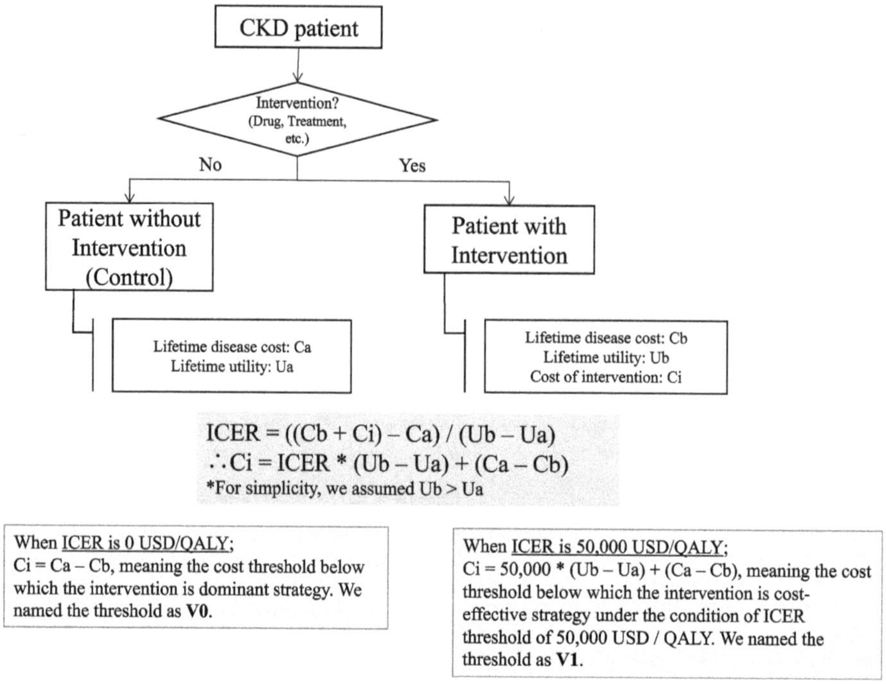

Fig. 4 Pictorial representation of definition of V0 and V1 values

The probabilistic sensitivity analysis revealed that life-years and utilities calculated with MSM-dg were shorter and lower, respectively, than those with MSM-kf in approximately two thirds of parameter sets. Costs calculated with MSM-dg were greater than costs calculated with MSM-kf in two thirds of cases. Regarding V0 and V1 values, the difference between both results distributed across zero almost equally. The vast majority of results (95%) were between − 91,300 USD and 75,700 USD (V0), and between − 108,300 USD and 98,600 USD (V1). The scatter plots of results of probabilistic sensitivity analyses are shown in Additional file 7: Figure S4.

Discussions

We compared two microsimulation models of CKD that are utilized within the field of health economics research: we called them MSM-dg and MSM-kf. First, we implemented simplified models. The Kaplan-Meyer curves of calculated results declined steadily, indicating that our implementations did not deviate from the reality so much.

We introduced two new parameters, V0 and V1, for our base-case settings comparison because directly analyzing cost-effectiveness of currently available therapy has scarce meaning. That is, currently available, partially-effective immunosuppressant therapy for IgAN [41] costs only 1200 USD [42, 43], which is too inexpensive to analyze cost-effectiveness with commonly-applied 50,000 USD/QALY threshold. We defined V0 as the difference between the total estimated costs of the control and intervention groups excluding the intervention cost. When the disease costs of the control group exceed those of the intervention group, V0 is positive and identical to the maximum present value of the cost of the intervention below which the intervention is dominant strategy over the control. Likewise, V1 represents the maximum present value of the intervention cost under the condition that the cost-effectiveness threshold is 50,000 USD/QALY. The threshold determining cost-effectiveness is a topic of health economics research [44] but is outside the scope of this study. Current effort on drug discovery focuses on innovative and expensive ones which should be examined cost-effectiveness. It is quite possible that such an expensive drug for stopping CKD would be invented in near future. From the viewpoint of payers or societies, it is very important to estimate the threshold below which an intervention is cost-effective for future CKD interventions in the era of increasing medical costs. In this context, V0 and V1 express this threshold.

In base-case analysis, MSM-dg results showed shorter life years and QALYs, and larger costs compared to MSM-kf. V0 were 86,870 USD by MSM-dg and 90,430 USD by MSM-kf, meaning that investigators who use MSM-dg will conclude an intervention is dominant strategy when the present value of the intervention cost is below 86,870 USD while those who use MSM-kf do so if the present value is below 90,430 USD. If the actual cost is between 86,870 and 90,430USD, conclusion becomes different due to selection of modeling method.

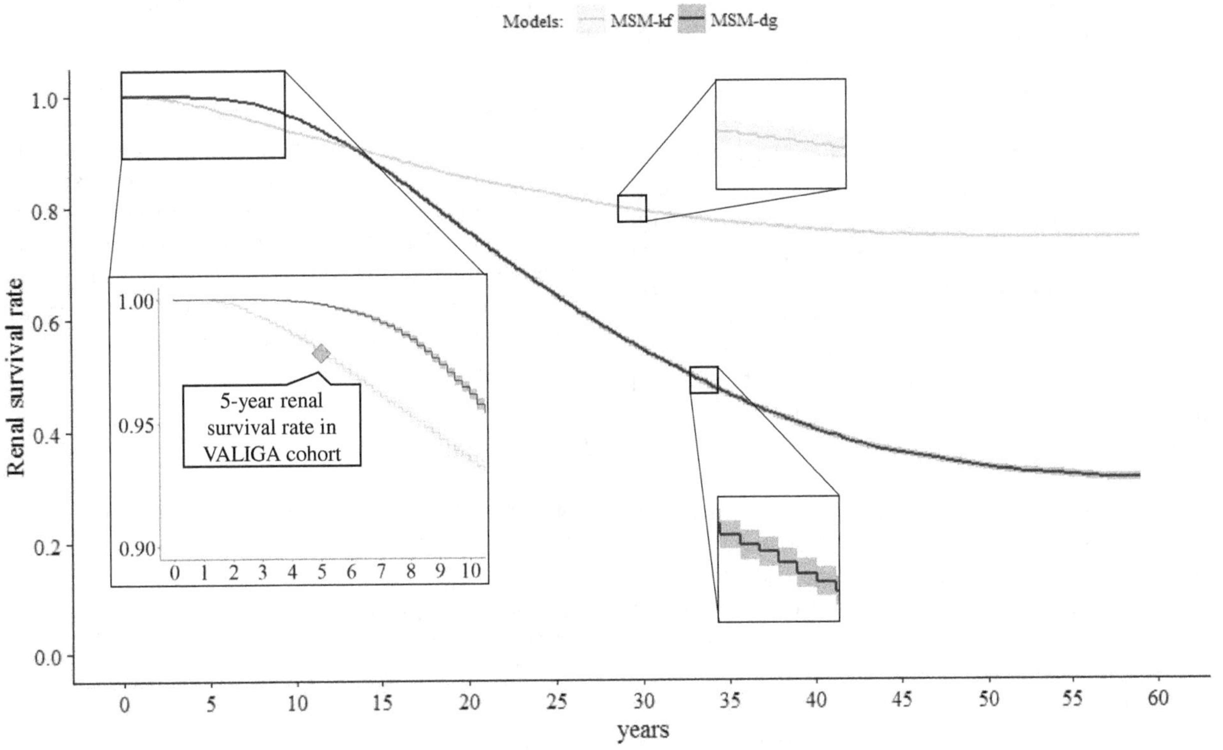

Fig. 5 Kaplan-Meier curve of renal survival rates calculated with MSM-dg and MSM-kf. The black line represents renal survival rate calculated with MSM-kf; gray line with MSM-dg. Light color bands represents 95% confidence intervals

Likewise, if the actual cost is between 132,290 USD and 146,250 USD, investigators conclude differently about cost-effectiveness of the intervention in the condition of ICER threshold is 50,000USD / QALY. This result indicates that the conclusion whether an intervention is dominant strategy or cost-effective is easily changed by the selection of their modeling method. In base-case setting, investigators who use MSM-kf will conclude the intervention is cost-effective more likely than those who use MSM-dg.

Our one-way sensitivity analysis showed that MSM-dg showed shorter results in life-years (by approximately 1.5–3.0 years) and utilities compared to MSM-kf but did larger results in costs in most cases. V0 and V1 values did not show specific tendencies, but the results calculated by MSM-dg were different from those by MSM-kf by approximately – 50,000 to 100,000 USD (V0) and – 100,000 to 150,000 USD (V1). These results imply that even if the initial parameters were uncertain, the tendencies were applicable with regard to calculated life years, utilities, and costs. Difference in V0 and V1 distributed largely, indicating that the threshold for an intervention to be dominant or cost-effective can fluctuate within these margins based on the selection of modeling method. These fluctuation margins are three to five times greater than the GDP per capita in the United States [45]; an amount that is difficult to ignore.

We performed probabilistic sensitivity analysis for proving generalizability of our findings. The analysis showed similar results to one-way sensitivity analysis.

Table 3 Calculation results of base cases. Standard deviations are shown in parentheses

	MSM-dg		MSM-kf	
	Immunosuppressant therapy	Control	Immunosuppressant therapy	Control
Life years (years)	76.35 (± 12.44)	73.89 (± 12.14)	78.80 (± 12.62)	75.80 (± 12.82)
Utility (years)	20.34 (± 4.08)	19.43 (± 4.06)	21.12 (± 4.08)	20.00 (± 4.33)
Cost (1000 USD)	199.98 (± 298.13)	286.85 (± 350.27)	122.99 (± 265.59)	213.42 (± 365.60)
V0 (1000 USD)	86.87		90.43	
V1 (1000 USD)	132.29		146.25	

MSM-dg Disease grade-based microsimulation, *MSM-kf* Kidney function-based microsimulation, *V0* boundary below which the intervention is dominant; *V1* boundary below which the intervention is cost-effective. V0 and V1 are defined in the main text

The differences between the V0 values calculated using MSM-dg versus MSM-kf were in the range of – 91,300 USD and 75,700 USD in 95% of the results while that of V1 values ranged from – 108,300 USD and 98,600 USD. These amounts are also difficult to ignore.

The reason for this difference can be partially explained by the characteristics of MSM-dg which ignored time-dependent variety of patients within a single health states. A cohort with eGFR of 55 mL/min/1.73m^2 (CKD G3a) at the beginning of a simulation, for instance, should have time-dependent transition probabilities to G3b because the fraction of patients with eGFR close to 45 mL/min/1.73 m2 (threshold between CKD G3a and G3b) will increase as the time goes, under the assumption of constant eGFR decline.

Policymakers can use cost-effectiveness studies to determine whether a given intervention is worth paying for. CKD is a common and lifelong disease with treatments available that may slow its progression to ESRD. Based on the results of our study, MSM-dg and MSM-kf based on different health states assumptions may produce different conclusions. In particular, compared to MSM-kf, MSM-dg showed shorter or smaller results in life-years and utilities, and estimated costs. The differences the between the V0 and V1 values were distributed bilaterally across zero, and the margins were relatively large. At a glance, MSM-kf emulates the real world more precisely from the clinical viewpoint. However, MSM-dg is easier to understand than MSM-kf, and it is more easily implemented using commercially available software. Simulation methods cannot avoid inaccuracy, and investigators must consider the biases inherent to the calculation methods they utilize. Our results may help clarify the biases derived from the selection of MSM-dg or MSM-kf for future CKD cost-effectiveness researchers.

This research has several limitations. First, we ignored major parameters affecting CKD progression such as race, ethnicity, and major cardiovascular risks for simplicity. Second, we did not consider kidney transplantation, which has a different cost structure than dialysis as RRT. Kidney transplantation is relatively inexpensive, and has become a considerable option for ESRD patients. This time we did not include kidney transplantation in our models to maintain simplicity, but it may be possible to include post-transplantation status into the models after reliable cost and utility data are accumulated. Third, we assumed constant eGFR decline rates, which is widely believed but sometimes pointed out to be incorrect. However, even when non-linear decline was assumed, our method of comparison could be applied even though it may become complicated, and similar difference would be possibly shown. Lastly, we only showed difference in calculation results, but we could not definitively determine which model is superior because of limited reliable accuracy indicators. Nevertheless, we believe this information is important.

Conclusions

MSM-dg, based on a conventional discrete state transition assumption, tends to show smaller results in utilities and larger ones in costs compared to more-realistic MSM-kf, based on the assumption of continuous state change in CKD disease modeling. The selection of a disease modelling method in cost-effectiveness researches of CKD intervention causes difficult-to-ignore fluctuations in their conclusions.

Additional files

Additional file 1: Figure S1. Implemented MSM-dg flowchart. Uniform random numbers were used for determination of live or death, and progression of CKD grade. Each period's costs and utilities were added after a state transition was determined. (PPT 192 kb)

Additional file 2: Figure S2. Implemented MSM-kf flowchart. Log-normal random numbers with reported mean and standard deviation values were used as the patient's constant eGFR decline rate. Similar to MSM-dg, a uniform random number was generated for determination of live or death. If the patient survives, his/her eGFR declined according to the previously assigned constant rate. Each period's costs and utilities were added after a state transition was determined. (PPT 174 kb)

Additional file 3: Figure S2. Supplementary documents describing parameter determination in detail. (DOC 128 kb)

Additional file 4: Python source code for models implementation. Python source code which implements MSM-kf and MDM-dg models. (TXT 9 kb)

Additional file 5: Python source code for models comparison. Python source code which implements models comparison. Users have to modify the code to import python code provided as Additional file 4 (Python source code for models implementation). (TXT 3 kb)

Additional file 6: Figure S3. a-e Results of one-way sensitivity analyses. (PPT 132 kb)

Additional file 7: Figure S4. a-e Results of probabilistic sensitivity analyses. (PPT 3755 kb)

Abbreviations

CKD: Chronic kidney disease; eGFR: Estimated glomerular filtration rate; ESRD: End-stage renal disease; ICER: Incremental cost-effectiveness ratio; IgAN: IgA nephropathy; MSM: Microsimulation; MSM-dg: Disease grade-based microsimulation; QALY: Quality-adjusted life-year; QOL: Quality of life; RRT: Renal replacement therapy; STM: State transition modelling

Acknowledgements

We would like to thank Drs. Genta Kato and Kazuya Okamoto, for their valuable advice in regard to technical and medical affairs. We gratefully acknowledge Ms. Kaori Shiomi, Yoko Hara, and Yuko Furusawa for secretarial assistance. We also thanks to Dr. Motoko Yanagita, Professor of Nephrology, graduate school of medicine, Kyoto University, for her generous advice and assistance in regard to affairs relating nephrology.

Funding

Financial support for this study was provided in part by a grant from Kyoto University and Advanced Science, Technology & Management Research Institute of KYOTO (ASTEM RI / KYOTO). The funding agreement ensured the authors' independence in designing the study, interpreting the data, writing, and publishing the report.

Authors' contributions

SH wrote the main manuscript text and prepared figures and tables. HT supervised programming implementation. RG supervised theoretical matters. TK leaded the discussion and the team. All authors reviewed, read and approved the final manuscript.

Competing interests

The authors declare that they have no competing interests.

Author details

[1]Division of Medical Information Technology and Administration Planning, Kyoto University Hospital, 54 Kawaharacho, Shogoin, Sakyo-ku, Kyoto 606-8507, Japan. [2]Department of Nephrology, Kyoto University Hospital, 54 Kawaharacho, Shogoin, Sakyo-ku, Kyoto 606-8507, Japan. [3]Graduate School of Business Administration, Keio University, 2-33-28 Hiyoshi Honcho, Kohoku-ku, Yokohama, Kanagawa 223-8526, Japan. [4]Keio Business School, Keio University, 2-33-28 Hiyoshi Honcho, Kohoku-ku, Yokohama, Kanagawa 223-8526, Japan.

References

1. Perlman RL, Finkelstein FO, Liu L, Roys E, Kiser M, Eisele G, et al. Quality of life in chronic kidney disease (CKD): a cross-sectional analysis in the renal research institute-CKD study. Am J Kidney Dis. 2005;45:658–66.
2. Chapter 11: Medicare expenditures for persons with ESRD: UNITED STATES RENAL DATA SYSTEM. Available from: http://www.usrds.org/2015/view/v2_11.aspx. Cited 6 Apr 2016.
3. Part 7. Stratification of Risk for Progression of Kidney Disease and Development of Cardiovascular Disease. Am J Kidney Dis. 39:S170–212. https://doi.org/10.1053/ajkd.2002.30946.
4. Walz G, Budde K, Mannaa M, Nurnberger J, Wanner C, Sommerer C, et al. Everolimus in patients with autosomal dominant polycystic kidney disease. N Engl J Med. 2010;363:830–40. https://doi.org/10.1056/NEJMoa1003491.
5. Jones C, Roderick P, Harris S, Rogerson M. Decline in kidney function before and after nephrology referral and the effect on survival in moderate to advanced chronic kidney disease. Nephrol Dial Transplant. 2006;21:2133–43. https://doi.org/10.1093/ndt/gfl198.
6. Wright JT Jr, Bakris G, Greene T, Agodoa LY, Appel LJ, Charleston J, et al. Effect of blood pressure lowering and antihypertensive drug class on progression of hypertensive kidney disease: results from the AASK trial. JAMA. 2002;288:2421–31.
7. Mennini FS, Russo S, Marcellusi A, Quintaliani G, Fouque D. Economic effects of treatment of chronic kidney disease with low-protein diet. J Ren Nutr. 2014;24:313–21. https://doi.org/10.1053/j.jrn.2014.05.003.
8. Erickson KF, Chertow GM, Goldhaber-Fiebert JD. Cost-effectiveness of tolvaptan in autosomal dominant polycystic kidney disease. Ann Intern Med. 2013;159:382–9. https://doi.org/10.7326/0003-4819-159-6-201309170-00004.
9. Harris A, Cooper BA, Li JJ, Bulfone L, Branley P, Collins JF, et al. Cost-effectiveness of initiating dialysis early: a randomized controlled trial. Am J Kidney Dis. 2011;57:707–15. https://doi.org/10.1053/j.ajkd.2010.12.018.
10. Weinstein MC, O'Brien B, Hornberger J, Jackson J, Johannesson M, McCabe C, et al. Principles of good practice for decision analytic modeling in health-care evaluation: report of the ISPOR task force on good research practices--modeling studies. Value Health. 2003;6:9–17.
11. Mazairac AH, de Wit GA, Grooteman MP, Penne EL, van der Weerd NC, den Hoedt CH, et al. Effect of hemodiafiltration on quality of life over time. Clin J Am Soc Nephrol. 2013;8:82–9. https://doi.org/10.2215/cjn.00010112.
12. Gorodetskaya I, Zenios S, McCulloch CE, Bostrom A, Hsu CY, Bindman AB, et al. Health-related quality of life and estimates of utility in chronic kidney disease. Kidney Int. 2005;68:2801–8. https://doi.org/10.1111/j.1523-1755.2005.00752.x.
13. Drummond MFSM, Claxton K, Stoddart GL, Torrance GW. Economic evaluation using decision-analytic modelling. Methods for the economic evaluation of health care Programmes. Oxford: Oxford University Press; 2015. p. 311–51.
14. Sonnenberg FA, Beck JR. Markov models in medical decision making: a practical guide. Med Decis Making. 1993;13:322–38. https://doi.org/10.1177/0272989x9301300409.
15. Siebert U, Alagoz O, Bayoumi AM, Jahn B, Owens DK, Cohen DJ, et al. State-transition modeling: a report of the ISPOR-SMDM modeling good research practices task Force-3. Med Decis Making. 2012;32:690–700. https://doi.org/10.1177/0272989x12455463.
16. Briggs A, Sculpher M. An introduction to Markov modelling for economic evaluation. PharmacoEconomics. 1998;13:397–409.
17. Heeg BM, Damen J, Buskens E, Caleo S, de Charro F, van Hout BA. Modelling approaches: the case of schizophrenia. PharmacoEconomics. 2008;26:633–48.
18. Chapter 1: Definition and classification of CKD. Kidney Int Suppl. 2013;3:19–62. https://doi.org/10.1038/kisup.2012.64.
19. Mitch WE, Walser M, Buffington GA, Lemann J Jr. A simple method of estimating progression of chronic renal failure. Lancet (London, England). 1976;2:1326–8.
20. Luo L, Small D, Stewart WF, Roy JA. Methods for estimating kidney disease stage transition probabilities using electronic medical records. EGEMS (Washington, DC). 2013;1:1040. https://doi.org/10.13063/2327-9214.1040.
21. Hoerger TJ, Wittenborn JS, Segel JE, Burrows NR, Imai K, Eggers P, et al. A health policy model of CKD: 1. Model construction, assumptions, and validation of health consequences. Am J Kidney Dis. 2010;55:452–62. https://doi.org/10.1053/j.ajkd.2009.11.016.
22. Japan nephrology s. Special issue: clinical practice guidebook for diagnosis and treatment of chronic kidney disease 2012. Nihon Jinzo Gakkai shi. 2012;54:1034–191.
23. Schwartz LM, Woloshin S, Wasson JH, Renfrew RA, Welch HG. Setting the revisit interval in primary care. J Gen Intern Med. 1999;14:230–5.
24. Skupien J, Warram JH, Smiles AM, Stanton RC, Krolewski AS. Patterns of estimated glomerular filtration rate decline leading to end-stage renal disease in type 1 diabetes. Diabetes Care. 2016;39:2262–9. https://doi.org/10.2337/dc16-0950.
25. Glassock RJ, Winearls C. Ageing and the glomerular filtration rate: truths and consequences. Trans Am Clin Climatol Assoc. 2009;120:419–28.
26. Imai E, Horio M, Yamagata K, Iseki K, Hara S, Ura N, et al. Slower decline of glomerular filtration rate in the Japanese general population: a longitudinal 10-year follow-up study. Hypertens Res. 2008;31:433–41. https://doi.org/10.1291/hypres.31.433.
27. Bartosik LP, Lajoie G, Sugar L, Cattran DC. Predicting progression in IgA nephropathy. Am J Kidney Dis. 2001;38:728–35. https://doi.org/10.1053/ajkd.2001.27689.
28. Skupien J, Warram JH, Smiles AM, Niewczas MA, Gohda T, Pezzolesi MG, et al. The early decline in renal function in patients with type 1 diabetes and proteinuria predicts the risk of end-stage renal disease. Kidney Int. 2012;82:589–97. https://doi.org/10.1038/ki.2012.189.
29. Cooper BA, Branley P, Bulfone L, Collins JF, Craig JC, Fraenkel MB, et al. A randomized, controlled trial of early versus late initiation of dialysis. N Engl J Med. 2010;363:609–19. https://doi.org/10.1056/NEJMoa1000552.
30. Blanchette CM, Liang C, Lubeck DP, Newsome B, Rossetti S, Gu X, et al. Progression of autosomal dominant kidney disease: measurement of the stage transitions of chronic kidney disease. Drugs Context. 2015;4:212275. https://doi.org/10.7573/dic.212275.
31. Orlando LA, Belasco EJ, Patel UD, Matchar DB. The chronic kidney disease model: a general purpose model of disease progression and treatment. BMC Med Inform Decis Mak. 2011;11:41. https://doi.org/10.1186/1472-6947-11-41.
32. Chapter 10: Immunoglobulin A nephropathy. Kidney Int Suppl. 2012;2:209–17. https://doi.org/10.1038/kisup.2012.23.
33. Tesar V, Troyanov S, Bellur S, Verhave JC, Cook HT, Feehally J, et al. Corticosteroids in IgA nephropathy: a retrospective analysis from the VALIGA study. J Am Soc Nephrol. 2015;26:2248–58. https://doi.org/10.1681/asn.2014070697.
34. Table 1a Complete life table, males, Ontario, Canada, 2009 to 2011: statistics Canada. Available from: http://www.statcan.gc.ca/pub/84-537-x/2013005/tbl/tbl7a-eng.htm. Cited 16 Mar 2016.
35. Table 1a Complete life table, females, Ontario, Canada, 2009 to 2011: statistics Canada. Available from: http://www.statcan.gc.ca/pub/84-537-x/2013005/tbl/tbl7b-eng.htm. Cited 16 Mar 2016.
36. Go AS, Chertow GM, Fan D, McCulloch CE, Hsu CY. Chronic kidney disease and the risks of death, cardiovascular events, and hospitalization. N Engl J Med. 2004;351:1296–305. https://doi.org/10.1056/NEJMoa041031.
37. Distribution of cause of death in dialysis patients who died in 2014 stratified by age group (in Japanese): the Japanese Society of Dialysis Therapy. Available from: http://docs.jsdt.or.jp/overview/index2014.html. Cited 19 Mar 2016.

38. Hirth RA, Chernew ME, Miller E, Fendrick AM, Weissert WG. Willingness to pay for a quality-adjusted life year: in search of a standard. Med Decis Making. 2000;20:332–42. https://doi.org/10.1177/0272989x0002000310.
39. Team RC. A language and environment for statistical computing. Vienna: R Foundation for Statistical Computing; 2015.
40. Kassambara A, Kosinski M, Biecek P, Fabian S. Drawing survival curves using 'ggplot2'. 2017. http://www.sthda.com/english/rpkgs/survminer/.
41. Pozzi C, Andrulli S, Del Vecchio L, Melis P, Fogazzi GB, Altieri P, et al. Corticosteroid effectiveness in IgA nephropathy: long-term results of a randomized, controlled trial. J Am Soc Nephrol. 2004;15:157–63.
42. Drugbank Version 5.0. Available from: https://www.drugbank.ca/. Cited 26 Dec 2016.
43. Canada's health expenditure: Spending on prescribed drugs increases, total growth remains slow: Canadian Institute for Health Information; 2016. Available from: https://secure.cihi.ca/estore/productFamily.htm?locale=en&pf=PFC3333. Cited 26 Dec 2016.
44. Marseille E, Larson B, Kazi DS, Kahn JG, Rosen S. Thresholds for the cost-effectiveness of interventions: alternative approaches. Bull World Health Organ. 2015;93:118–24. https://doi.org/10.2471/blt.14.138206.
45. Indicators: The World Bank. Available from: http://data.worldbank.org/indicator/. Cited 11 Oct 2016.
46. Honeycutt AA, Segel JE, Zhuo X, Hoerger TJ, Imai K, Williams D. Medical costs of CKD in the Medicare population. J Am Soc Nephrol. 2013;24:1478–83. https://doi.org/10.1681/asn.2012040392.

Permissions

All chapters in this book were first published in MI&DM, by BioMed Central; hereby published with permission under the Creative Commons Attribution License or equivalent. Every chapter published in this book has been scrutinized by our experts. Their significance has been extensively debated. The topics covered herein carry significant findings which will fuel the growth of the discipline. They may even be implemented as practical applications or may be referred to as a beginning point for another development.

The contributors of this book come from diverse backgrounds, making this book a truly international effort. This book will bring forth new frontiers with its revolutionizing research information and detailed analysis of the nascent developments around the world.

We would like to thank all the contributing authors for lending their expertise to make the book truly unique. They have played a crucial role in the development of this book. Without their invaluable contributions this book wouldn't have been possible. They have made vital efforts to compile up to date information on the varied aspects of this subject to make this book a valuable addition to the collection of many professionals and students.

This book was conceptualized with the vision of imparting up-to-date information and advanced data in this field. To ensure the same, a matchless editorial board was set up. Every individual on the board went through rigorous rounds of assessment to prove their worth. After which they invested a large part of their time researching and compiling the most relevant data for our readers.

The editorial board has been involved in producing this book since its inception. They have spent rigorous hours researching and exploring the diverse topics which have resulted in the successful publishing of this book. They have passed on their knowledge of decades through this book. To expedite this challenging task, the publisher supported the team at every step. A small team of assistant editors was also appointed to further simplify the editing procedure and attain best results for the readers.

Apart from the editorial board, the designing team has also invested a significant amount of their time in understanding the subject and creating the most relevant covers. They scrutinized every image to scout for the most suitable representation of the subject and create an appropriate cover for the book.

The publishing team has been an ardent support to the editorial, designing and production team. Their endless efforts to recruit the best for this project, has resulted in the accomplishment of this book. They are a veteran in the field of academics and their pool of knowledge is as vast as their experience in printing. Their expertise and guidance has proved useful at every step. Their uncompromising quality standards have made this book an exceptional effort. Their encouragement from time to time has been an inspiration for everyone.

The publisher and the editorial board hope that this book will prove to be a valuable piece of knowledge for researchers, students, practitioners and scholars across the globe.

List of Contributors

Emmanuelle Sylvestre, Guillaume Bouzillé, Cécil His-Mahier, Christine Riou and Marc Cuggia
INSERM, U1099, F-35000 Rennes, France
Université de Rennes 1, LTSI, F-35000 Rennes, France
CHU Rennes, CIC Inserm 1414, F-35000 Rennes, France
CHU Rennes, Centre de Données Cliniques, F-35000 Rennes, France

Emmanuel Chazard
Département de Santé Publique, Université de Lille EA 2694, CHU Lille, F-59000 Lille, France

Hee-Jin Lee, Yaoyun Zhang, Jun Xu, Cui Tao and Hua Xu
School of Biomedical Informatics, The University of Texas Health Science Center at Houston, Houston, TX, USA

Min Jiang
Pieces Technologies, Dallas, TX, USA

Aravindhan Ganesan
Faculty of Pharmacy and Pharmaceutical Sciences, University of Alberta, Edmonton, Canada

Theinmozhi Arulraj
Faculty of Pharmacy and Pharmaceutical Sciences, University of Alberta, Edmonton, Canada
School of Life Sciences, University of Hyderabad, Hyderabad, India

Tahir Choulli
Department of Mathematical and Statistical Sciences, Faculty of Science, University of Alberta, Edmonton, Canada

Khaled H. Barakat
Faculty of Pharmacy and Pharmaceutical Sciences, University of Alberta, Edmonton, Canada
Li Ka Shing Institute of Virology, University of Alberta, Edmonton, Canada

Jade Kettlewell
Division of Rehabilitation and Ageing, School of Medicine, University of Nottingham, D1409, Medical School, Queens Medical Centre, Nottingham NG7 2UH, UK

Julie Phillips
Division of Rehabilitation and Ageing, School of Medicine, University of Nottingham, B114, Medical School, Queens Medical Centre, Nottingham NG7 2UH, UK

Kate Radford
Rehabilitation Research (Long Term Conditions), Division of Rehabilitation and Ageing, School of Medicine, University of Nottingham, B102, Medical School, Queens Medical Centre, Nottingham NG7 2UH, UK

Roshan dasNair
Clinical Psychology & Neuropsychology, Division of Psychiatry & Applied Psychology, C22, Institute of Mental Health, Jubilee Campus, University of Nottingham, Nottingham NG7 2TU, UK

Rachel F. Eyler
Department of Pharmacy Practice, University of Connecticut School of Pharmacy, 69 North Eagleville Road, Storrs, CT 06269, USA

Sara Cordes
Department of Psychology, Boston College, 300 McGuinn Hall, 140 Commonwealth Ave, Chestnut Hill, MA 02467, USA

Benjamin R. Szymanski
Department of Chronic Disease Epidemiology, Yale School of Public Health, 60 College Street, New Haven, CT 06510, USA

Liana Fraenkel
Department of Medicine, Section of Rheumatology, Yale University School of Medicine, 300 Cedar Street, TAC #525, New Haven, CT 06520, USA
VA Connecticut Healthcare System, West Haven, CT 06516, USA

Kuo Yang, Guangming Liu, Ning Wang and Jian Yu
School of Computer and Information Technology and Beijing Key Lab of Traffic Data Analysis and Mining, Beijing Jiaotong University, Beijing 100044, China

Runshun Zhang
Guanganmen Hospital, China Academy of Chinese Medical Sciences, Beijing 100053, China

Jianxin Chen
Beijing University of Chinese Medicine, Beijing 100029, China

Xuezhong Zhou
School of Computer and Information Technology and Beijing Key Lab of Traffic Data Analysis and Mining, Beijing Jiaotong University, Beijing 100044, China
Data Center of Traditional Chinese Medicine, China Academy of Chinese Medical Sciences, Beijing 100700, China

Xinyuan Zhang and Cui Tao
School of Biomedical Informatics, The University of Texas Health Science Center at Houston, Huston, TX, USA

Shiqi Wang and Jie Liu
Department of Dermatology, Peking Union Medical College Hospital, Chinese Academy of Medical Sciences and Peking Union Medical College, Beijing, China

Qiu-Yue Zhong, Bizu Gelaye and Michelle A. Williams
Department of Epidemiology, Harvard T.H. Chan School of Public Health, Boston, MA 02115, USA

Elizabeth W. Karlson
Department of Medicine, Division of Rheumatology, Immunology and Allergy, Brigham and Women's Hospital and Harvard Medical School, Boston, MA, USA

Sean Finan
Children's Hospital Informatics Program, Boston Children's Hospital, Boston, MA, USA

Paul Avillach
Department of Epidemiology, Harvard T.H. Chan School of Public Health, Boston, MA 02115, USA
Children's Hospital Informatics Program, Boston Children's Hospital, Boston, MA, USA
Department of Biomedical Informatics, Harvard Medical School, Boston, MA, USA

Jordan W. Smoller
Department of Epidemiology, Harvard T.H. Chan School of Public Health, Boston, MA 02115, USA
Psychiatric and Neurodevelopmental Genetics Unit, Massachusetts General Hospital, Boston, MA, USA

Tianxi Cai
Department of Biostatistics, Harvard T.H. Chan School of Public Health, Boston, MA, USA

Duaa Aljabri
Department of Health Sciences Research, Mayo Clinic, Jacksonville, FL, USA

Adrian Dumitrascu and M. Caroline Burton
Division of Hospital Internal Medicine, Mayo Clinic, Jacksonville, FL, USA

Launia White
Division of Biomedical Statistics and Informatics, Mayo Clinic, Jacksonville, FL, USA

James Naessens
Department of Health Sciences Research, Mayo Clinic, Rochester, MN, USA

Mahmud Khan, Sudha Xirasagar and Ronnie Horner
Department of Health Services Policy and Management, University of South Carolina, Columbia, SC, USA

Mary E. Cooley and Manan M. Nayak
The Phyllis F. Cantor Center, Dana-Farber Cancer Institute, 450 Brookline Avenue, Boston, MA 02115, USA

Janet L. Abrahm, Ilana M. Braun and Joanna Paladino
Department of Psychosocial Oncology and Palliative Care, Dana-Farber Cancer Institute, 450 Brookline Avenue, Boston, MA 02115, USA

Donna L. Berry
The Phyllis F. Cantor Center and the Department of Medicine, Dana-Farber Cancer Institute, 450 Brookline Ave, LW-512, Boston, MA 02115, USA

Michael S. Rabin
Lowe Center for Thoracic Oncology, Dana-Farber Cancer Institute, 450 Brookline Avenue, Boston, MA 02115, USA

David F. Lobach
Klesis Healthcare and Department of Family Medicine, Durham, NC 27705, USA

Department of Family Medicine, Duke University Medical Center, 2100 Erwin Road, Durham, NC 27710, USA

Paolo Fraccaro, Richard Williams and Niels Peek
NIHR Greater Manchester Primary Care Patient Safety Translational Research Centre, The University of Manchester, Manchester, UK
Health eResearch Centre, Farr Institute for Health Informatics Research, London, UK
Centre for Health Informatics, Division of Informatics, Imaging and Data Science, The University of Manchester, Manchester, UK

Sabine N. van der Veer and Lamiece Hassan
Health eResearch Centre, Farr Institute for Health Informatics Research, London, UK
Centre for Health Informatics, Division of Informatics, Imaging and Data Science, The University of Manchester, Manchester, UK

Grahame Wood and Smeeta Sinha
Renal Clinic, Salford Royal NHS Trust, Salford, UK

Markel Vigo
School of Computer Science, The University of Manchester, Manchester, UK

Iain Buchan
Microsoft Healthcare, Microsoft Research, Cambridge, UK

Panagiotis Balatsoukas
Centre for Health Informatics, City University, London, UK

Zhaoyi Chen and Mattia Prosperi
Department of Epidemiology, College of Public Health and Health Professions & College of Medicine, University of Florida, 2004 Mowry Road, Gainesville, Florida 32610-0231, USA

Victoria Y. Bird
Department of Urology, University of Florida, Gainesville, Florida, USA

Rupam Ruchi and Mark S. Segal
Division of Nephrology, Hypertension, & Renal Transplantation, University of Florida, Gainesville, Florida, USA

Jiang Bian
Department of Health Outcomes and Biomedical Informatics, University of Florida, Gainesville, Florida, USA

Saeed R. Khan
Department of Pathology, Immunology, and Laboratory Medicine, Gainesville, Florida, USA

Marie-Carmelle Elie
Department of Emergency Medicine, University of Florida, Gainesville, Florida, USA

Amy M. Kwon
Big Data Science, Division of Economics & Statistics, College of Public Policy, Korea University, Sejong, Korea

Haihong Guo, Xu Na and Jiao Li
Institute of Medical Information / Medical Library, Chinese Academy of Medical Sciences & Peking Union Medical College, Beijing, China

Joseph Thobias
College of Informatics and Virtual Education, University of Dodoma, Dodoma, Tanzania

Achilles Kiwanuka
Medical Research Council/Uganda Virus Research Institute and London School of Hygiene & Tropical Medicine Uganda Research Unit, Entebbe, Uganda

Šefket Šabanović, Majnarić Trtica Ljiljana and Aleksandar Včev
Department for Internal Medicine, Family Medicine and the History of Medicine, Faculty of Medicine, Josip Juraj Strossmayer University, Osijek, Croatia, Huttlerova 10b, 31 000 Osijek, Croatia

František Babič, Michal Vadovský and Ján Paralič
Department of Cybernetics and Artificial Intelligence, Technical University of Košice, Faculty of Electrical Engineering and Informatics, Letná 9/B, 042 00 Košice, Slovakia

Andreas Holzinger
Medical University Graz, Institute for Medical Informatics/Statistic, Auenbruggerplatz 2/V, 8036 Graz, Austria

Pantelis Natsiavas and Vassilis Koutkias
Institute of Applied Biosciences, Centre for Research & Technology Hellas, Thermi, Thessaloniki, Greece

Janne Rasmussen and Jan Petersen
MedCom, Odense, Denmark

Maja Voss-Knude
Sundhed.dk, Copenhagen, Denmark

Kostas Votis and Dimitrios Tzovaras
Information Technologies Institute, Centre for Research & Technology Hellas, Thermi, Thessaloniki, Greece

Luigi Coppolino and Luigi Romano
Department of Engineering, University of Naples "Parthenope", Naples, Italy

Paolo Campegiani
Bit4id S.r.l, Naples, Italy

Isaac Cano
IDIBAPS, Hospital Clinic de Barcelona, Universitat de Barcelona, Barcelona, Spain

David Marí
eHealth R&D Unit, EURECAT, Barcelona, Spain

Giuliana Faiella and Fabrizio Clemente
Fondazione Santobono Pausilipon, Naples, Italy

Marco Nalin
Telbios S.r.l, Milan, Italy

Evangelos Grivas
Eulambia Advanced Technologies Ltd, Athens, Greece

Oana Stan
CEA, LIST, Point Courrier 172, 91191 Gif-sur-Yvette Cedex, France

Erol Gelenbe
Department of Electrical and Electronic Engineering, Imperial College of Science, Technology and Medicine, London, UK

Jos Dumortier
Time.lex, Brussels, Belgium

Ioannis Komnios
Exus Software Ltd, London, UK

Shusuke Hiragi
Division of Medical Information Technology and Administration Planning, Kyoto University Hospital, 54 Kawaharacho, Shogoin, Sakyo-ku, Kyoto 606-8507, Japan
Department of Nephrology, Kyoto University Hospital, 54Kawaharacho, Shogoin, Sakyo-ku, Kyoto 606-8507, Japan

Hiroshi Tamura and Tomohiro Kuroda
Division of Medical Information Technology and Administration Planning, Kyoto University Hospital, 54 Kawaharacho, Shogoin, Sakyo-ku, Kyoto 606-8507, Japan

Rei Goto
Graduate School of Business Administration, Keio University, 2-33-28 Hiyoshi Honcho, Kohoku-ku, Yokohama, Kanagawa 223-8526, Japan
Keio Business School, Keio University, 2-33-28 Hiyoshi Honcho, Kohoku-ku, Yokohama, Kanagawa 223-8526, Japan

Index

N

P

R

S

T

V

www.ingramcontent.com/pod-product-compliance
Lightning Source LLC
LaVergne TN
LVHW080658210926
848485LV00003B/395